"Nigel Dawes has produced a work of both historical and practical value, placing the role of abdominal palpation in diagnosis and healing in its rightful position. The text is a thorough exploration of palpation utilized in the traditional Japanese healing arts."

—*Peter Yates L.Ac. Former chair of Acupuncture and clinic director, New College for Holistic Health, Education and Research, New York*

"Nigel's text is a welcome addition to an all-too-scant body of works on the Japanese tactile diagnosis, Fukushin. This work introduces a strong emphasis on tactility formed through years of practice and extensive training in physical therapies and Shiatsu. His approach is accessible to therapists of many backgrounds."

—*Gretchen De Soriano, MSc University of Oxford, Founder of the Kampo Apprentice Course in Japanese Herbal Medicine, founding member of the International Society of Japanese Kampo Medicine, the British Acupuncture Council and the Register of Chinese Herbal Medicine*

"Fukushin and Kampo launches a new era for the international growth of Kampo medicine despite its restricted practice in Japan. It is much more than the clearest introduction in English to the art of Kampo palpation and formula correspondence. It is a body-mind cultural primer and history of the abdominal palpatory traditions in Japan. The book shines with Kampo clarity, thought and techniques and is enhanced with first rate history, cultural, and professional philosophical concerns."

—*Jeffrey Dann Ph.D., LAc. Developer of Koshi Balancing: an integrated acupuncture and manual medicine approach to structural acupuncture and hara-visceral work*

"There are few things in my life as a physician which enriched my diagnostic skills more than the unique abdominal diagnosis Fukushin from Japanese Kampo Medicine! Given the author's depth of practical experience and thorough research, this work fills a gap and allows comprehensive study for Western practitioners."

—*Dr. Heidrun Reißenweber-I*.............*sident of the Internat*.............*dicine*

Fukushin and Kampo

by the same author

Kampo
A Clinical Guide to Theory and Practice, Second Edition
Keisetsu Otsuka
Translated by Gretchen De Soriano and Nigel Dawes
Foreword by Dan Bensky
ISBN 978 1 84819 329 1
eISBN 978 0 85701 286 9

of related interest

Structural Energetics in Zero Balancing Bodywork
Alan Hext
Foreword by Fritz Frederick Smith, MD
ISBN 978 1 84819 375 8
eISBN 978 0 85701 332 3

**Seitai (Lymphatic) Shiatsu, Cupping and Gua
Sha for a Healthy Immune System**
Richard Gold
Foreword by Ted Kaptchuk
Photographs by Kenneth Goff
ISBN 978 1 84819 364 2
eISBN 978 0 85701 323 1

Tuina/Massage Manipulations
Basic Principles and Techniques
Edited by Li Jiangshan
ISBN 978 1 78592 997 7
eISBN 978 0 85701 046 9

Shiatsu Theory and Practice
Carola Beresford-Cooke
ISBN 978 1 84819 308 6
eISBN 978 0 85701 260 9

FUKUSHIN AND KAMPO

Abdominal Diagnosis in Traditional Japanese and Chinese Medicine

Nigel Dawes

Foreword by Dr. Kenji Watanabe

Photographs and Line Drawings by
Kurt Ossenfort

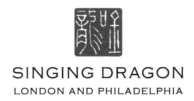

SINGING DRAGON
LONDON AND PHILADELPHIA

First published in Great Britain in 2021 by Singing Dragon,
an imprint of Jessica Kingsley Publishers
An Hachette Company

1

Copyright © Nigel Dawes 2021
Foreword copyright © Dr. Kenji Watanabe 2021
Photographs and line drawings copyright © Kurt Ossenfort 2021

A CIP catalogue record for this title is available from the
British Library and the Library of Congress

ISBN 978 1 84819 367 3
eISBN 978 0 85701 326 2

Printed and bound by CPI Group (UK) Ltd, Croydon, CR0 4YY

Jessica Kingsley Publishers' policy is to use papers that are natural,
renewable and recyclable products and made from wood grown in
sustainable forests. The logging and manufacturing processes are expected
to conform to the environmental regulations of the country of origin.

Jessica Kingsley Publishers
Carmelite House
50 Victoria Embankment
London EC4Y 0DZ

www.singingdragon.com

Contents

Foreword

Kenji Watanabe

In Asian traditional medicine, diagnosis is made by four procedures, i.e., Inspection (looking), Listening and Smelling Examination, Inquiry, and Palpation. Tongue Diagnosis belongs to Inspection, and Pulse Diagnosis (脈診 Myakushin) and Abdominal Diagnosis (腹診 Fukushin) belong to Palpation.

In Sino-Japanese Traditional Herbal Medicine (漢方 Kampo) pattern diagnosis (証 Sho) is made, using these four diagnostic procedures, amongst which abdominal diagnosis is the core of these procedures in Japanese Kampo medicine.

The origin of Kampo medicine is, of course, ancient Chinese medicine. It was transmitted via the Korean peninsula. The oldest description concerning the medicine from the Korean peninsula appears in NIHON SHOKI 日本書記 ("The Chronicles of Japan") in 720 AD, in which the Japanese emperor, INGYO 允恭, became ill and asked one of the three ancient Kingdoms of the Korean peninsula, SHIRAGI 新羅 (Silla), to send a doctor. The doctor came in 414 AD and cured the illness of the emperor. Later, Japan began trading directly with successive Chinese dynasties and medical books were imported directly from China.

Then gradually, a distinctive Japanese style of the medicine came to be formed, especially during the Edo (Tokugawa) period (1603-1868), when this "Japanization" progressed intensively, during which time Fukushin was established. Although Fukushin had been described in the Shang Han Lun (傷寒論), a medical textbook from the Han dynasty in China, it was not commonly used in practice. It is understood that medicine of that era was reserved for high society, and the doctor was not allowed to touch such noble persons directly, according to the strict influence of Confucianism.

However, in modern Kampo medicine, Fukushin has become the cornerstone of treatment.

As Dr. Dawes describes in this book, Fukushin was first mentioned during the Edo period. It started as a treatment (Anpuku 按腹) during the Muromachi era (1336 – 1573), which was a kind of hands-on healing of disease. Then Dosan Manase (1507-1594) started the Goseiha (後世派) School Fukushin. The oldest Fukushin book, 百腹図説 Zusetsu (written in 1602), which means "100 illustrations of Fukushin", is preserved in the library of Keio University. I have had a chance to take a look at it. It is still vividly colored and well preserved.

Then Todo Yoshimasu (1702-1772) is thought to have established the Koho School (古方派 Koho-Ha) of Fukushin, however, he did not leave a book of Fukushin. Todo-style Fukushin was published in 1800 by Bunrei Inaba (稲葉克文禮) as Fukusho Kiran 腹証奇覧 ("Extraordinary Views of Abdominal Patterns"), and supplemented by Shukuko Wakuta in his book, Fukusho Kiran Yoku (腹証奇覧翼), published in 1809.

These two books are still well read by Kampo doctors nowadays in Japan.

The purpose of Fukushin is not only as a diagnostic procedure, but also to provide the indication for treatment. For example, Kyo Kyo Ku Man 胸脇苦満 (Hypochondriac painful fullness) is the abdominal sign indicating the formula: Sho Saiko To 小柴胡湯 (Minor Bupleurum Combination). Shin Ka Hi Ko 心下痞硬 (Epigastric Obstruction Resistance) is the finding indicating Hange Sha Shin To 半夏瀉心湯 (Pinellia Combination). Also, the Oketsu 瘀血 (Blood Stasis) finding is very important when prescribing Keishi Bukuryo Gan 桂枝茯苓丸 (Cinnamon and Hoelen Combination). In this sense, Fukushin is essential in the practice of Kampo medicine.

The author, Dr. Nigel Dawes, studied acupuncture and Kampo in Japan. His teacher was a student of Dr. Yasuo Otsuka (1930-2009), a famous Kampo doctor in Japan who passed away in 2010. He has continued to practice acupuncture and Kampo in New York and also teaches Kampo through his NY Kampo Insitute, offering classes in the US and abroad, including Canada, Europe, Israel and Australia. He is a great leader of Kampo medicine in the USA and has influence all over the world.

I myself studied Kampo from Dr. Yasuo Otsuka and inherited his clinic, the Otsuka Kampo Clinic, in Tokyo. Nigel and I share the same dream which is to introduce Kampo and Fukushin to practitioners in the US and other countries. I have supported Nigel and other Kampo practitioners in the US and UK in starting the North American Kampo Consortium (NAKC).

I hereby offer my congratulations for the publication of his life's work on Fukushin. At the same time, I appreciate Dr. Dawes' achievement in providing us with an authentic Fukushin book in English. I am convinced that this book will be read and used practically amongst practitioners of Kampo, not only in the US, but all over the world.

Kenji Watanabe, MD, PhD, FACP
Director, Otsuka Kampo Clinic
Visiting Professor, Center for Kampo Medicine,
Keio University School of Medicine

Author's Preface

Anyone familiar with the practice of Traditional Japanese Medicine (hereafter referred to as TJM), which in the context of this book I am defining as disciplines that include *Hari* 針 (Acupuncture), *Kyu* 灸 (Moxibustion), *Kampo* 漢方 (Herbal Medicine) and various physical therapies such as *Shiatsu* 指圧 (Acupressure), *Sotai Ho* 操体法 (Neuromuscular Therapy), *Seitai Ho* 整体法 (Structural Therapy) and others, will be aware of the privileged status enjoyed by palpation in both diagnosis and treatment.

The direct use of touch in sensory assessment and therapeutic techniques has always been highly valued by Japanese physicians through the ages. It is perhaps no wonder that from medieval times until the present day, blind practitioners of manipulative therapies as well as Acupuncture have flourished in Japan. In fact, it is estimated that roughly 30 percent of all licensed Acupuncturists in Japan today are blind, so the notion that acquired, non-visual sensory skill can directly inform clinical decision-making at the highest level is neither alien nor undervalued in the Japanese sensibility.

In TJM the most vital examples of palpatory examination include Pulse Diagnosis (*Myakushin* 脈診) and Abdomen Diagnosis (*Fukushin* 腹診) as well as the palpation and diagnosis of channels and collaterals (*Keiraku Shin* 経絡診). According to *Kampo* literature (Otsuka, 2010), it is said that illnesses of external etiology and manifestation (such as acute febrile disease) can be diagnosed on the pulse whilst those of internal cause and nature (chronic constitutional disease) can be assessed through the abdomen.

The subject matter of this book concerns itself with how the abdomen has come to play such a pivotal role in the practice of TJM and, within the context of Sino–Japanese Herbal Medicine (*Kampo* 漢方) in particular, why and in what precise clinical manner it has remained one of the cornerstones of the diagnostic process.

This fact should perhaps not be so surprising. After all, the abdomen represents the body's anatomical center, housing as it does the vital organs as well as forming its myofascial and structural core. In Asian systems of medicine, it is also the source of Vital energy (*Seiki* 生氣) acting as a crucible for the transmutation of innate or "Pre-Heaven Energy" (*Gen Ki* 元気) and acquired or "Post-Heaven Energy" (*Ko Ten No Ki* 後天之気).

It also represents a metaphysical cauldron in which the vital organs play a pivotal role, each acting as repository and catalyst for specific manifestations at the psychic and emotional level.

It is in this context that East Asian cultural references to the abdomen (*Hara* 腹) and the corresponding area in the lower back (*Koshi* 腰) are repeatedly used in all manner of traditional Japanese practices and disciplines from the fine arts to the martial arts and equally so in the medical arts. It is from these areas of the body that the Vital energy originates and thus they are seen and experienced as the primary source of power, health and psychic, emotional and physical vigor in human beings.

Throughout the history and development of Traditional East Asian Medical systems, the abdomen has thus occupied a pivotal role in both diagnostic and treatment paradigms. In more recent times, however, its significance in the clinic has dwindled and many practitioners, especially in modern China, rarely use it in practice.

This, happily, has not been its fate in Japan where, from the *Edo* period (*Edo Jidai* 江戸時代, 1603–1868) onward in particular, Acupuncturists as well as *Kampo* and *Shiatsu* practitioners have developed highly sophisticated methods of using the abdomen in clinical assessment and practice. The esteemed *Edo* period practitioner from the Classical School (*Koho-Ha* 古方派), *Yoshimasu Todo* (吉益東洞, 1702–1773) aptly summarizes this predilection in his well-known saying, "*Hara* is the source of life and also the origin of all diseases" (Yasui, 2007).

A contemporary example of such an abdominal palpation method is that employed by modern herbalists (mostly MDs) in Japan, who use a detailed and highly specific form of Abdominal Diagnosis (*Fukushin* 腹診) to obtain critical clinical information, which strongly influences the selection of specific herbal prescriptions.

This book will present the author's interpretation and adaptation of one of these methods of abdominal palpation currently practiced within the modern Classical School (*Koho-Ha* 古方派) *Kampo* tradition as developed by Dr. *Otsuka Keisetsu* (大塚敬節 1900–1980), itself based on various classical sources that will be referred to in the course of this text.

There are other surviving historical traditions of abdominal palpation and diagnosis deriving from different currents within the broader development of *Kampo* as a whole in Japan. For example, in addition to the Classical School mentioned above of which Dr. *Otsuka* is seen as the main modern proponent, there preceded it the Later Generation School (*Gosei-Ha* 後世派), which also survives into the modern era, retaining its own unique system of abdominal diagnosis. In the 19th century, yet another *Kampo* school evolved, the Eclectic School (*Secchu-Ha* 折衷派), in an effort to synthesize the teachings of both the preceding factions by seeking to further develop and refine abdominal theory and practice, integrating some of the European medical teachings that had begun filtering into Japan by that period.

Where possible, this book will include references to all these various traditions of abdominal diagnosis reflecting the different historical currents of *Kampo*, but will inevitably focus on that of the Classical School and the teachings of Dr. *Otsuka* in particular as well as offering some of the author's own insights and experience on the subject.

Chapter 1 ("Context") will begin by outlining a clear definition of abdominal diagnosis in which various cultural, linguistic and historical references will be made. It will be important for readers to distinguish the particular significance of the abdomen in the Japanese mindset, which will go some way to explaining the survival of this ancient clinical practice into the modern era despite its decline in currency in other East Asian cultures. The chapter will continue with a discussion of the clinical significance of the abdomen with regard specifically to the practice of TJM and more particularly *Kampo*. This section will deal with outlining the broad significance of the use of the abdomen in both diagnostic and treatment paradigms including the significance of *Fukushin* in Constitutional, Disease and Formula patterns.

Chapter 2 ("History") will start with a brief treatment of other disciplines in which the abdomen plays a pivotal role in both diagnosis and treatment. This will include some examples from the practice of *Shiatsu*, most notably from the work of *Masunaga Shizuto* (増永静人, 1925–1981), whose *Zen Shiatsu* style incorporated extensive use of the abdomen, as well as from various styles of Japanese Acupuncture, in particular Meridian Therapy (*Keiraku Chiryo* 経絡治療), a 20th century movement founded by *Yanagiya Sorei* (柳谷素霊, 1906–1959) based on the classics as manifest in contemporary Japan by such masters as *Denmei Shudo* 首藤傳明 (1932–). The final section of this chapter will deal with a thorough analysis of the history and development of abdominal diagnosis in the *Kampo* tradition. It will trace its origins to the Classical period of the *Han* dynasty (漢朝, 206 BCE–220 CE) in ancient China, through to its transmission into the Japanese mainland in the 6th century CE and its cultural transformation during the Japanese *Edo* period (1603–1868), right up to the present time and its integration into modern medical practice. This chapter is devoted to revealing the profound cultural impact on the practice of abdominal diagnosis during its transmission through almost 2000 years of history and across continents and cultures.

Chapter 3 ("Methodology") will deal with the technical aspects of the abdominal exam itself. Illustrative and descriptive accounts of the various sequences involved in performing the exam will be given in an attempt to demonstrate the practical skills necessary to achieve an effective outcome. Details will be offered on the aspects of technique which require special attention, along with the pitfalls of incorrect methodology. Naturally, learning the unique skills required to gain confidence and proficiency with this exam does not come from a book and requires years of dedicated learning with an experienced teacher, but the basics are nonetheless offered in this chapter.

Chapter 4 ("Interpretation") concerns itself with the clinical findings obtained from the exam. Each finding will be clearly identified within the nomenclature of the *Kampo* system into the principal Abdominal Conformations (*Fukusho* 腹証) that can be identified by the exam. These will be clearly illustrated in each case. Each presenting pattern will then be discussed in terms of its morphology, charting methodology and clinical interpretation in relation to possible herbal formulas that may correspond in each case. Herb "families" and groupings of classical herbal formulas will be identified and correlated to each abdominal finding. Additionally, with respect to each abdominal pattern, there will be discussion of both associated constitutional typing as well as patterns of pathology expressed in typical *Kampo* terms according to Vital energy (*Ki* 氣), Blood (*Ketsu* 血) and Fluids (*Sui* 水). The main purpose of this chapter is to present each abdominal pattern from the perspective of practical herbal prescribing as well as from a patho-mechanistic perspective. Chapter 4 will include a "Summary of findings" section, in which the details presented in Chapter 4 will be reviewed and summarized with illustrations.

Chapter 5 will outline why I believe the use of abdominal diagnosis in the practice of *Kampo* is not only as relevant today as it was at its inception almost 2000 years ago, but also how its skillful use can elevate clinical practice to new heights with correspondingly successful outcomes for patients.

Fukushin is, I believe, an intrinsic and indispensable component of East Asian Medical practice in general and of TJM in particular—

one that, sadly, the majority of contemporary practitioners are either unaware of or untrained in. It is my sincere hope, through this work, to contribute to the continued appreciation for, and informed practice of, this most essential of manual skills, whose continued transmission through the centuries is testimony to its practical use and significance in successful treatment outcomes.

I cannot imagine my own practice now without palpation of the abdomen. I am so grateful and fortunate to have been introduced to it in the early 1980s in Japan, first through my *Shiatsu* studies and subsequently through my study and practice of Acupuncture and *Kampo* medicine. Over the years it has become the cornerstone of my clinical work and teaching and has developed into a passion of mine. I am privileged to share it with you in this work, which represents over 30 years of study and practice of this art.

Nigel Dawes
Brooklyn, New York
2018

Acknowledgements

The topic of this text has been an interest of mine since my very first encounter with the use of the abdomen in clinical practice in early 1983 in Japan. Though at that time I had no idea that one day I might publish a book on the subject, I realize now, at the moment of its completion, that I owe so much gratitude to a countless number of individuals and experiences that have all in one way or another contributed to this work. I would like to acknowledge just a few that come readily to mind.

For my critical thinking and writing skills, such as they are, I gratefully acknowledge all my inspirational teachers and fellow students at the University of Cambridge in England where I completed my master's degree in Comparative Literature back in 1982. It is one thing to study a particular discipline and even become quite adept at it; it is quite another to organize one's thoughts about it in a critical manner and put them down on paper. These skills I owe to that early part of my education at the hands of such gifted supervisors as Dr. Robert Lethbridge (French 19th/20th century literature) and Dr. Geoffrey Walker (Spanish Golden Age literature).

For my *Shiatsu* education I thank my very first teacher in Japan, Edward Bailey, and my main *Shiatsu* mentor during the five years I spent in Japan, *Suzuki Takeo* 鈴木竹雄. His weekly classes and treatments made a huge impression on me and introduced me to the world of *Zen Shiatsu* which I use to this day in my practice. I would also like to thank my friend Nigel Reid, himself a ten-year disciple of *Suzuki sensei*'s, without whose in-class fluent translation from the Japanese, learning would have been so much harder! I thank also all my fellow students who shared that particular journey known to foreigners studying TJM during that heady time in Tokyo in the 1980s! My thanks also go to the several other *Shiatsu* teachers I have had the good fortune to spend time with either in Japan or later in Europe including *sensei's Kimura Susumu, Endo Ryokyu, Sasaki Kazunori, Kishi Akinobu* and others. I thank also *Kun Somboon*, my Thai Massage teacher at Wat Po in Bangkok where I lived for six months in 1985.

For my Acupuncture education I would like to thank first of all my very good friend Peter Yates without whom I likely would never have made it into my first Acupuncture class back in 1983. An accomplished martial artist and practitioner himself, he introduced me to the International Institute of Oriental Medicine (IIOM) in Tokyo where, alongside him and several other keen foreigners at the time, we studied under *Suzuki Todo*, to whom I am so grateful for my basic Acupuncture training. I'm lucky to have spent time also in those years as an apprentice of Dr. *Nagura* in his clinic in *Shinjuku* (Tokyo) as well as extended visits to other clinics in the Tokyo area including a short stint in Korea under Dr. *Yom*. I am also incredibly indebted to all the many excellent doctors and interpreters I studied with in my intensive six months in Beijing, China in 1987 after leaving Japan. There are too many names to include here, but I would acknowledge one in particular with whom I did extensive study—Dr. *Gao Li Shan*, at the time attending physician at *Guang An Men* hospital in Beijing.

For my *Kampo* training I am very grateful to my first teacher at the International Institute of Oriental Medicine (IIOM) in Tokyo, Peter Townsend, who helped lay the foundations of my then growing interest in Herbal Medicine. It wasn't until later that Gretchen De Soriano, a friend and colleague of mine from that same time in Japan, who had studied at *Kitasato* Institute in Tokyo as a private student of Dr. *Otsuka Yasuo*, became my primary *Kampo* teacher on my return to London in 1988. To her I owe great gratitude and respect and I was honored to have worked with her on the translation of *Otsuka Keisetsu*'s text: *Kampo Igaku*, which we published together in 2010 (see "Selected Bibliography").

A final thanks in regard to my training goes to *Yamada Koun* 山田耕雲, my *Zen* teacher at the *San Un Zendo* in *Kamakura*, near Tokyo where I lived for the last two years of my time in Japan. I am humbled and deeply grateful for his teaching and wisdom.

In the writing and preparation of this book I would like to thank the following for their incredibly hard work, continual inspiration and unending support:

Yuri Matsumoto, whose tireless editing of the text, in particular the Japanese *Kanji* terms and proper names, represents a monumental task in itself and one that, without doubt, I myself was unequipped to accomplish. In addition, *Yuri* acted graciously as the model for all the drawings and photographs. In short, this book could not have happened without her help and inspiration. Thank you, dear Yuri for your indomitable fortitude and canny ability to handle anything that came along—such is your tiger-like nature!

Kurt Ossenfort, whose beautifully simple and expressive abdomen drawings bring the text to life along with his minimalist black and white photographs that capture the exam sequence perfectly. Thank you, my friend, for giving light and life to the words in such inimitable style.

I am also greatly indebted to Dr. *Kenji Watanabe*, whose Foreword to this text is warmly appreciated. *Kenji* had previously contributed to Gretchen and my translation of Dr. *Otsuka*'s text (see above) and I am so grateful for his expert opinion and support. His own *Kampo* lineage is directly linked to that of the Otsuka family through marriage, as well as having been himself a Kampo student of Otsuka Yasuo, whose clinic he inherited and now runs in Tokyo. Dr. Watanabe's contribution to the modern Kampo lexicon in terms of research, teaching and practice is well-known and hugely respected and I am honored to count him as a friend and colleague.

I would like in addition to acknowledge the several individuals who generously wrote endorsements for this book, all of whom have longtime associations with the traditional medical system of Japan in all its many forms:

Stephen Brown, a friend and colleague who was born in Japan, studied acupuncture and Shiatsu there in the late 1970's and early 80's, and came to Seattle in the US where he now practices and teaches. Stephen is well-known in the field for his clinical work in Meridian Therapy as the principal western disciple of Shudo Denmei as well as for his teaching, writing and editorial work at the North American Journal of Oriental Medicine.

Jeffrey Dann, a long-time friend and respected colleague in the field whose eclectic background includes a PhD in Medical Anthropology as well as martial, healing and fine art study in Japan and 45 years in practice. He is one of the pioneers of Traditional Japanese Medicine in the West and has always been a staunch advocate of the importance of direct experience through touch in practice.

Gretchen De Soriano, my esteemed teacher, of whom I have already spoken, who not only inspires as a practitioner and teacher of Kampo, but who more recently has brought the interdisciplinary study of Medical Anthropology to bear in her work, adding the critical perspective of culture, language and history into the study and practice of traditional medical disciplines such as Kampo.

Dr. Gregory Plotnikoff, a friend and colleague practicing Internal Medicine who studied Kampo with Kenji Watanabe at Keio University in Tokyo and who now runs Minnesota Personalized Medicine, an Integrated Medicine clinic using a systems biology approach to integrative healthcare.

Dr. Heidrun Reißenweber-Hewel, a colleague from Germany practicing Internal Medicine, Kampo and Acupuncture who also spent an extended period of time in Japan studying Kampo Medicine. She is the recent President (now President Emeritus) of the International Society of Japanese Kampo Medicine with a very active membership of Kampo doctors from around the world (including myself).

Yorai Sella, my close friend from many years of shared teaching in Israel over the last 30 years, a seasoned Clinical Psychologist and East Asian Medicine practitioner dedicated to an Integrated Medical paradigm, whose book: "From Dualism to Oneness in Psychoanalysis – a Zen Perspective on the Mind-Body Question" speaks for itself.

Peter Yates, my good friend whom I met in Tokyo in 1983 and who encouraged me to take up East Asian Medicine studies. An unassuming talent and genuine healer and teacher, Peter is an amazingly gifted acupuncturist with a vast practical knowledge of the body through a lifetime of strength-training, internal and external martial arts, meditation and health practices. His example has influenced my own development, and that of many others, profoundly.

Additional thanks go to my dear friend Dr. Boaz Mourad who, at short notice was sequestered to do an impromptu photo shoot on a hike in Joshua Tree National Park, the result of which is the author portrait on the back cover. Boaz you rock!

Finally, I am lucky to have had a truly supportive and where necessary, long-suffering and generous editor, Claire Wilson and her equally professional and supportive assistant editor, Maddy Budd, as well as senior production editor Emma Holak at Singing Dragon (Jessica Kingsley Publishers). A big thank you also to the professional indexer on this and many other projects at Singing Dragon, Sybil Ihrig, an esteemed colleague and Kampo student of mine. Thank you, Claire, Maddy, Emma, and all your excellent team for believing in this project. I hope it was worth the wait!

1

CONTEXT

"Hara is that state (Verfassung) in which the individual has found his primal centre and has proven himself by it. When we speak of the state of an individual we mean something that concerns him in his entirety, that is, something that transcends the duality of body and soul…with Hara the world looks different, it is as it is, always different from what one wants it to be and yet always in harmony. Self-will causes suffering. Suffering denotes deviation from the Great Unity and reveals the truth of the Whole. The ordinary eye does not see this—the Hara sense apprehends it and only when will, feeling, and intellect are "comprehended" in Hara do they cease to resist what is, and instead, through it, serve the "way" in which all things are contained. To discover that way, to recognize it and thereafter never to lose it is tantamount to genuine striving for Hara."

Hara: The Vital Center of Man, Durkheim, K.G., Original publ. 1956, Transl. Von Kospoth, S., publ. Inner Traditions, 2004.

DEFINITION OF *FUKUSHIN*

"The Ancients had a saying: Diseases reside in the abdomen. Hence, [the physician] must search [the abdomen] to find the [regions of] congestion and stagnation."

From the Author's Preface to *Extraordinary Views of Abdominal Patterns: Fukusho-Kiran, Inaba Katsu Bunrei*, 1800, Transl. Kageyama, J., publ. The Chinese Medicine Database, 2018.

1. Language and terminology

In the Japanese written language, there is a single ideogram 腹, used to denote the abdomen. However, this character can be pronounced in several ways depending on the context and when combined with other characters can have subtle and often distinctly different meanings.

Firstly, there is the phonetic "sounding out" of the character itself. One pronunciation can be *Fuku*, which generally means "bag" or "sack" such as one might be handed in a store to carry things in. This refers in the medical context specifically to the abdomen—literally the abdominal sac which houses or "carries" the vital organs. In this context the usual term employed is *Fukubu* 腹部, the second of the two ideograms referring to the portion of the body in which this "sac" is located, that is to say the entire abdominal area, both upper and lower.

It is here that we find the context for the meaning of the term *Fukushin* 腹診, usually translated as "Abdominal Diagnosis," which constitutes the subject matter of this book. *Fukushin* is therefore defined for the purposes of this material as a palpatory technique performed on the abdomen by which one may obtain sensory information used in the diagnostic process in *Kampo* practice. The skilled *Kampo* practitioner is able by means of this abdominal exam to classify their findings into an identifiable Abdominal "Pattern" (*Fukusho* 腹証), which in turn will correspond with a specific Formula "Pattern" (*Yakusho* 薬証) or at least a "family" of formulas, thereby streamlining the clinical differentiation process. This method of determining a treatment strategy by identifying a specific Abdominal Conformation is central to *Kampo* practice and is referred to as "matching pattern and formula."

In *Kampo* practice it is usual to privilege such tactile sensory findings over those obtained through other means such as patient questioning so that in the *Kampo* system as a whole *Fukushin* has a hierarchically significant role in clinical decision-making as we shall see.

A further linguistic differentiation related to this anatomical definition is the sub division of the abdominal area, *Fukubu*, into the Stomach (upper abdomen), known both as *Ibukuro* 胃袋, literally the stomach organ, a medical term also used in butchery as in "tripe," or more commonly in the vernacular as *Onaka* お腹, the term used most often when talking about one's "tummy" in everyday Japanese (literally "honorable middle").

Examples may include symptoms such as *O Naka Ga Itai Desu* お腹が痛いです, "My tummy hurts," or states such as *O Naka Ga Sukimashita* お腹が空きました (*Suita* 空いた—informal), "I'm hungry," or *O Naka Ga Ippai Desu* お腹がいっぱいです, "I'm full," or anatomical references to the stomach area such as *O Naka Wo Shita Ni Nette Kudasai* お腹を下に寝てください, "Please lie down on your tummy."

However, the very same ideogram 腹, pronounced as either *Fuku* or *Naka* in the examples cited above, can also be pronounced phonetically as *Hara* in Japanese depending on the context. The term *Hara* however has an altogether different, though related, meaning. In the purely physical sense *Hara* can equally well refer to one's belly just as *O Naka* in the above examples such as in the phrases *Hara Ga Itai* 腹が痛い, "My stomach hurts," or *Hara Ga Hetta* 腹が減った, "I'm hungry."

But to return for a moment to the abdominal divisions into upper and lower, we find that when it comes to specifically identifying the area below the navel the language takes an interesting turn away from the physical and toward the energetic or metaphysical.

Saika Tanden 臍下丹田, for example, refers to the energetic center located in the lower abdomen and literally translates as "Elixir Field" or "Cinnabar Field," an alchemic reference used extensively in East Asian Medical and martial practices to describe the locus of the transformation of *Sei* 生, "essence," into *Ki* 気, "Vital energy," whilst *Tanden* 丹田 (*Dan Tian* in Chinese) describes the general area of what the classic text "The Inner Cannon of the Yellow Emperor" (*Ko Tei Nai Kyoh* 黄帝内経, *Huang Di Nei Jing* in Chinese) terms: "the movement of *Ki* between the Kidneys." The specific anatomical location at which this energetic transformation is said to actually occur corresponds to the Acupuncture Point CV6, "Sea of Qi" (*Kikai* 気海, *Qihai* in Chinese), located three finger widths below the navel on the midline along the pathway of the Conception Vessel (*Nin Myaku* 任經, *Ren Mai* in Chinese).

Thus the term *Hara* can often take on less concrete and more metaphysical connotations in the language, including expressions of emotion such as *Hara ga tatsu* 腹が立つ (literally "the abdomen stands up") meaning to get angry, or in descriptions of character traits such as *Hara ga futoi* 腹が太い (literally "fat belly") referring to someone who has a generous nature, or conversely *Hara Guroi* 腹黒い (literally "black belly") suggesting someone with a dark or sinister nature.

It is also a term used in relationship to one's very essence, such as in the phrase *Hara wo watte hanasu* 腹を割って話す (literally "breaking open the *Hara* and talking") meaning to open one's heart to somebody, or *Hara o kukuru* 腹を括る (literally "tying up the *Hara*") meaning to commit wholeheartedly or to knuckle down to something. The notion of binding the *Hara* is literally expressed by the word *Haramaki* 腹巻, originally a term used to describe Samurai armor (put on from the front and tied at the back), but in modern times one that refers to an article of clothing that wraps around the belly (like a sash) to protect it or keep it warm. In *Kampo*, during the *Edo* period in particular, women planning to get pregnant who were considered to have a Cold Constitution (*Hie Sho* 冷え症), were advised to wear a specially designed *Haramaki*, with a pouch on the inside, into which a metal box containing lighted coals could be placed to warm the *Hara*, in order, it was believed, to increase the chances of conception by improving blood flow to the uterus.

There is also the phrase *Hara o saguru* 腹を探る (literally "to investigate the *Hara*") meaning to see into someone's soul and reveal their truth or to read someone's mind. Perhaps the art of *Fukushin* can be appreciated from this perspective—as that of trying to "divine the truth" or get to the "heart of the matter" in diagnostic terms by touching, connecting to and sensing the *Hara* of another and by using one's own *Hara* in the process.

Though sometimes translated as "mind," the concept of *Hara* lends symbolic and concrete meaning to the way in which the Japanese privilege direct sensory experience that is, literally, "gut-felt," rather than the more abstract "heart-felt" more common in Western culture and language. This singular prejudice for implicit trust in the innate value of sensory experience, in this case emanating from the gut or *Hara*, goes some way to explaining why, in TJM, the role of the abdomen has maintained such an elevated status in terms of both diagnosic and treatment practices.

So it is that the practice of *Fukushin* in the *Kampo* tradition has a particular linguistic bias. It would be important in this regard therefore to distinguish the terms *Fukushin* and *Harashin* from one another, both descriptive terms (using the same Japanese character) but each one characterizing distinct and different traditions of abdominal diagnostic techniques. It could be said, for example, that the former is used to describe a more concrete, physical exam involving assessment of skin and muscle temperature, tonus and reactivity as well as percussion for tympanic or succussion sounds, palpation of aortal pulsations and so on. The latter, however, might be better described as an "energetic" assessment of the abdomen in terms of Excess (*Jitsu* 実) and Deficiency (*Kyo* 虚) in the flow of Energy (*Ki* 気) in specific areas, meridians or points.

Certainly, within the various disciplines that make up TJM, these terms are used to consciously emphasize such differences between the physical and metaphysical aspects that they each imply.

For example, in *Shiatsu* the term *Harashin* is always used whilst in *Kampo* we tend to use the term *Fukushin*, a linguistic preference that clearly points to the relative physicality or meta-physicality of the discipline involved, in this case abdominal palpation and diagnosis.

It is worth noting here the textual and historical origins of the different linguistic qualities associated with sensory descriptions of the abdomen. Those terms that are described above as having more concrete, physical connotations derive principally from the "Treatise on Cold Damage" (*Sho Kan Ron* 傷寒論, *Shang Han Lun* in Chinese), the canonical text for *Kampo* herbalists, whilst those that have more abstract, energetic associations derive from the "Classic of Difficulties" (*Nan Gyo* 難 経, *Nan Jing* in Chinese), the single most influential classical text for Japanese Acupuncture practitioners.

Simply put, *Fukushin* belongs to the Classical School (*Koho-Ha* 古方派) *Kampo* tradition of concrete physical findings in the abdomen that correspond directly to internal medicine diagnostics and matching classical herbal formulas whilst *Harashin* corresponds to the practice of gathering clinical evidence used to correct imbalances in the flow of *Ki* at the meridian level using manipulative therapies such as *Shiatsu*, *Sotai* and *Seitai* as well as *Hari Kyu* (see references to these therapies in the Preface).

Thus, the language here is specific and deliberate. In *Kampo* practice we talk of *Fukushin* rather than *Harashin* (though as we have seen it is almost impossible to entirely separate the two).

2. Form and function

The Japanese notion that one's spiritual, emotional and physical "center" is literally housed in the belly is testimony to a deep and intrinsic understanding of the way in which form and function are inexorably related.

Anyone visiting Japan cannot miss being struck by the national obsession with golf, for example. This, in spite of the fact that golf is an exclusive sport, open to the few due to its prohibitive cost, though "practiced" by the many. At bus stops, for example, on the train platform or in the street at almost any time of day it is not uncommon to see people of all ages practicing their golf swing with imaginary clubs (such as umbrellas). This is perhaps the most visible vernacular example of the attention paid to precise and almost obsessively detailed outward form and its relationship to, in this case, the power and accuracy of a golf swing.

Such examples of body–mind dynamics are perhaps more traditionally seen in the martial arts (*Budo* 武道), where no matter the particular discipline, the primary educational goal is always to develop a mature understanding of proper form and movement from which power and effectiveness can flow. In all traditional Japanese martial arts (and by extension the healing and fine arts) one's "Form" (*Kata* 型), along with one's Physical Posture (*Shisei* 姿勢), reveal the depth or otherwise of one's spirit and intention and thereby one's skill and effectiveness in any given endeavor.

This notion of what can be implied by what is seen is manifest in the twin concept in Japanese of *Omote* 表 ("Surface" or "Outside") implying what is visible and obvious, and *Ura* 裏 ("Bottom" or "Inside") implying that which is hidden or subtle, and can be applied to almost any aspect of life in Japan.

For example, geographically, the East side of Japan is *Omote* (the outward face of the country, most well-known amongst foreigners, including the major cities of Tokyo, Kyoto and Osaka), whilst the West is *Ura*, the so-called "inner Japan" much less traveled or known to outsiders. Similarly, the "inside" of Japan, meaning the (mountainous) countryside (*Inaka* 田舎), would relate to *Ura* whilst the coastal urban sprawl (80% of Japanese live near the coast) would constitute the *Omote*. The association implied here is that in order to truly penetrate the Japanese culture one must seek the *Ura* but necessarily begin with the *Omote*.

The dialectic that defines the relationship between the obvious "Outside" and the hidden "Inside" in Japanese culture is clearly evident in the philosophy and practice of TJM also. For example, in the theory of the Eight Parameters (*Hakko Ben Sho* 八綱弁証), used in Pattern Differentiation (*Zui Sho Chi Ryo* 随証治療), two of these eight principles are defined as either Exterior (*Hyo* 表) or Interior (*Ri* 裏), referring to disease manifestations that occur either on the surface of (*Gai* 外) or inside (*Nai* 内) the body. Similarly, in etiology, Disease Patterns (*Byo Sho* 病証) can be categorized as Root (*Hon* 本) or Branch (*Hyo* 標) and in the same way as described above with regard to *Ura/Omote* in respect to the culture, in medicine it is often the case that in order to understand and treat the root of any disease, we must often attend to the branch first.

To return to the martial arts, the *Omote* is represented by the *Shisei* 姿勢, the outward Physical Posture, through which may be perceived the *Kokoro* 心 meaning "Heart" or inner spirit of the person, here representing the *Ura*.

In human anatomy, an analogous relationship expressed in terms of *Omote/Ura* could be defined by the *Koshi* 腰 (lower back and hips), the outward structural source of support and motive power in the human body, and the *Hara* 腹 (belly), the innate source of mental, emotional and psychic energy at the core of such power.

Indeed, the sign of an accomplished and mature individual, someone who is grounded and secure "in their center," is characterized by the Japanese expression *Hara ga dekiru* 腹ができる meaning literally to have "completed" or "finished one's belly." In this phrase, *Hara* may also be written with the character 肚 instead of the typical 腹 as this immediately associates its meaning with mastery and maturity and is deeply rooted in the *Samurai* 侍 culture. Indeed, someone referred to as *hara ga dekita hito* 肚ができた人 (literally "one with an accomplished belly") would be considered none other than a "Master."

As we have seen in the case of the term *Hara*, so too with the term *Koshi* there are many linguistic references that help to appreciate its fullest meaning. *Koshi o ireru* 腰を入れる means literally to "put your back into something," indicating the will or resolve to achieve it. Conversely *Yowa goshi* 弱腰, meaning "weak *Koshi*," suggests negativity or a lack of determination, and such a person may be called *Koshinuke* 腰抜け, "spineless" or cowardly. A physically strong *Koshi* for the Japanese is associated with a strong will, with having literally a strong and balanced center (of gravity), which is ultimately visible in the proper postural alignment of the person.

I am reminded of a very well-known Japanese *Sumo* 相撲 wrestler who came to dominate the ranks of the *Yokozuna* 横綱 (the highest rank) during the 1980s. His name was *Chiyonofuji* 千代の富士, nicknamed "the wolf," and as such, he personified the polar opposite of *Koshinuke*, embodying instead the fearless posture of someone who would surely be described as *Kenka Goshi* 喧嘩腰 (literally "fighting waist"), that is, seriously ready for a fight, or defiant and gnarly, like a wolf.

At this point, I cannot resist a quote from an excellent article on this topic by the founder of "The *Koshi* Balancing Method," Jeffrey Dann PhD., L.Ac., an accomplished Acupuncturist, martial artist, dancer, *Sotai* master and friend:

> In the body-mind construct of Japanese culture we might understand Hara both as immovable stability (the Yang force within the Yin abdomen) the visceral center that holds the body-mind focused; and Koshi as the power vector of the structural musculoskeletal center (the Yin structure within the Yang posterior), that puts driving power, and rotational adaptability into movement. (2005)

This description brilliantly summarizes, not only the relationship between form and function in the Japanese mindset, but also in this case the specific correlation and interdependence of inner and outer, back and front—of *Ura* and *Omote*—in the context of the human body.

With this in mind it is not difficult to appreciate the positive image in Japanese culture attributed to a strong and ample "belly." For such an outward form is automatically associated with inner vitality, and its cultivation in martial, meditative and artistic disciplines could be said to characterize their most essential pursuit.

Cultural examples of this bias abound in Japan—one need only think of the national sport *Sumo* 相撲 to observe how strength (both physical and mental) is associated with size, in particular the size of the *Hara* and *Koshi*. Indeed, the staple diet of all wrestlers

(*Rikishi* 力士)—literally "men of power"—is *Chankonabe* ちゃんこ鍋 (a *nabemono* or "one-pot stew" made with large quantities of protein-rich foods including fish, meat and vegetables, eaten in huge quantities along with beer and rice or noodles to further increase the calorific value), served for lunch (*Sumo* wrestlers have no breakfast) after which a siesta is advised to further increase the weight-gaining potential of this regimen. As compared with the image of strength in the West, where the upper body is developed and the waist and hips are tight and narrow, the Japanese corollary is one where weight and power are visibly concentrated in the waist, hips and belly.

Another powerful cultural reference demonstrating the significance of the abdomen, in this case related more to character and personality traits rather than physical strength, can be found in certain Buddhist iconography in Japan. A notable example is the image of *Hotei* 布袋 (*Budai* in Chinese), one of the 7 Gods of Fortune (*Shichifukujin* 七福神) in Japanese mythology. Often nicknamed "the laughing Buddha," his large belly and smiling face are readily associated with contentment and generosity and as has been noted, the image of a big *Hara* is immediately linked to that of a broad mind and kind heart in the Japanese sensibility.

As for the realm of medicine, in both practitioners and patients, strong *Hara* and strong *Koshi* imply deep reserves of compassion, resolve, intelligence and skill housed in a robust, healthy constitutional envelope (the body). This perceived relationship between form and function has vital implications in the realms of prognosis, diagnosis and treatment in the TJM paradigm as we shall see.

3. Seeing and touching

In the context of the *Ura/Omote* definitions as described above, it can be argued that *Koshi* represents the "seen," *Hara* the "unseen" vital centers of man (this is a reference to the text *Hara: The Vital Center of Man*, Durckheim, K. G., publ. Inner Traditions, 2004 (originally published in Germany 1956).

It is typical in fact in TJM diagnosis for the back to be used more often in observational diagnosis whilst the abdomen is always palpated. This suggests that the *Yang* portions of the body, defined by the posterior anatomy (in particular the back), can often provide useful visual diagnostic clues related to structural imbalances and their corresponding skeletal and myofascial distortions visible to the trained eye. By contrast the *Yin* areas of the body, as defined by the anterior anatomy (in particular the abdomen), must inevitably be palpated in order to ascertain potential imbalances in the viscera that necessarily rely upon subtle and skillful tactile investigation.

In the realm of TJM, this juxtaposition of *Omote* and *Ura* represented by *Koshi* and *Hara* raises inevitable questions as to the relative hierarchy of the visual and the tactile within the diagnostic paradigm of East Asian Medicine as a whole.

There is clear textual evidence from Chinese sources, dating back to the early *Han* dynasty (206 BCE–220 CE), that observation in diagnosis was considered the most valued sensory skill over and above the others, namely smelling, listening, touching and asking. Yet it is also the case that both in ancient China as well as ancient Greece, touch was often hailed as the primary, most immediate sense and the most reliable for ascertaining veracity in manifest phenomena.

In her compelling article "Tactility and the body in early Chinese Medicine" (*Science in Context* 18(1), 7–34 (2005)) Elizabeth Hsu refers to this in some detail:

> …in ancient Greece, touch was considered the "primary form of sense" that belonged to all animals (Aristotle, De Anima, cited in Lloyd 1996, 135). Touch and smell, in particular, due to the bodily proximity they involved, were subordinated to vision and hearing, senses which enabled perception at a greater distance (Synnott 1991). In the hierarchy of senses, vision became associated with the superior masculine, and touch with the inferior feminine (Classen 1997). In this way, touch became associated with the erotic and affective (Gilman 1993). On the other hand, touch has also been respected for the authoritative knowledge it generates and the divine

powers it can transmit. While optical illusions are easily produced, veracity is often ascertained through touch: in the bible, Thomas did not trust his eyes when he saw Christ, who had been crucified and buried, he had to touch Christ's wounds to be assured of the veracity of resurrection (Immerwahr 1978); and in the Sistine Chapel, God, by touching Adam's finger, intends to transmit the breath of life (Boyle 1998). (pp.28–29)

She goes on to provide references (Billeter 1984, 26–27) to the "ocular metaphor" easily discernible in the occident, especially in Greek philosophy, seen in words like "idea" (*Eidos* meaning "image") or "theory" (*Theorein* meaning "to look"). She quotes the same author as stating, "In Chinese texts, the 'ocular metaphor' is remarkable, precisely, for its very absence" (p.30).

In fact, the main thrust of her article is to suggest a primary protagonist in the evolution of scholarly medical knowledge in pre-dynastic China (3rd and 2nd centuries BCE) was indeed "tactile perception prompted by tactile exploration of living bodies" (p.7).

However, I think the suggestion here is not so much that we should assume a hierarchy of one sense over another in the ancient Chinese sensibility, but that at the very least, as she offers us in another reference, "…seeing and hearing, looking and listening, in interaction with each other, were thought to produce knowledge" (p.31).

Indeed, in TJM diagnostics, the practice of relying on evidence derived exclusively from one or other of our senses is firmly discouraged. Inevitably, the diagnostic process must include as much sensory input and interpretation as possible utilizing all five of the senses.

That said, returning to post-Enlightenment medical theory, it cannot be denied that the visual inspection of cadavers has been central to the development of anatomy in modern Europe, which itself in turn has become the cornerstone of modern allopathic medicine. In many respects, this process of elevating the role of the visual in advancing medical knowledge, particularly in the post-modern era where technology has become so focused on observable data, has necessarily subjugated the role of touch in modern medical education and practice.

So much so in fact, that to rely on empirical evidence derived through direct palpation, something much valued in former times, is today considered "quasi-" or "un-"scientific and is to be actively mistrusted and consigned to the (inferior) "subjective" category of clinical data. One might even claim that what has become known today as "scientific fact" is synonymous with what has been "seen with one's own eyes" (and confirmed by others in similar fashion) rather as it might have been in the cadaver classes of 19th century Europe where to "observe" dissection was the surest way to gain understanding of anatomy.

Returning to the context of the abdomen and touch within the history and development of TJM, there can be no doubt that by the *Edo* period in Japan, there was already a profound cultural sense of the importance of *Hara* and *Koshi* in relationship to health and disease. As I have already suggested, the visual appearance of the abdomen was firmly related to one's general constitutional and mental/emotional strength. But it was equally understood by people of that time that, in order to specifically locate and diagnose illness, the abdomen must be palpated by a practitioner skilled in the art of *Fukushin* and in the interpretation of the findings provided by the abdominal examination.

So how shall we summarize the clinical significance of the use of the abdomen in diagnosis and treatment?

FUKUSHIN IN DIAGNOSIS AND TREATMENT

"The Abdomen is the root of life; thus, the hundred diseases take root therein. For this reason, the examination of diseases must (involve) examination of the abdomen. The external signs are secondary."

From "Variety of Assembled Formulas" Ruijuho 類聚
方 (1764) by *Yoshimasu Todo* 吉益東洞 (1702–1773)

1. The abdomen in the diagnostic hierarchy of *Kampo*

In the *Kampo* tradition, the interpretation of abdominal findings greatly influences the diagnostic and treatment process, and in terms of the hierarchy of clinical evidence, *Fukushin* is often considered "the last word" in clinical assessment and decision-making.

This is to say that not only does tactile evidence tend to be positively privileged in the *Kampo* diagnostic but also, considering the two main tactile sources of assessment—the pulse and the abdomen—it is always the abdomen that dominates clinical thinking and action when it comes to Herbal practice. As Dr. *Otsuka* is careful to remind us:

> In acute febrile disease, there are striking variations during the course of the illness, to which the pulse can sensitively respond, while the abdomen Sho (pattern) cannot respond as quickly. In endogenous-induced (internal damage) illnesses, the disease stages pass slowly and Kyo (Deficiency) and Jitsu (Excess) can be diagnosed by the abdomen Sho (pattern). (*Kampo: A Clinical Guide to Theory and Practice*, Otsuka, K., Transl. De Soriano, G. and Dawes, N., 1st edn. publ. Churchill Livingstone, 2010; 2nd edn. publ. Singing Dragon, 2017)

It is certainly the case that in TJM disciplines whose diagnostic is expressed in terms of patterns of Excess (*Jitsu* 実) or Deficiency (*Kyo* 虚) at the meridian (exterior) level, such as in the practice of Acupuncture, pulse findings tend to predominate. However, organ level (interior) patterns, such as those diagnosed in *Kampo*, are always assessed primarily using abdominal findings.

I would add here that, in a similar way to the abdomen, changes on the tongue also do not occur quickly. Using the familiar language of *Yin* and *Yang*, we might characterize the pulse as a *Yang* diagnostic indicator compared with both the tongue and abdomen that belong to *Yin*. This comparison would suggest that findings on the tongue or abdomen will likely reflect chronic Disease Patterns, and in terms of disease progression and treatment evaluation, would be unlikely to demonstrate evidence of sudden change. This is contrary to the pulse, which can change in an instant. It also would indicate that it is much more likely for the tongue and abdomen findings to concur, even when the pulse may not.

An example of this would be that if, in the *Fukushin* exam, the Lower Abdominal Oketsu Point (*Sho Fuku Kyu Ketsu* 小腹急結) is found (see Chapter 3 for a clear description of this finding), the likelihood of the tongue exam showing similar signs of Blood Stasis is very high. For example, the tongue body would likely show some purple or dusky hue in general or purple petechiae in particular, as well as distended sublingual veins, also purple or dark in color. The relative degree of sublingual vein distention on either side may even match exactly the degree of intensity of the abdominal *Oketsu* point on the same side (left or right) of the lower abdomen. In this way, the frequent correspondence of tongue and abdomen findings in the diagnostic process is clinically very useful and accounts for their privileged place in the diagnostic hierarchy of *Kampo* practice.

2. The purpose of the abdominal exam

According to Dr. *Otsuka* (quoted above), "The aim of Fukushin in Kampo is to determine the Kyo and Jitsu of the patient." This would seem to suggest that the exam is used primarily to assess the relative strength of the patient's constitution (and therefore their potential for resistance against disease). Such an assessment could prove invaluable in terms of both predicting prognosis as well as in informing dosing, intensity and duration of treatment approaches.

However, whilst constitutional assessment is indeed strongly influenced by abdominal palpation, as discussed extensively below, there are also individual findings on the abdomen that point to specific Formula Patterns that correspond to them. This becomes a critical factor in the diagnostic process as it will influence directly the precise choice of formula in any given clinical situation.

In *Kampo* practice, therefore, the abdomen is used in identifying and categorizing both of the following aspects of pattern diagnosis (discussed later in this chapter):

- Constitutional Patterns (*Tai Shitsu Sho* 体質証)

- Disease Patterns (*Byo Sho* 病証)

Indeed, a *Kampo* diagnosis cannot be said to be complete unless it makes reference to both of these aspects of assessment. They will each be the subject of detailed discussion in subsequent parts of this chapter, but for the moment a clinical example may be useful:

If the *Fukushin* exam were to reveal the first finding listed in Chapter 3 as #1a Lax and Powerless Abdomen *Fuku Bu Nan Jyaku Mu Ryoku* 腹部軟弱無力, with its accompanying description, then we would likely be tempted to classify the Constitutional Pattern (*Tai Shitsu Sho* 体質証) of such a person as one of Weakness (*Kyo Sho* 虚証) and probably Coldness (*Hie Sho* 冷え症). This in turn would imply a person whose general metabolism was always sluggish, otherwise known in TJM as a *Yang* Deficient Type (*Yo Kyo Sho* 陽虚証). Such an individual will always tend to experience poor circulation, have cold limbs, feel tired and sluggish, have a poor appetite, gas and loose stools. In fact, these latter digestive symptoms are even classified as a subset of the Weak, Cold Type known in *Kampo* as *I Cho Kyo Jyaku* 胃腸虚弱 (literally "Weak and Powerless Stomach and Intestines"). Such symptoms in this case belong, not necessarily to a specific Disease Pattern such as hypothyroidism or IBS for example in biomedicine, or Spleen *Yang* Deficiency (*Hi Yo Kyo Sho* 脾陽虚証) in *Zang-Fu* Organ theory (*Zo Fu Setsu* 臓腑説) in Chinese Medicine, but rather to a constitutional tendency.

However, if alongside this constitutional abdominal finding, we were also to find the following Abdominal Conformations listed by # in Chapter 3, then the totality of abdominal findings in this example would reveal a mixture of constitutional and symptomatic evidence which, when considered as a whole, would likely conform to a particular Formula Pattern (Yakusho 薬証):

- #4 Epigastric Obstruction (*Shin Ka Hi* 心下痞)

- #7 Epigastric Splash Sound (*Shin Ka Bu Shin Sui On* 心下部振水音)

- #10 Epigastric Pulstations (*Shin Ka Ki* 心下悸)

Indeed, such an abdomen precisely matches the pattern of the following *Taiyin* Stage (*Tai In Byo* 太陰病) formula described by Dr. *Otsuka* thus: *Ninjin To* 人参湯 (*Ren Shen Tang* in Chinese) aka *Ri Chuh To* 理中汤 (*Li Zhong Tang* in Chinese)—Ginseng and Ginger Combination.

> This formula is used to warm "cold on the inside" (*Ri No Kan* 裏の寒), when the digestive organs are weak (hypofunctioning) (*Kyo Jyaku* 虚弱), the complexion (*Kesshoku* 血色) is poor and there is a lack of *Sei Ki* 生気 (Essential *Qi*). The tongue has no coat and is wet, the urine is clear and copious, the four limbs easily "become icy" (*Hieru* 冷える), the saliva is thin and collects in the mouth, the feces are soft and there is a tendency towards diarrhea. There may also be complaints of dizziness, vomiting and stomach pain.
>
> There are two types of abdominal *Sho* (腹証): the first is the Lax and Powerless Abdomen (*Fuku Bu Nan Jyaku Mu Ryoku* 腹部軟弱無力), when the Splash Sound (*Shin Ka Bu Shin Sui On* 心下部振水音) is present. In the second *Sho*, the abdominal wall is thin, delicate and rigid (*Hi Jyaku* 菲弱), like a sheet of veneer when pressed.
>
> (Otsuka, 1956)

The above example demonstrates that the combined Constitutional and Formula Pattern findings are both considered essential in the final diagnostic assessment of such a patient. The diagnostic pattern itself, a combination of both a Constitutional Pattern (*Tai Shitsu Sho* 体質証) and a Disease Pattern (*Byo Sho* 病証), is expressed in the *Kampo* dialectic as the formula name used to treat such a pattern. Thus, in the example given the diagnosis would be: the Ginseng and Ginger Pattern (*Ren Shen Tang Sho* 人参湯証). Indeed, the use of a formula name in this way to characterize a pattern of diagnosis is standard in the *Kampo* diagnostic system as we will see.

Ultimately then, the purpose of the *Fukushin* exam in the *Kampo* diagnostic process is to arrive at a definition of the Abdominal Pattern (*Fukusho* 腹証) for each case at hand. The clinical narrative that accompanies this finding will automatically direct the practitioner toward a matching Formula Pattern (*Yakusho*薬証) which, in turn, will define therefore both the diagnosis and treatment of that patient.

This direct correlation between a pattern of diagnosis (in this example that of an abdominal pattern) and the treatment strategy itself is a distinctive feature of *Kampo* and can be summarized in the phrase "Matching Pattern and Formula" (*Ho Sho So Tai* 方証相対) used by *Todo Yoshimasu* 吉益東洞 (1702–1773) in the late *Edo* period. More on this later.

For now, let's consider some of the Constitutional, Disease and Formula Patterns that can be revealed by the abdominal exam.

3. *Fukushin* Constitutional Patterns (*Tai Shitsu Sho* 体質証)

As previously discussed, one of the primary clinical implications of the abdominal exam is to afford the practitioner a sense of the relative strength of the patient's constitution, expressed in terms of Strong (*Jitsu Sho* 実証) or Weak (*Kyo Sho* 虚証) as follows:

Strong Constitutional Type (*Jitsu Tai Shitsu Sho* 実体質証)

The definition of constitutional strength as epitomized by a *Jitsu* type, is that they have abundant *Yang Qi* (*Yo Ki* 陽気). The health implications in this case are that their resistance to disease is typically strong, their response to therapeutic stimuli of any kind is dynamic and they tolerate strong treatment methods (such as Sudorific, Emetic and Purgative actions in Herbal Medicine or longer treatment times, more needles and stronger needle stimulation in Acupuncture).

In terms of disease tendencies, *Jitsu* types will suffer intense and severe symptomology (though more likely acute than chronic), they will tend towards Excess Patterns (*Jitsu Sho* 実証) in general, including Heat Patterns (*Netsu Sho* 熱証), *Qi* Stasis (*Ki Tai Sho* 気滞証) and *Qi* Counterflow Patterns (*Ki Nobose Sho* 気のぼせ証),

Blood Stasis (*Oketsu Sho* 瘀血証) and Blood Counterflow Patterns (*Ketsu Nobose Sho* 血のぼせ証) and Fluid Accumulation (*Tan In Sho* 痰飲証) and Fluid Counterflow Patterns (*Sui Nobose Sho* 水のぼせ証).

There are the following two subdivisions in *Jitsu* types:

1. Amongst the *Jitsu* types there is the *Yang* within *Yang* (*Yo Chu No Yo* 陽中の陽) who tend to be tighter, drier and hotter by nature with robust, boisterous, at times hyperactive energy and intense affect, usually known as Strong Blood Types (*Jitsu Ketsu Taishitsu Sho* 実血体質証). They literally have an abundance of blood in their system and in many ways are reminiscent of the "Sanguine" types as defined by medieval European Humoral Medicine. In *Kampo*, they are considered likely to suffer from Excess Patterns of Blood Stasis with Blood Counterflow and Heat symptomology (which will be identified later). They will require formulas that crack, invigorate, cool and at times detoxify the Blood.

2. The *Yin* within *Yang* (*Yo Chu No In* 陽中の陰) types tend to be more corpulent, more heavy-set and watery (Damp) and thus relatively less hot by nature with a more calm, stable affect though equally full of energy potential so that they are known as Strong Water Types (*Jitsu Sui Taishitsu Sho* 実水体質証). They literally have an abundance of fluid in their system and are more reminiscent of the "Phlegmatic" types in Humoral Medicine. In *Kampo* they are likely to manifest Excess Patterns of Fluid Accumulation with Water Counterflow and Damp symptoms (discussed later). They will require formulas to drain, dry, resolve and regulate fluids.

Weak Constitutional Types (*Kyo Tai Shitsu Sho* 虚体質証)

Kyo types, on the other hand, suffer from a lack of *Yang Qi* (*Yo Ki* 陽気). Their resistance to disease is poor, their response to stimuli is either sluggish or hyper-reactive, they are cold, easily fatigued and they cannot tolerate strong methods of treatment, requiring instead more gentle approaches (such as regulating, warming and tonifying herbs, shorter needling times with gentle stimulation and fewer needles in Acupuncture along with Moxibustion). In terms of disease tendencies, *Kyo* types will suffer milder, less acute symptoms (though likely chronic and recalcitrant), they will tend towards Deficient Patterns (*Kyo Sho* 虚証) including Deficiency Cold Patterns (*Kyo Kan Sho* 虚寒証), *Qi* and *Yang* Deficient Patterns (*Ki/Yo Kyo Sho* 気 / 陽虚証) and Patterns of Deficient Counterflow (*Kyo Nobose Sho* 虚のぼせ証) either of Blood (*Ketsu* 血) or Fluids (*Sui* 水).

There are the following two subdivisions in *Kyo* types:

1. Amongst the *Kyo* types there is the *Yin* within *Yin* (*In Chu No In* 陰中の陰) who tend to be (like their #2 *Yo Chu No In* 陽中の陰 counterparts above) more corpulent, wet (Damp) and colder by nature though they always feel tired and heavy with a reserved and at times passive affect and thus can be called Weak Water Types (*Kyo Sui Taishitsu Sho* 虚水体質証). As weak "Phlegmatic" types they have too much fluid in the system along with a lack of *Yang Qi* (*Yo ki* 陽) that leads to Deficient Patterns of Fluid Accumulation (*Kyo Sui Tai Sho* 虚水証). They will require formulas that regulate fluids but also tonify *Qi* (*Ki* 気) and warm *Yang* (*Yo* 陽).

2. *Yang* within *Yin* (*In Chu No Yo* 陰中の陽) types, (like their #1 *Yo Chu No Yo* 陽中の陽 counterparts above), tend to be thinner, tighter and drier and though their energy may appear to be dynamic; they lack root or substance and easily become unstable and strained, leading to fatigue and anxiety. They are referred to in *Kampo* as Weak Blood Types (*Kyo Ketsu Taishitsu Sho* 虚血体質証). As weak "Sanguine" types, they are deficient and dry and lack sufficient moistening Constructive (Nutritive) *Qi* (*Ei Ki* 營氣), which leads to Deficient Patterns of *Qi* and Blood (*Ki Kyo/Ketsu Kyo Sho* 気虚 / 血虚証) with accompanying Counterflow (*Nobose* のぼせ) symptoms.

It should be noted here that there is also the Moderate or "Middle" constitution (*Chu Tai Shitsu Sho* 中体質証), which indicates a person who is neither Weak nor Strong.

Constitutional assessment in *Kampo* is a process of getting to know the patient's build, affect, behavior and other characteristics including their tendencies for illness as well as their typical response to treatment. Clearly, such a process takes time and an accurate assessment of constitution may take weeks or months to establish and will always be subject to ongoing re-evaluation.

Nonetheless, from a practical standpoint, each formula used in *Kampo* can be categorized as either for the Strong (*Jitsu Taishitsu Sho* 実体質証), Weak (*Kyo Taishitsu Sho* 虚体質証) or Moderate (*Chu Taishitsu Sho* 中体質証) Constitutional Type. Such a system of categorization is highly useful clinically as it often serves to influence specific decision-making in the treatment process.

For example, in an External Cold Pattern (*Hyo Kan Sho* 表寒証), where the patient is suffering all the symptoms of *Taiyang* Stage Disease (*Tai Yo Byo* 太陽病) such as Evil Cold/Wind (*Okan/Fu* 悪寒/風), Chills (*Samu Ke* 寒気) and Fever (*Netsu* 熱), Floating Pulse (*Fu Myaku* 浮脈), Sweating (*Hakkan* 発汗) or Absence of Sweating (*Mukan* 無汗), Headache (*Zu Tsu* 頭痛) and so on, if that patient is known to have a Weak Constitution then *Mahuang* Combination (*Ma O To* 麻黄湯) or any other *Mahuang*-based formula will be forbidden and Cinnamon Combination (*Keishi To* 桂枝湯) or its derivatives must be used instead. This is a classic example of where constitutional assessment can take precedence in determining the treatment approach as opposed to only the Disease Pattern (*Byo Sho* 病証) by itself.

As difficult and complex as it may be to reliably assess patient constitution, the abdomen can provide both visual and tactile information that can be immediately useful in beginning to establish the basis of a person's constitutional tendencies. Here are some examples.

Visual signs on the abdomen

The color of the abdominal wall may point to the nutritional status of the patient: pale often indicating Cold (*Hie Sho* 冷え症) or Blood Deficient (*Ketsu Kyo Sho* 血虚証) tendencies, typical of Weak Types (*Kyo Taishitsu Sho* 虚体質証) whilst a darker or dusky color might point towards a tendency for Blood Stasis (*Oketsu* 瘀血) more common in Strong Type individuals (*Jitsu Taishitsu Sho* 実体質証).

The shape of the abdomen often points to strength or weakness: well-musculated and with good color and luster, whether large or small, is suggestive of a Strong Type whilst the thin-walled, lax or sometimes tight, overstrained abdomen, again either small or large, is more likely the Weak Type.

In terms of the costal angle, a sharp or an acute angle is more commonly found in Weak Types while Strong individuals will often have a more dull or obtuse angle.

If the peristaltic movement is visible at the surface of the abdomen this is always a sign of Weakness where the abdominal wall will always be thin and malnourished.

Tactile signs on the abdomen

STRONG TYPES (*JITSU SHO* 実証)

If the overall tone and strength of the abdominal wall is good, there is ample adipose tissue and the skin is firm and feels warm and elastic, whether in a smaller or larger body frame, this suggests a Strong Type (*Jitsu Sho* 実証). These types will often dislike pressure applied to the abdomen.

Amongst the Strong Type Constitutions, there is the *Yang* within *Yang* (*Yo Chu Yo Sho* 陽中の陽証), described above, who will tend to have firm, tight and well-defined musculature with very little body fat. The skin will feel warm, elastic and responsive, and the muscles dense and firm. A body image that may capture this type would be that of a 100m professional sprinter.

The *Yin* within *Yang* Strong Type (*Yo Chu No In Sho* 陽中の陰証), also mentioned above, has a more rounded, smooth body profile with less clearly defined musculature, though nonetheless powerful. The skin will be cooler and softer though there will be plenty of strength at a deeper level when pressed. Here the body image that comes to mind is that of a professional swimmer.

WEAK TYPES (*KYO SHO* 虚証)

On the other hand, when the abdomen is either thin, tight and non-elastic, or there are conversely large amounts of lax, cool, atonic muscle and adipose tissue that have no strength or vitality to them, then this suggests the Weak Type (*Kyo Sho* 虚証). These types will always like both pressure and heat applied to their abdomens.

Amongst the Weak Type Constitutions, there is the *Yin* within *Yin* (*Yin Chu No Yin Sho* 陰中の陰証), described above, who will tend to have lax, flaccid and poorly defined, atonic musculature. The skin surface will be puffy, loose and cold and there will be an absence of "strength in the depths" (*Fuku Bu Nan Jyaku Mu Ryoku* 腹部軟弱無力). There is a tendency for obesity and Toxic Water Accumulation (*Sui Doku* 水毒) in this type of person.

The *Yang* within *Yin* (*In Chu No Yo Sho* 陰中の陽証) constitution, described above, will tend to have a much smaller, tighter abdomen, which is "Delicate and Rigid" (*Hi Jyaku* 菲弱). It will show "Strained Resistance" (*Ko Kyu* 拘急) on the surface, including tension in the rectus abdominis muscle (*Ri Kyu* 裏急), but will feel hollow or empty underneath. The skin and fascia are extremely thin, dry and poorly nourished and the abdomen often feels tight and hollow (*Kin Cho* 緊張) like a drum. There is a tendency for being underweight and for Blood Stasis (*Oketsu* 瘀血) in this type of person.

Summary of constitutional findings

These basic visual and tactile qualities can easily be perceived from the very beginning of the exam as described in Figures 3.2a and 3.2b, and 3.2c. From the first moment of touching the patient, the practitioner can quickly form an impression of whether the person is basically Strong or Weak. Then, according to the differential assessments offered above, the Strong and Weak abdomens can be further subdivided into *Yin* and *Yang* respectively, allowing for further categorization into Cold (Water) Types and Hot (Blood) Types respectively.

Kampo therefore distinguishes four basic Abdominal Patterns in terms of constitutional assessment, using language already identified above as follows:

1. *Yang* within *Yang* Constitution (*Yo Chu No Yo Taishitsu Sho* 陽中の陽体質証)—the Strong, Dry/Hot (Excess *Yang*) Blood Type.

2. *Yin* within *Yang* Constitution (*Yo Chu No In Taishitsu Sho* 陽中の陰体質証)—the Strong, Damp (Excess *Yin*) Water Type.

3. *Yang* within *Yin* Constitution (*In Chu No Yo Taishitsu Sho* 陰中の陽体質証)—the Weak, Chilly/Dry (Deficient *Yin*) Blood Type.

4. *Yin* within *Yin* Constitution (*In Chu No In Taishitsu Sho* 陰中の陰体質証)—the Weak, Damp/Cold (Deficient *Yang*), Water Type.

Once the practitioner is able to distinguish clearly between these four basic abdominal types, this will provide a clear starting point for more comprehensive clinical interpretation. They will then be ready to proceed with the rest of the exam and attempt to establish findings which relate to Disease Patterns (*Byo Sho* 病証) in addition to the Constitutional Pattern (*Taishitsu Sho* 体質証) already determined. This process will be discussed comprehensively in the "Morphology, charting and interpretation" section in Chapter 4.

Let us now discuss Disease Patterns (*Byo Sho* 病証) as they reflect on the abdomen.

4. *Fukushin* Disease Patterns (*Byo Sho* 病証)

The traditional classification of Disease Patterns (*Byo Sho* 病証) in *Kampo* was originally made based on a literal description of the primary symptoms that characterized the illness. This is a significant feature of *Kampo* diagnostics as it demonstrates that the patient's subjective experience is carefully considered in relation to reaching a decision about the disease diagnosis.

In fact, many traditional disease names included both subjective and objective language in their definition in the same way, as we shall see below, that the Formula Patterns (*Yakusho* 薬証) also comprise the findings (*Sho Ken* 所見), including both patient (symptoms) and practitioner (signs), in the body of clinical evidence or Pattern (*Sho* 証) that defines them.

For example, if a patient complained in the past of "Sudden Turmoil" (*Kaku Ran* 霍乱), they would likely have had acute, urgent diarrhea and stomach pain possibly characteristic of an infectious disease such as cholera, whereas "Sudden Turmoil in the Uterus" would have referred to hysteria (originating from the Greek word for uterus). In fact, traditionally in *Kampo*, panic attacks were known as: "Running Piglet Syndrome" (*Hon Ton Sho* 奔豚証), a phrase originally used in the "Prescriptions from the Golden Cabinet" (*Kin Ki Yo Ryaku* 金匱要略), probably to evoke either the physical sensation of out-of-control pigs scattering in panic (related to symptoms like palpitations and "butterflies in the stomach") or the emotional state (anxiety) associated with the unsettling noise of a squealing herd of pigs.

Similarly, if someone had complained of "Wasting Thirst" (*Sho Katsu* 消渇), they would likely have been suffering from diabetes mellitus in modern terminology just as the patient with "Weakness and Fatigue" (*Kyo Ro* 虚労) could well have had pulmonary tuberculosis ("consumption"). Someone with "Fifty-Year Shoulder" (*Go Ju Kata* 五十肩) most probably had a frozen shoulder, whilst a woman who may have complained of a syndrome originally referred to in the past as "The Way of the Blood" (*Chi No Michi Sho* 血の道

症) could be said today to be experiencing the symptoms of peri-menopausal syndrome.

In some cases a single symptom was used to define what in modern medicine might be differentiated into multiple disease names such as "cough" (*Gai Gyaku* 咳逆), which could in the past have referred to bronchitis, bronchiecstasis, bronchitic asthma, asthmatic bronchitis, emphesema and any number of pulmonary diseases which are characterized by the shared symptom of coughing. In the same way, a diagnosis of "diarrhea" (*Ri Shitsu* 痢疾), in traditional terms, could refer to any number of modern gastro-intestinal diseases which manifest that particular symptom such as colitis, diverticulitis, Crohn's disease and irritable bowel syndrome.

In diagnostic terms, it is therefore highly unwise in *Kampo* practice to rely on biomedical disease names alone when considering treatment options and the selection of formulas, and whilst traditional *Kampo* disease names are at least helpful in terms of identifying some of the main symptoms experienced by the patient, neither system of disease nomenclature and classification, old or new, provides a differential diagnosis that can be relied upon exclusively for determining appropriate treatment.

For example, in the case of "diarrhea" (*Ri Shitsu* 痢疾) mentioned above, though a valid diagnostic term, it does not by itself reveal the nature of the pattern involved in terms of whether it may be Excess (*Jitsu Sho* 実症) or Deficient (*Kyo Sho* 虚症), Hot (*Netsu Sho* 熱症) or Cold (*Kan Sho* 寒症) or any combination thereof, all of which are essential differential aspects of *Kampo* diagnosis. Nor does the name alone identify whether the basic pathological nature of the disease involves dysfunction at the level of *Qi* (*Ki* 気), Blood (*Ketsu* 血) or Fluids (*Sui* 水) and neither does it give any clue as to the Etiology (*Byo In* 病因) of the problem, which in the *Kampo* diagnostic must be differentiated into External (*Gai In* 外因) versus Internal (*Nai In* 内因) causes.

Thus in *Kampo* formula classification, each formula is associated not only with the respective constitutional type to which it is suited (as mentioned above), but also with whether it is a formula used to treat Patterns of Excess or Deficiency; Heat or Cold and combinations thereof.

Furthermore, each formula in *Kampo* is classified according to whether it belongs essentially to the category of *Qi* Formulas (*Ki Yaku* 気薬), Blood Formulas (*Ketsu Yaku* 血薬) or Fluid Formulas (*Sui Yaku* 水薬).

Finally, formulas are classified also according to whether they treat Exterior Patterns (*Hyo Sho* 表症) or Interior Patterns (*Ri Sho* 裏症) or both. For example, Cinnamon Combination (*Keishi To* 桂枝湯) is classified in *Kampo* as a formula for the Weak (Dry) Constitutional Type. It is considered a formula both for Exterior and Interior Patterns of Deficiency and is very clearly classified as a *Qi* Formula (*Ki Yaku* 気薬). *Dang Gui* Four Combination (*Shi Motsu To* 四物湯) is also classified as a formula for the Weak (Dry) Constitutional Type although only for Interior Patterns of Deficiency, in this case of Blood. Hoelen Five Formula (*Go Rei San* 五苓散) on the other hand is classified as a formula for the Strong (Wet) Constitutional Type. It is considered a formula for both Exterior and Interior Patterns of Excess and is classified as a Water Formula.

This kind of detailed differential diagnostic categorization explains why, when consulting contemporary *Kampo* literature that often lists diseases by their modern biomedical name according to a typical systems approach, multiple *Kampo* formulas will be indicated in the treatment of any one such named disease. Thus, as has been mentioned, a disease name such as colitis for example, with a main symptom of "diarrhea," must in fact be carefully differentiated according to the factors listed above in order to match an appropriate formula for treatment in *Kampo*.

For example, there can be diarrhea caused by External or Internal factors; the nature of the diarrhea may belong to a pattern of Excess or Deficiency; Heat or Cold and may be categorized as belonging primarily to *Qi*, Blood or Fluid disharmony or some combination thereof. This example of diarrhea and its differentiation and treatment with varying *Kampo* formulas will be discussed below in the "*Fukushin* formula patterns" (*Yakusho* 薬証) section.

For the moment it is enough to note that the *Kampo* diagnostic clearly does not rely on disease and symptom names alone when it comes to selecting a formula for treatment. Fortunately, in place of the disease category itself (whether traditional or modern), *Kampo* focuses rather on defining what is referred to as the Disease Pattern (*Byo Sho* 病証) in order to determine the correct treatment. This pattern or syndrome is best defined by the clinical "proof" or evidence that identifies and is uniquely associated with it. Indeed, the *Kampo* diagnostic process is one in which the practitioner is constantly attempting to match this clinical evidence, gathered from careful inspection, palpation and questioning of the patient, with an already existing treatment "unit" in the form of a Formula Pattern (*Yakusho* 薬証).

One of the factors most hierarchically privileged in this clinical endeavor is the subtle and judicious use of Abdominal Diagnosis (*Fukushin* 腹診). Amongst the many aspects of the differential diagnostic process already mentioned, including the Constitutional Pattern as well as patterns of Exterior/Interior, Excess/Deficiency, Hot/Cold, Qi/Blood/Fluids, the pulse, the tongue, the patient's subjective complaints, the name of the disease and so on, it is often the abdominal pattern that can help clarify the correct "Matching of Pattern and Formula."

In fact, it can be said of the *Kampo* diagnostic system as a whole that an accurate reading of the Abdominal Pattern (*Fukusho*) in any given disease is tantamount to identifying the correct formula for treatment of that disease.

Another way of saying this is that each and every specific Formula Pattern (*Yakusho*) used in the *Kampo* treatment system includes its own unique Abdominal Pattern (*Fukusho*) as one of its primary identifying features.

As testimony to this direct correlation between abdomen and Formula Patterns we need only refer to a landmark text from the *Edo* period (1800) written by *Inaba Katsubunrei, Extraordinary Views of Abdominal Patterns (Fukusho Ki Ran)*. Until very recently this seminal work was unavailable in the English language, but happily we now have a translation by Jay Kageyama, publ. The Chinese Medicine Database, 2018. This text systematically presents a detailed abdominal description along with illustrations for each of more than 75 commonly used *Kampo* formulas. It provides clear testimony to the fact that, in the *Kampo* process of "matching of pattern with Formula," the abdominal pattern often provides the key to both diagnosis and treatment rather than the disease name or pattern alone.

Let us now explore this concept of "Matching Pattern and Formula" and the role of *Fukushin* within it in more detail.

5. *Fukushin* Formula Patterns (*Yakusho* 薬証)

It can be said of the *Kampo* system that, uniquely perhaps, it considers the Formula Pattern (*Yakusho* 薬証) to comprise a clinical narrative that correlates precisely with that of the corresponding Disease Pattern (*Byo Sho* 病証) associated with it, thereby rendering the name of the formula synonymous with the name of the disease it is designed to treat.

Since each formula used in *Kampo* is associated with its own distinctive and unique clinical pattern made up of objective signs determined by the practitioner (including pulse, tongue and abdomen), subjective symptoms (as reported by the patient), as well as the constitutional type for which it is best suited, it is the formula name therefore that constitutes the diagnosis itself, which necessarily includes at the same time the Disease Pattern associated with it.

It is not altogether unusual, for example, for a *Kampo* practitioner to refer in his or her patient charting to their "Cinnamon Combination (*Keishito* 桂枝湯) patient," meaning a patient who has been diagnosed with the *Keishito* Pattern (*Keishito Sho* 桂枝湯証), aka the diagnosis, and thus has been duly prescribed the *Keishito* Formula (*Keishito Yaku* 桂枝湯薬), aka the treatment.

Those familiar with the work of Samuel Hahnemann (1755–1843), the German physician who created the practice of homeopathy, will recognize here a similarity with the way in which his "homeopathics" or remedies are each directly associated with the symptom patterns they are designed to treat. He posited a "drug picture" for each remedy so that the name of the remedy itself operates clinically as a kind of diagnostic categorization as well as the treatment modality itself. "I saw an interesting *Nux Vomica* patient in the clinic today" would not be an unusual start to a case discussion amongst Classical homeopaths, any of whom would immediately be able to paint a clinical picture in their minds of the detailed signs and symptoms such a patient must have presented with in order to have been prescribed that particular remedy.

So too in *Kampo*, when the name of a particular formula is invoked, there comes with it an immediate, detailed and almost visceral association with a highly specific set of signs and symptoms uniquely and exclusively associated with that formula, and only that formula. It is in this sense therefore that *Kampo* considers the Classical Formula "unit" to function both as a diagnostic label and a treatment method, thus precluding the necessity to articulate the diagnosis in any more abstract or theoretical manner.

In the *Kampo* system, therefore, we might say that the individualizing of the treatment process is done at the Formula level by carefully matching a correct existing formula with the patient at hand. In Traditional Chinese Medicine (TCM), in contrast, in fact a post-war modern version of Classical Chinese Medicine, this process is rather individualized not at the Formula level but at the individual herb level, by compounding each herb one at a time into a new formula designed to suit the patient presentation, symptom by symptom.

In *Kampo*, the practice of individualizing treatment using pre-existing classical formulas most likely started in the *Edo* period in Japan. Some historical scholars and *Kampo* researchers have suggested that one reason for the start of this "formula-based" approach to individualizing treatment in Japan was because, during that time period (1600s–1800s), the supply and availability of abundant raw herb materials was not guaranteed. Most had to be imported from China and this process was not always reliable. This led, some have argued, to the deliberate reduction in dosage used in any given formula, in order to economize on usage and ensure a reliable supply of raw materials.

It has been suggested by Watanabe *et al.* in an article entitled "Pattern Classification in Kampo Medicine" (publ. *Evidence Based Complementary and Alternative Medicine*, 2014) that "usage of different amounts of herbs was described in a book by Kaibara in 1712. According to this book, the amount of each herb used in Japan was 1/5 to 1/3 that used in China."

This may indeed have accounted for a practical reason as to why doctors in the *Edo* period became wedded to the individualizing of treatment according to formula matching and not individual herb matching. After all, formulas from the Eastern (Later) *Han* dynasty (*Higashi Kan* 東漢, 25–220 CE) texts, the "Treatise on Cold Damage" (*Sho Kan Ron* 傷寒論) and "Prescriptions from the Golden Cabinet" (*Kin Ki Yo Ryaku* 金匱要略), are mostly small, comprising only between three and seven or eight herbs in total. Furthermore, the herbs used in them are mostly not uncommon and so would have been more readily available in Japan at that time.

Be that as it may, it was undoubtedly during the *Edo* period that *Kampo* identified and established the specific clinical characteristics of each formula, based on the classics, that then came to be known as the Formula Pattern (*Yakusho*). This practice inevitably led in the later *Edo* period to *Todo Yoshimasu*'s practice of "Matching of Pattern and Formula" already alluded to.

Let us now return to the example (above) of diarrhea as a main complaint in order to illustrate the way in which this whole process of differential diagnosis is followed in *Kampo* practice, and also where the abdominal pattern, once identified, can often help point directly to the formula to be selected for treatment—in other words how it illustrates the matching of pattern with formula.

ACUTE DIARRHEA

In cases of acute, sudden-onset diarrhea, when likely there is a micro-organism involved (virus, bacterium or parasite) this is considered an Exterior Pattern (*Hyo Sho* 表証) in *Kampo*. As such, according to the clinical evidence, a differentiation will be made using the Six Stage Pattern theory (*Roku Byo Sho* 六病位証) deriving from the *Han* dynasty text "Treatise on Cold Damage" (*Sho Kan Ron* 傷寒論) by *Zhang Zhong Jing* written in 219 CE. Typically, the acute stage will fall into one of the *Yang* Stages (*Yo Byo* 陽病) as follows.

If, in addition to sudden onset of diarrhea, the pulse is Floating (*Fu Myaku* 浮脈) and there are accompanying signs of Evil Cold/ Wind (*Okan/Fu* 悪寒／風), Chills (*Samu Ke* 寒気), Fever (*Netsu* 熱), Sweating (*Hakkan* 発汗) or Absence of Sweating (*Mukan* 無汗), Headache (*Zu Tsu* 頭痛) and so on this is considered the Greater *Yang* Disease Stage (*Tai Yo Byo Sho* 太陽病証). If the pulse is Floating, Tight (*Kin Myaku* 緊脈) and Strong (*Jitsu Myaku* 実脈) it is the Exterior Cold Excess Pattern (*Hyo Kan Jitsu Sho* 表寒実証), and if in addition the diarrhea is watery, there is thirst, a desire to drink, but nausea is experienced when water is drunk, with reduced urinary output, edema (especially facial) and an abdomen that is well-nourished (a sign of a strong constitution), Full and Distended (*Fuku Man* 腹満, see Chapter 4) along with a Water Splash Sound (*Shin Ka Bu Shin Sui On* 心下部振水音, see Chapter 4) then the diagnosis is the Hoelen Five Formula Pattern (GRS—*Go Rei San Sho* 五苓散証).

If, on the other hand, the pulse is Floating and Weak (*Kyo Myaku* 虚脈) it belongs to the Exterior Cold Deficiency Pattern (*Hyo Kan Kyo Sho* 表寒虚証) in the Greater *Yang* Disease Stage. If, in addition the abdomen is thin, Tight and Powerless (*Fuku Bu Kin Mu Ryoku* 腹部緊無力, see Chapter 4)—a sign of a weak constitution—with Empty Distension (*Kyo Fuku Man* 虚腹満, see Chapter 4), overall abdominal muscle tension (*Fuku Choku Kin Ren Kyu* 腹直筋攣急) and specifically tension in the rectus abdominis muscle called "Inside Spasm" (*Ri Kyu* 裏急, see Chapter 4) and the diarrhea is accompanied by severe spasms and cramps in the abdomen then this is the Cinnamon and Peony Combination Pattern (KSTS— *Keishikashakuyakuto* 桂枝加芍薬湯).

These formula examples are likely associated with treating acute diarrhea caused by enteroviruses according to modern biomedical models.

If, however, there is a sudden onset of diarrhea that is urgent and "explosive" with fetid, unformed stools and peri-anal irritation and burning, often called "Hot Diarrhea" (*Netsuri* 熱利) in *Kampo*, accompanied by Tidal Fever (*Cho Netsu* 潮熱), extreme Thirst (*Ko Katsu* 口渇), dehydration (possibly with delirium) where the pulse is Deep (*Chin Myaku* 沈脈), Rapid (*Saku Myaku* 数脈) and Surging (*Ko Myaku* 洪脈) and the entire abdomen is Full (*Fuku Man* 腹満, see Chapter 4) and the Lower Abdomen is Full and Hard (*Sho Fuku Ko Man* 小腹鞕満, see Chapter 4) then this is the Bright *Yang* Disease Stage (*Yo Mei Byo* 陽明病), which is a pattern of Interior Heat Excess (*Ri Netsu Jitsu Sho* 裏熱実証).

This stage may well correspond to the acute diarrhea associated with severe bacterial infections such as cholera and typhoid or more commonly salmonella (food poisoning) and so on in modern biomedicine. Such patients today would likely be taking antibiotics and possibly be hospitalized, however the traditional approach used to treating such conditions in Kampo would have been to "flush out" the pathogen by causing strong purgative formulas.

Such formulas would have included Major Rhurbarb Combination (DJT—*Dai Joki To* 大承気湯); Minor Rhubarb Combination (SJT—*Sho Joki To* 小承気湯), Persica and Rhubarb Combination (TJT—*Tokaku Joki To* 桃核承気湯) and Rhubarb and Moutan Combination (DBT—*Daio Botanpi To* 大黄牡丹皮湯) amongst others.

If the diarrhea has lingered several days following a sudden onset, the pulse is no longer floating but may have become Wiry (*Gen Myaku* 弦脈) and there are Alternating Chills and Fever (*Orai Kannetsu* 往来寒熱), a Bitter Taste in the mouth (*Koku* 口苦) or a loss of sense of taste, Nausea (*Kio* 喜), appetite loss, Dizziness (*Gen Un* 眩暈) or a feeling of pressure and fullness in the head, Chest Discomfort (*Kyo Hi* 胸痺) and a White Coating (*Haku Tai* 白苔) that has formed on the tongue then this is considered the Lesser *Yang* Disease Stage (*Sho Yo Byo* 少陽病). The abdominal finding will either be Hypochondriac Painful Fullness (*Kyo Kyo Ku Man* 胸

脇苦満, see Chapter 4), the *Ku Man* being a reference to a bloated, uncomfortable feeling in the chest and hypochondrium sometimes called "Bitter Fullness," or Hypochondriac Obstruction Resistance (*Kyo Ka Hi Ko* 脇下痞硬, see Chapter 4) where *Hi Ko* refers to a feeling of stuffiness along with localized tension, rigidity and resistance. This is the Minor Bupleurum Combination Pattern (SSK—*Sho Saiko To* 小柴胡湯) in *Kampo* including modifications of it specifically to treat diarrhea in the *Shaoyang* Stage such as Bupleurum and Hoelen Combination (SRT—*Sai Rei To* 柴苓湯) and Bupleurum and Magnolia Combination (IRT—*I Rei To* 胃苓湯).

CHRONIC DIARRHEA

In cases of Chronic Diarrhea, the symptoms typically come and go episodically, and are often related to various environmental factors such as diet, stress levels, weather conditions and in some cases, ongoing pathogenic factors such as chronic viral infections (e.g. HIV) or parasites. In *Kampo*, there are also cases believed to be related to constitution such as those involving Coldness (*Hie Sho* 冷え症) and Weak Gastro-Intestinal Function (*I Cho Kyo Jyaku* 胃腸虚弱).

As such, these are considered Internal Patterns of Deficiency (*Ri Kyo Sho* 裏虚証) in *Kampo* and, according to the clinical evidence, a differentiation will be made either using the theoretical principles governing diagnosis in internal medicine previously discussed, namely *Yin/Yang* (*In/Yo* 陰 / 陽), Hot/Cold (*Netsu/Kan* 熱 / 寒), *Qi*/Blood/Fluids (*Ki/Ketsu/Sui* 気 / 血 / 水) or, in cases of chronic pathogenic activity, the Six Stage Pattern theory (*Roku Byo Sho* 六病位証), which in chronic patterns will fall into one of the three *Yin* Stages (*In Byo* 陰病) as follows.

Diarrhea is one of the principal symptoms of all three *Yin* Stages, whose mechanism belongs to the damage done to the body's Internal *Yang* (*Ri Yo* 裏陽) by the penetration of Cold (*Kan* 寒). In particular, the function of digestion is impaired by this damage to its *Yang* (function) and thus peristaltic action, breakdown of food, absorption rates and transit time are all affected leading to loose, watery or unformed stools. Of clinical significance in such cases is the absence of mucous or blood in the stool, both pointing to a pattern of Cold (*Yang* Deficiency) rather than Heat (*Yang* Excess).

Further complaints are of borbyrygmus (*Fuku Chu Rai Mei* 腹中雷鳴, literally "Abdominal Thunder"), as gas collects in the intestines due to sluggish movement. If enough gas accumulates, causing stasis, it can lead to abdominal pain which over time can produce local inflammation or Heat (*Netsu*). Inflammation of this type will typically give rise to the complaint Intestinal Colic (*Sen Tsu* 疝痛, literally "Mountain of Pain"). Thus, it is important in *Kampo* to ascertain the presence or absence of pain which accompanies diarrhea, as this will determine the degree of "warming" action required in the corresponding formula.

When the rectum is the site of the inflammation the pain is called "Inside Acute Heavy After" (*Ri Kyu Ko Jyu* 裏急後重), which refers to a spasm of pain followed by a bearing-down sensation (tenesmus).

In the language of the "Treatise on Damaging Cold" (*Sho Kan Ron* 傷寒論), there is the diarrhea of the Greater *Yin* Stage (*Tai In Byo* 太陰病) and that of the Lesser *Yin* Stage (*Sho In Byo* 少陰病). Both stages involve *Yang* Deficiency and Cold and therefore loose stools, but in each stage the abdominal presentations are different as are the pulse and some other signs even though the tongue will be similar.

For example, in Greater *Yin* Stage diarrhea, there is undigested food in the stool which is loose and poorly formed. Diarrhea will likely occur in the morning and especially after eating. The Abdominal Conformation (*Fukusho* 腹証) will include a Water Splash Sound (*Shin Ka Bu Shin Sui On* 心下部振水音), Subjective Epigastric Discomfort (*Shin Ka Hi* 心下痞), Pulsations (*Shin Ki* 心悸) and a tendency for the abdomen to be Lax and Powerless (*Fuku Bu Nan Jyaku Mu Ryoku* 腹部軟弱無力) though also bloated from Deficiency Fullness (—*Kyo Fuku Man* 虚腹満). The patient will often feel nauseous and even vomit (clear fluid) because of this sensation of abdominal fullness. They will also display general lassitude, pallor and even anemia as their absorption rates are decreased. The tongue is puffy and moist. This is the Pattern (*Sho* 証) for Ginseng and Ginger Combination (*Ninjinto* 人参湯 aka *Richuto* 理中湯).

Other formulas used to treat diarrhea also based on Ginseng (*Ninjin* 人参), like Ginseng and Ginger Combination, in what would equate to a Greater *Yin* Stage pattern in *Kampo* terms, include Four Major Herb Combination (*Shikkunshito* 四君子湯) and Six Major Herb Combination (*Rikkunshito* 六君子湯) both of which are commonly used in Japan as adjunct treatments for diarrhea, poor absorption (with weight loss), anorexia and other symptoms associated with stomach and other forms of intestinal cancer and side-effects from its treatment. Compared with Ginseng and Ginger Combination with which they are similar, these two formulas treat patterns of Internal *Qi* Deficiency (*Ri Ki Kyo* 裏気虚) rather than cold itself reflected in the fact that the patient feels less chilly, has less likelihood of watery diarrhea and has a tongue which is flaccid with teethmarks but not puffy or swollen. Another diarrhea formula in this category would include Ginseng and Astragalus Combination (*Hochuekkito* 補中益気湯) when exhaustion, muscle weakness, hemmorhoids and lowered immunity are part of the pattern.

There are also several formulas for Greater *Yin* Stage diarrhea that do not use the herb Ginseng such as:

- Magnolia and Ginger Combination (*Heiisan* 平胃散), which is often used to treat erratic bowel movements where diarrhea is a common symptom along with excessive gas accumulation and abdominal fullness

- Cinnamon and Peony Combination (*Keishikashakuyakuto* 桂枝加芍薬湯), which treats abdominal cramps and pain with loose stool where the abdomen is less lax but rather Tight and Hard (*Kin Cho* 緊張) with rectus abdominis (muscle) Tension (*Ri Kyu* 裏急), no Splash sound and a generally tighter, thinner but nonetheless weak abdominal wall

- Minor Cinnamon and Peony Combination (*Shokenshuto* 小建中湯), which derives from the previous formula by adding Maltose (*Koi* 膠飴) used where the abdominal wall is especially thin and weak and the patient has lost weight

- Cinnamon and Ginseng Combination (*Keishininjinto* 桂枝人参湯), which is often used when there is diarrhea but also a low grade fever as in the case of chronic pathogenic activity in the gut (either viral or parasitic)

- Motility issues in the intestines in *Kampo* in *Yang* Deficient, Cold patterns where gas has accumulated and there may be episodes of explosive diarrhea along with abdominal pain are often treated with Major Zanthoxylum Combination (*Daikenchuto* 大建中湯)

In the case of Lesser *Yin* Stage diarrhea, the stool is usually completely unformed and watery and occurs especially on waking in the early morning (called "cock crow" diarrhea in TJM, a reference to its early morning occurrence). There may be repeated bouts during the day. The *Fukusho* is always Lax and Powerless (*Fuku Bu Nan Jyaku Mu Ryoku* 腹部軟弱無力) and is not distended with gas and fluids as in the Greater *Yin* Stage. Both stages, however, share the Water Splash Sound, the Epigastric Subjective Discomfort and the Pulsations (see above); however, in this case there is also the finding of Lower Abdomen Lacking Benevolence (*Sho Fuku Fu Jin* 小腹不仁). The patient will feel completely exhausted, experience icy cold extremities and often need to lie down, curl up and cover up. In this stage, the pulse is described as Minute (*Bi Myaku* 微脈) or Impalpable (*Fuku Mayaku* 伏脈) and the entire body metabolism is waning rather than just the intestinal function alone. The Constitution is one of Coldness (*Hie Sho* 冷え症) and the limbs are icy cold. This is the *Sho* for Vitality Combination (*Shinbuto* 真武湯).

Other classic Lesser *Yin* Stage formulas to treat diarrhea include:

- Aconite, Ginger and Licorice Combination (*Shigyakuto* 四逆湯)

- Ginseng Ginger and Aconite Combination (*Ninjinbushito* 人参附子湯)

- Ginseng, Licorice and Aconite Combination (*Shi Gyaku Ka Ninjin To* 四逆加人参湯)

In all three examples, the abdominal pattern is the same as that of Vitality Combination as is the nature of the diarrhea.

In cases of chronic diarrhea where the body strength has not begun to wane and actually the pattern is one of accumulation rather than deficiency, there will be evidence on the abdomen of Epigastric Obstruction Resistance (*Shin Ka Hi Ko* 心下痞硬) in an abdomen that is either Average (*Chu* 中) or Strong (*Jitsu* 実) and shows no other signs of deficiency. In such cases of diarrhea one of the Drain the Epigastrium (*Sha Shin To* 瀉心湯) formula families is often selected such as Pinellia Combination (*Hangeshashinto* 半夏瀉心湯), Pinellia and Ginger Combination (*Sho Kyo Sha Shin To* 生姜瀉心湯) when there is more belching, nausea and hiccup, and Pinellia and Licorice Combination (*Kanzo Sha Shin To* 甘草瀉心湯) when there is more abdominal discomfort and spasmodic cramping.

The above examples of formulas that may be used to treat different presentations in which diarrhea may be the main complaint are offered here, not as an exhaustive list of treatment possibilities—indeed there are many more in *Kampo*—but rather as an example of the detail and complexity of the traditional methods of differential diagnosis according to Formula Pattern (*Yakusho*) used in the *Kampo* tradition.

Amongst these methods which include differentiation according to the Six Stages of Disease, *Qi*, Blood and Fluid, disease name and Formula Patterns, perhaps one of the most reliable and commonly referenced methods is that of *Fukushin*.

It would be useful at this point therefore to entertain a brief history of *Fukushin* in TJM, its origins, development and how it came to assume such a privileged place in the hierarchy of *Kampo* diagnostics and practice. In so doing I will also make some comparisons to other disciplines within TJM that have also developed their own unique forms of abdominal palpation for use in diagnosis and treatment, notably Acupuncture (*Hari*) and Massage (*Shiatsu*).

2

HISTORY

"Do not seek to follow in the steps of the men of old; seek what they sought"

From *Kyoroku Ribetsu No Kotoba* ("Words given to *Kyoroku* as he parts", 1693), by Matsuo Chuemon Munefusa 松尾忠右衛門宗房, better known by his pen name Basho 芭蕉 (1644–1694), quoting the words of the famous Bhuddist priest *Kukai* (774–835) to one of his disciples.

FUKUSHIN IN OTHER TJM DISCIPLINES

"What is known as a bush or shrub has no trunk, has no focus at its core (Chuh Shin 中心). With no central trunk its branches and twigs lend themselves merely to being collected simply for firewood bundles. The scope of Chinese Medicine (Kampo 漢方) is vast, and erring in the method of your investigations, you will find yourself with bundles of twigs, like a bush...there are various methods of treatment for any illness, and applying those skills to treat an illness is called healing and is a splendid thing, but if your core is hollow you will constantly be asking yourself: 'what if this...' or, 'how about that...' like reaching blindly into a beggar's sack (Ko Jiki Bukuro 乞食袋), and hoping to find

treasure. First, to develop your central core, it is necessary to be discerning."

Kampo: A Clinical Guide to Theory and Practice, Otsuka, K.,
Transl. De Soriano, G. and Dawes, N., 1st edn. publ. Churchill
Livingstone, 2010; 2nd edn. publ. Singing Dragon, 2017

I myself combine the use of Acupuncture, *Shiatsu* and *Kampo* in my practice. Each of these disciplines has its own rich and varied history in TJM and when it comes to the use of palpation in diagnosis and treatment, each has developed its own style of *Fukushin*. In many respects, these varying expressions of abdominal palpation have evolved separately through time and, as Dr. *Otsuka* advises us in the quote above, each requires an extensive period of study and practice to become fluent in. According to his advice we would do well to deepen our understanding of one discipline at a time before attempting to incorporate a new one.

One of the issues related to *Fukushin* as practiced in different TJM disciplines is a potential lack of correlation between findings. As has been suggested in Chapter 1, the interpretation of findings on the abdomen may vary greatly according to the discipline through which they are obtained. For example, findings on the abdomen in the practice of Acupuncture or *Shiatsu* will likely be interpreted within the framework of Excess (*Jitsu* 実) or Deficiency (*Kyo* 虚) in the flow of Vital energy (*Ki* 氣), in the channels and collaterals. As such, these findings will guide the practitioner in his or her selection of points and channels to be palpated or needled—the "treatment plan"; this will then dictate which are to be reduced/drained (*Sha* 瀉) or tonified/reinforced (*Ho* 補)—the "treatment method."

In the case of *Kampo*, however, as we have already established, findings on the abdomen point directly to a formula or group of formulas to be considered, thus constituting both the treatment plan and method all in one.

With this in mind, and paying heed to Dr. *Otsuka*'s quote as mentioned, it might be assumed not to be a good idea to try and mix abdominal findings from different disciplines in TJM as they might seem at times to conflict. At the very least we should probably not expect them to concur with one another as they are reflecting different focuses in terms of categorizing imbalance and disharmony.

This said, in my case, I do palpate each patient using different methods of *Fukushin* according to the different disciplines I myself practice. How exactly I integrate my findings from these various sources is still a work in progress and is anyway beyond the scope of this book. However, I would like to offer here a brief history and analysis of the use of abdominal diagnosis in both *Shiatsu* and Acupuncture practice both by way of underlining the diversity of palpatory exam techniques that exist in TJM and also to illustrate the possible influences they undoubtedly have had on the development of *Fukushin* in the *Kampo* tradition.

1. The abdomen in Finger Pressure Massage (*Shiatsu* 指圧)

This is quite possibly the oldest form of massage in the world, forming part of a complete system of breathing, self-massage, exercise and therapeutic techniques known collectively as *Dao Yin Anmo* 導引 按蹻 (*Do In An Kyo* in Japanese). The system is likely derived from the Yogic tradition in India as part of Ayurvedic medicine and may have included aspects of ancient Arabic medicine also.

The "Inner Canon of the Yellow Emperor," (*Ko Tei Nai Kyo* 黄帝 内経), discussed in the section "the abdomen in acupuncture" below, includes many references to the use of massage as an intrinsic part of Chinese Medicine along with Acupuncture, Moxibustion, Cupping, Herbs, Diet, Exercise and other health practices. Later on, during the *Tang* dynasty (618–907 CE) in China, some of the techniques from the *Anmo* system were extrapolated to create a new system of bodywork which came to be known as *Tuina* (推拏), literally meaning to "push" (推) and to "pull" (拏), which gradually replaced *Anmo* and survives as the main form of Chinese bodywork today.

In Japan, from the 6th century CE onward, *Anma* became quite established and required a three-year training to practice professionally as an *Anmashi* 按摩師, or massage therapist. In the *Edo* period (1603–1868), the profession of *Anma* began to be associated with blind practitioners as it was one of the professions they were able to study and practice, often to a very high degree of skill, as opposed to Acupuncture or Herbal Medicine education which required the kind of extensive textual study only accessible to the sighted. Notwithstanding, Acupuncture itself also developed a strong following amongst blind practitioners, which continues to this day in Japan where it is estimated that as many as 25 percent of all licensed individuals are blind.

Also in the *Edo* period, the practice of *Ampuku* 按腹 (literally "Palpate the Abdomen") emerged as another expression of bodywork, in this case focused exclusively on the palpation of the abdomen. First mentioned in 17th century Japan by Ota Shinsai 太田晋斎, this discipline involves initial tactile examination of the abdomen to establish a diagnosis, followed by various techniques of pressure and manipulation of the abdominal area and sometimes corresponding areas on the back. It still survives in modern Japan, though, like *Anma*, is relatively rare in comparison to modern day *Shiatsu* (see below). But as a discipline uniquely focused on the assessment and palpation of the abdomen, it provides yet another clear historical reference to the significance placed on this area of the body by Japanese health practitioners. As *Ota* claims in his book *Ampuku Zukai* 按腹図解 (publ. 1827):

> If we do Ampuku Therapy, it will smooth out the basic stagnation of the basic Ki, producing harmony among the organs, making the flow of blood smooth, the bones and joints more flexible, the muscles less tense, the skin moist, the appetite will be good, urine and stool will come easily, the power of the Ki will increase, one's memory will improve...

Interestingly, Japanese *Ampuku* is not unique amongst massage traditions that focus exclusively on the abdomen. For example, traditional Mayan abdominal massage (popularized by Rosita Arvigo, a naturopathic doctor who studied with Mayan Healer Don Alijio

Panti) is used in particular in problems of the female reproductive system. *Chi Nei Tsang*, a Taoist abdominal massage system (introduced to the West by *Mantak Chia*), is used to release blockages in the flow of blood, lymph and energy from the abdomen, and in more recent times the *Wurn* Technique (developed by Belinda and Larry Wurn, physical therapist and licensed massage therapist respectively) involves specific pelvic floor massage through the abdomen that claims to remove adhesions often involved in various reproductive and urogenital problems as well as post-surgical. In the osteopathic tradition too, there has been great interest in the use of the abdomen in visceral manipulation techniques such as those developed by Jean-Pierre Barral. In contemporary Japan, there exist other expressions of bodywork developed in the modern era all of which continue to use the abdomen as the core for diagnostic assessment and treatment, notably both *Sotai Ho* 操体法, a form of neuromuscular therapy, and *Seitai Ho* 整体法, another form of structural therapy.

As for the practice of *Anma* and *Ampuku*, they both declined from the late *Edo* period on as Western Medicine began to dominate modern Japan from the later part of the 19th century. As new techniques of massage and manipulation began arriving into Japan from Europe in the early 20th century, the medical role of *Anma* was displaced and ultimately lost, except, that is, for one particular clinical discipline within the *Do In An Kyo* system as a whole—the use of static pressure applied to specific points and meridians. This had in fact originally been developed by *Ota Shinsai* (see above) but as a technique in its own right it eventually became known as *Shiatsu* (指圧, literally "Finger Pressure") by the beginning of the 20th century. Its popularity grew quickly from the 1920s onward as it incorporated a hybrid approach to bodywork including classical pressure techniques alongside stretch and manipulation borrowed from modern physiotherapeutic disciplines.

The following definition of Shiatsu is taken from *The Theory and Practice of Shiatsu* published by the Japanese Ministry of Health in 1957:

Shiatsu technique refers to the use of the thumb, fingers and palm of one's hands to apply pressure to particular sections on the surface of the body, and for maintaining and promoting health. It is also a method of contributing to the healing of specific illness.

It has been licensed as a profession since the 1950s in Japan separately from Acupuncture and requires three years of postgraduate education. Some *Shiatsu* therapists are also trained and licensed in the use of Moxibustion (*Kyu* 灸).

In the last hundred years there have been many well-known *Shiatsu* practitioners in Japan, some starting their own schools such as *Namikoshi Tokujiro* (浪越 徳治郎 1905–2000) who some have credited with coining the term *Shiatsu*. (In fact, it seems that a book by *Tamai Tempeki* 玉井天碧 published in 1939 entitled *Shiatsu Ho* 指圧法 ["Finger Pressure Method"] is a more likely candidate for this credit.)

Most have incorporated the use of *Fukushin* as the main tool for assessment in guiding the treatment approach in any given situation. Some have even made the palpation of the abdomen the cornerstone of their style of practice such as *Kuzome Naoichi* whose *Hara Shiatsu* 腹指圧 style has become well-known in Japan and internationally.

But one practitioner and teacher in particular is known for his development of a style referred to as *Zen Shiatsu* 禅指圧, in which the role of the abdomen in assessment and treatment is considered paramount. His name was *Masunaga Shizuto* 増永静人 (1925–1981). Amongst his many books, his *Zen Shiatsu: How to Harmonize Yin and Yang for Better Health* (publ. Japan Publications, 1977) remains his most influential and, due to its English translation facilitated by one of his students, *Ohashi Wataru* 大橋渉 (1944–) (who himself later became a well-known *Shiatsu* practitioner and teacher in the USA), has reached a worldwide audience.

My own arrival in Japan in 1982 was the year after *Masunaga's* death, but I had the good fortune to meet and become the student of one of his primary disciples, *Suzuki Takeo* 鈴木竹雄, who at the time had taken over as head of *Masunaga's Iokai* 医王会 (literally Medicine King Institute) in Tokyo (he later left and continued practice and teaching on his own). I thus came to study the *Zen Shiatsu* style myself and learned the practice of *Fukushin* (usually termed *Harashin* in *Shiatsu* circles—for an explanation of this difference see Chapter 1) and though the context and clinical interpretation of the findings in this discipline are vastly different from those used in the *Kampo* tradition, I have nonetheless incorporated the methodology and techniques from it for use in the *Fukushin* exam presented in this book.

It is worth noting that *Masunaga's* abdominal chart (Figure 2.1), illustrating the diagnostic reflex areas on the abdomen and back for each of the organ and meridian systems, shows remarkable similarity to the abdominal chart first published in 1685 in the *Shindo Hiketsu Shu* 鍼道秘訣集 (Compilation of Secrets of Acupuncture) by *Misono Isai* 御薗意斎 (see Figure 2.3 below). This is just another example of the interdisciplinary influences amongst practitioners of massage, Acupuncture and *Kampo* throughout Japanese history.

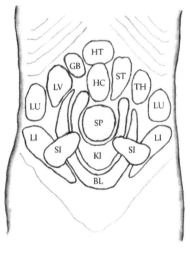

2.1

On the issue of interdisciplinary practice in TJM, I would argue that the touch sensitivity developed in the course of *Shiatsu* training can, at times, surpass that of Acupuncture and *Kampo* practitioners and thus can provide a strong basis for attempting to acquire the necessary tactile skills to perform *Fukushin* accurately and with success. It is perhaps no surprise that in Japanese Acupuncture schools, *Shiatsu* study is an absolute requirement during the first two years of training (as it was in my case).

Certainly, therefore, I owe a great deal to the practice of *Shiatsu* in terms of the development of both the Form (*Kata* 型) and Physical Posture (*Shisei* 姿勢) of the *Fukushin* exam I now use in my *Kampo* practice. I believe it highly likely, in terms of the historical development of *Anma*, *Ampuku* and *Shiatsu* alongside that of Acupuncture and *Kampo*, that there has been a good measure of interdisciplinary exchange over the centuries whereby each has learned from the other even as they have continued to develop along their own distinctive paths throughout history.

Meanwhile, what of the role of the abdomen in the various Acupuncture disciplines within the framework of TJM?

2. The abdomen in Acupuncture (*Hari* 針)

Acupuncture is generally held to have originated in China although precise origins and dates still remain unclear. References to pointed stones (*Bian Shi* 砭石) used to massage and puncture the body date back almost 6000 years although they could have been used for bloodletting, lancing boils or other minor surgery. Silk scrolls recovered from the *Ma Huang Dui* (馬王堆) archaeological site in China in 1973 (which was sealed in 198 BCE) refer to a system of meridian pathways although Acupuncture itself is not directly mentioned. But the first concrete and extensive textual reference to the theory and practice of Acupuncture is found in the "Inner Canon of the Yellow Emperor" (黄帝内経—*Huang Di Nei Jing* in Chinese; *Ko Tei Nai Kyo* in Japanese), thought to date from 100 BCE. It is a text in two parts: the "Basic Questions" (素問 *Suwen* in Chinese; *Somon* in Japanese), which covers the theoretical foundations and diagnostic principles of Chinese Medicine; and the "Spiritual Pivot" (靈樞 *Ling Shu* in Chinese; *Rei Shu* in Japanese), which specifically details Acupuncture theory, diagnostics and treatment and includes various references to the abdomen.

The first clear and systematic treatment of the abdomen in an Acupuncture text however appears in the "Yellow Emperor's Classic of 81 Difficult Questions" (黃帝八十一難經 *Huang Di Baishiyi Nanjing* in Chinese; *Ko Tei Hachijuichi Nan Gyo* in Japanese). Written in the Later or Eastern *Han* dynasty (25–220 CE), it has multiple references to the abdomen in terms of its use in diagnosis and treatment and has become the single most influential source text for *Fukushin* in the Acupuncture tradition. It also includes a simple diagram of the abdomen showing the energetic reflex areas associated with each of the internal viscera and their respective elemental associations (Figure 2.2).

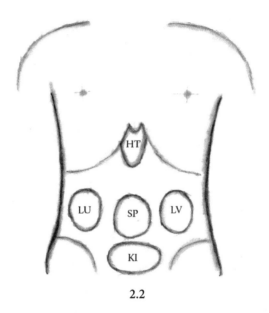

2.2

With the advent of Chinese medical knowledge into Japan from the 6th century CE onwards, the use of the abdomen in diagnosis and practice in Acupuncture remained heavily influenced by the information drawn from the "Classic of Difficulties," right up to the late *Muromachi* period (*Muromachi Jidai* 室町時代, 1336–1573) and into the *Azuchi-Momoyama* period (*Azuchi Momoyama Jidai* 安土桃山時代, 1573–1600). During that time, *Misono Isai* 御薗意斎 (1557–1616) aka *Joshin Matsuoka*, who was a court doctor of

Emperors *Oogimachi-Tenno* 正親町天皇 (crowned 1557–1586) and *Goyozei-Tenno* 後陽成天皇 (crowned 1586–1611), wrote several texts which have not survived, though the *Shindo Hiketsu Shu* 鍼道秘訣集 (1685) "Compilation of Secrets of Acupuncture"), written by one of his students, provides significant testimony to the teacher's work almost a hundred years prior.

In this text he mentions Isai's father and teacher, *Misono Mubunsai* 御薗夢分斎 (birth and dates unknown), founder of the *Mubun* style (*Mubunryu* 夢分流) which is famous in Japanese Acupuncture and massage circles for its well-documented map (Figure 2.3) of the abdomen based on, but distinct from, the *Nan Jing* 難經 map (Figure 2.2). The text references a method of abdominal palpation and treatment, developed by *Mubunsai*, using the "Hammer" or "Striking Needle" (*Da Shin* 打鍼) technique, whereby a large needle (*Uchibari* 打鍼) is struck by a small mallet (*Kozuchi* 小槌) at multiple points over the surface of the abdomen to clear pathogenic accumulations (*Ja Ki* 邪気). These accumulations were defined as obstructions (hardness) in the flow of *Ki* 気 known as *Kori* こり, and were differentiated according to whether they belonged to Fullness (*Shaku* 積) or Emptiness (*Ju* 聚).

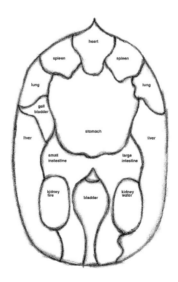

2.3

It is clear then that the *Mubunryu* style focused exclusively on the abdomen for both diagnostic and treatment purposes and that this practice was well established throughout the Middle Ages in Japan. In fact, *Mubun's* teacher was *Taga Hoin* 多賀法印 (a high-ranking monk from *Daitokuji* 大德寺 temple in Kyoto) whose school produced a book on abdominal diagnosis "The Way of Abdominal Diagnosis" (*Fukushin No Ho* 腹診の法), said to be based on techniques already taught in the early *Muromachi* period or possibly even earlier during the *Kamakura* period (1185–1333).

Indeed, an anecdotal reference to the practice of *Fukushin* is provided by *Fujiwara Sadaie* 藤原定家 (1162–1241), better known as *Teika* (an alternate pronunciation of his name in Japanese), who was an imperial court poet, scribe, calligrapher and scholar of the early *Kamakura* period (1185–1333). He repeatedly referred to abdominal palpation in his personal diary, the *Meigetsuki* 明月記 ("The Record of the Clear Moon"). For example, "I called the chief doctor of the Tenyakunokami (Imperial Hospital), Tanba Tadamoto, and let him diagnose my abdomen" (July 5, 1213); and "I called Shinjakubo, a monk doctor, and let him palpate my abdominal disease" (Aug. 17, 1226). Thus, there are clear references to the role of the abdomen in medical practice that appear consistently throughout the Middle Ages in Japan from the 13th to 16th centuries.

What is noticeable, returning to the *Shindo Hiketsu Shu* for a moment, is that the period in which it was written (17th century) seems to have marked a significant move away from the meridian-based model derived from the *Nan Jing* and towards a more anatomically based one that began to take hold in Japan as the first European anatomy texts began arriving by the mid *Edo* period. A highly significant quote from the text itself reads, "This school does not take into account the 12 meridians or the 15 collaterals for needling. It focuses on the 5 organs and 6 bowels as the basis for diagnosis and it ignores trivial matters."

This suggests that by the time it was written in 1685, clear distinctions were already being made in the use of the abdomen in diagnosis and treatment across the different disciplines of TJM. In fact this quote is more characteristic of the *Koho-Ha* 古方派 (Classical School) faction, called the *Shang Han Lun* faction (傷寒論) by *Otsuka Keisetsu* 大塚敬節 (1900–1980—more on him later), who were mostly herbalists, as opposed to what he called the *Nan Jing* faction (難経), which included the *Mubun* School and others of the *Gosei-Ha* 後世派 (Later Generation School) faction, who were mainly Acupuncturists (more on this in the *Kampo* history section below).

Indeed, by the early part of the *Edo* period (1603–1868), the divergent trajectory of Acupuncture and herbal development in terms of their incorporation of the abdomen into their respective diagnostic and treatment frameworks seemed already set in motion.

Notwithstanding, what *Otsuka* has called the *Nan Jing* faction has survived more than 400 years into the modern era, embodied by prominent physician and Acupuncturist such as *Manaka Yoshio* 間中善雄 (1911–1989) and *Kobayashi Shoji* 小林詔司 (1942–) who both echoed the *Mubunryu* style in terms of their focus on the abdomen in assessment and treatment. In *Manaka*'s case (like those who influenced him such as *Akabane Kobe* 赤羽幸兵衛 and those he himself came to influence including *Miki Shima* and Stephen Birch), this involved abdominal palpation to establish imbalances in the 8 Extraordinary Channels and, using his Ion-Pumping cords, to drain excess from stagnant areas and redistribute *Ki* 気 to areas of depletion.

In the case of *Kobayashi*, still in practice today, his treatment style has become known as *Shaku Ju Chiryo* 積聚治療, a direct reference to the work of *Mubunsai* himself (see above), once again involving careful and systematic assessment and treatment of the abdomen, something *Kobayashi* refers to in English as "Core Therapy."

Other Japanese Acupuncturists in the modern era have developed their own unique styles of *Fukushin* which can ultimately also trace their origins to medieval Japan. For example, *Matsumoto Kiiko* 松本岐子, an internationally renowned teacher based in Boston in the USA, has developed her own method of *Fukushin* based on the family-style lineage of her teacher, *Nagano Kiyoshi* 長野潔 (who died in 2003). This system is clearly referenced in her book *Hara*

Diagnosis: Reflections on the Sea (Matsumoto, K., Birch, S., *et al.*, publ. Paradigm Publications, 1988).

Another Acupuncture system that emerged in the 20th century and has gained wide acceptance in the West is known as Meridian Therapy style (*Keiraku Chiryo* 経絡治療). Developed by *Yanagiya Sorei* 柳谷素霊 in 1927 with the philosophy of espousing a "return to the classics," this system drew its inspiration from the "Classic of Difficulties" (see above) at a time when traditional Acupuncture was being replaced by "scientific" Acupuncture in Japan with its narrow focus on anatomical and neurological mechanisms. This style, in addition to the pulse, also focuses on palpation of the abdomen in diagnosis, using quite a light touch to locate *Kori* and indurations on the surface of the abdomen as well as temperature differences to help determine Excess and Deficient Patterns.

The most senior contemporary Meridian Therapy style practitioner in *Yanagiya's* lineage, (whose original group was formed in the 1930's and included the likes of *Okabe Sodo, Inoue Keiri, Honma Shohaku* and others) is *Shudo Denmei* 首藤傳明 (1932–) who is currently still in practice in his late 80s. He is the author of the book *Japanese Classical Acupuncture: An Introduction to Meridian Therapy,* publ. Eastland Press, 1990, which is translated by my colleague and friend, Stephen Brown. Other senior practitioners in this style include *Okada Akizo, Ikeda Masakazu* and *Kuwahara Kuei*, all of whom have taught internationally, each with their own different "take" on the abdomen and its uses in practice. I myself practice this particular style of Acupuncture and its related abdominal palpation system, though again it is quite distinct from the *Kampo* system of *Fukushin* I am presenting in this book.

Yet another prominent contemporary Acupuncture style in which the abdomen once again features large in diagnosis is *Toyo Hari* 東洋はり, a system founded by Fukushima Kodo 福島弘道 (1911–1992). Blinded in the army in Manchuria, he tried to join the ranks of the Meridian Therapy group (see above) but was initially refused on account of his blindness. He was later accepted into the Meridian Therapy group and trained in that style by *Inoue*.

Perhaps because of his blindness, however, in much the same way as one of the earliest and best-known blind Acupuncturists from the *Edo* period, *Sugiyama Waichi* 杉山和一 (1614–1694), he became one of the most prominent 20th century practitioners in Japan, and the *Toyohari* Association has become an international force in Acupuncture education and practice. In this style, the palpation of the abdomen is done using an extremely light touch.

These are just some of the styles of Acupuncture, old and new, that incorporate the use of the abdomen in their practice and from this brief analysis two facts are hopefully self-evident:

1. *Fukushin* has survived from medieval times and is used comprehensively across multiple styles of contemporary Acupuncture.

2. Acupuncture *Fukushin* styles belong to the *Nan Jing* faction as compared with the styles used in *Kampo*, which belong to the *Shang Han Lun* (see above).

I would like now to offer a slightly more comprehensive historical overview of the development of *Fukushin* within the practice of *Kampo* itself.

HISTORY AND DEVELOPMENT OF *FUKUSHIN* IN THE *KAMPO* TRADITION

Kampo 漢方 (also pronounced *Kanpo*) literally means: "Chinese Medicine." The character *Kan* 漢 (*Han* in Chinese) refers to the *Han* dynasty (206 BCE–220 CE) and for the Japanese, *Kan* tends, as a pronoun, to designate all things Chinese—for example, *Kango* 漢語 (The Chinese language) versus *Kokugo* 国語 (the Japanese language). *Po* 方 means method, skill or way and in this context is suggestive of the particular methods or skills specifically related to medical practices that originally derived from China. So perhaps the more accurate translation of the word *Kampo* might be "Chinese Medical Techniques."

The term *Kampo* was probably first used by *Sohaku Asada* 浅田宗伯 (1813–1894) somewhere around the end of the *Edo* period (1603–1868) and the beginning of the *Meiji* period (1868–1912) and according to his definition seems to have been used to identify the practice of *Koho* 古方 (Classical) Herbal Medicine from China as embodied in the *Han* dynasty classic "On Cold Damage" (傷寒論 *Shang Han Lun*) by *Zhang Zhong Jing* 張仲景 (219 CE). In fact many, including *Otsuka Keisetsu*, have often identified the *Koho-Ha Kampo* lineage as synonymous with *Shang Han Lun* medicine. Yet strictly speaking, the term *Kampo* has been used historically to distinguish between *Waho* 和方 (Traditional Japanese Folk Medicine) and later on, of course, *Rampo* 蘭方 (Western biomedicine).

To summarize, although in the modern era including up to the present day, many in Japan have tended to associate the term *Kampo* uniquely and exclusively with the practice of Herbal Medicine, the fact is that it dates back all the way to the 10th century CE and the publication of the *Ishimpo* (see below) and therefore represents a generic term that can legitimately be used to describe any and all forms of "Chinese Medical Practice." For the purposes of the following section, which will focus on Herbal Medicine, we will more accurately use the term *Kampo Yaku* 漢方薬 (*Kampo* Herbal Medicine).

1. Classical origins (*Han* dynasty, 206 BCE–220 CE)

The classical origins of *Kampo Yaku* pre-date in fact even the *Han* dynasty and derive from the *Yin* 殷 (1600–1046 BCE) and *Zhou* 周 (1046–256 BCE) dynasties of ancient China. But though there is some surviving evidence of various shamanistic practices and other herbal medical knowledge from that time, scholars generally agree that it wasn't until the *Han* dynasty that such theories and practices began to be systematized and recorded in any organized and enduring manner.

The great surviving classics from that time include the *Huang Di Nei Jing* 黄帝内経 and *Nan Jing* 難経, both referenced above in the

Acupuncture section of this chapter. As has already been suggested, these two classics have strongly influenced the development of Acupuncture in Japan and to a large extent have been ignored by some *Kampo* herbalists, especially the *Koho-Ha* faction, as they contain very few direct references to pharmacology itself.

Meanwhile, during the same period, the two great Chinese classics of Herbal Medicine were also written—the *Shang Han Lun* 傷寒論 and the *Shen Nong Ben Cao Jing* 神農本草経 (exact date unknown: Later *Han* dynasty, 25–220 CE), the first recorded Chinese pharmacopeia, referencing 365 medicinal substances from the animal, plant and mineral kingdoms. During the following 1500 years, many revised versions of this basic pharmacopeia were written in the *Sui* 隋 (581–618), *Tang* 唐 (618–907) and *Song* 宋 (960–1279) dynasties respectively, right up to the *Ming* 明 dynasty (1368–1644) when the "Compendium of Materia Medica" (*Ben Cao Gang Mu* 本草綱目 1590) was written by *Li Shi Zhen* 李時珍 (1518–1593), which included 1892 items and has remained one of the standard reference texts in Herbal Medicine to this day.

But it was not the pharmacognosy of old China alone that was to have the greatest influence on the development of *Kampo Yaku* in Japan, but rather the practical manuals of medicine, involving detailed therapeutics and the differentiated application of formulas in a clinical setting. The Treatise on Cold-induced and Miscellaneous Diseases (*Shang Han Za Bing Lun* 傷寒雜病論) (219 CE) was the first and most potent example of such a text (see reference above). Composed of the *Shang Han Lun* itself, a treatise on Febrile Disease, and the *Jin Gui Yao Lue* 金匱要略, a manual of Internal Medicine, this text has had, perhaps more than any other, the most profound and enduring influence on Japanese *Kampo* medicine.

It is estimated that today in modern China, as many as 25 percent of all traditional herbal practitioners still identify with the *Shang Han Lun* school, especially in colder regions such as *Chengdu*. Herbal formulas from the *Han* dynasty in which the *Shang Han Lun* was written are referred to in Chinese as *Jing Fang* 经方 (Classical Formulas). However, the dominant style of practice in modern times since the 1950s has become Traditional Chinese Medicine (TCM), which in fact is a recent hybrid of differing styles of herbal practice, predominantly based on texts and herbal formulas from the *Ming* dynasty (1368–1644) and later. The role of *Shang Han Lun* medicine within this new medical system has tended to be limited to the treatment of febrile disease and many of the *Jing Fang* formulas have lost currency and are much less used these days in China, replaced by *Shi Fang* 时方 (Contemporary Formulas) and *Jin Fang* 今方 (Modern Formulas).

The situation in contemporary Japan, however, is radically different, where study of the *Shang Han Lun* still dominates *Kampo* education and *Jing Fang* formulas taken from it and from its sister text, the *Jin Gui Yao Lue* (referenced above), still form the basis for the majority of *Kampo* prescriptions.

There have been many suggested explanations as to why, after almost 1500 years of sustained transmission of an incalculable breadth of medical knowledge from the Chinese mainland into Japan, the predominant influences on the Japanese medical culture have remained those of the very earliest classical texts, their theoretical models and the formulas they used in practice. In many ways in fact, *Kampo* medicine today might be described as the fusion of the very old (*Koho*) with the very new (*Rampo*) in medicine, with less attention being paid in practical terms to the intervening centuries and their changing medical models.

Some historians have claimed that *Kampo*'s adherence to the use of *Jing Fang* has been due in part to the fact that these formulas only contain small numbers of (mostly common) herbs which made them more practically available in Japan where the consistent supply of crude drugs (mostly from China) was hardly assured over the centuries. Others have pointed to several periods in history during which Japan was relatively isolated from the outside world, notably during the *Tokugawa* 德川 (*Edo*) period, so that the many medical advances and changes that may have occurred in mainland China during those periods did not always succeed in transmitting to the Japanese culture to any great or enduring extent.

The fact remains, however, that the practical methodology of disease assessment and treatment set out in the *Shang Han Lun* has held enduring appeal for Japanese physicians when it comes to the art of traditional medical practice. The way in which diagnosis is directly linked to treatment in the *Shang Han Lun*, without recourse to complex philosophical and theoretical explanation, has been held up by successive generations of *Kampo* practitioners as the epitome of simplicity and elegance in practice.

By the *Edo* period, as we shall see, this emphasis on matching assessment findings directly to formula prescribing led to the pattern-based treatment method: *Ho Sho I Chi* 方証一致 for which *Kampo* is so well-known today. The *Edo* doctors, especially those from the *Koho-Ha* faction, painstakingly reinvented a detailed clinical narrative (called the *Sho* 証) for each of the *Jing Fang* formulas, taken from the *Shang Han Lun*, adding many signs and symptoms to each *Sho* from their own clinical experience. In particular, these additions included references to both patient constitution (*Taishitsu Sho* 体質証) and of course to abdominal patterns (*Fukusho* 腹証). Both these terms have already been discussed in Chapter 1.

Reference to these *Fukusho* originally appeared throughout the *Shang Han Lun* and *Jin Gui Yao Lue* though they are mixed into the body of the text in reference to specific Formula Patterns and treatment strategies and are not explained individually. For example, in clause 54 of the *Shang Han Lun*, by *Zhang Zhong Jing*, Transl. and Ed. *Hong Yen Hsu*, publ. Oriental Healing Arts Institute, Los Angeles, 1981 it states:

> If the *Shang Han* 傷寒 (condition) persists for five to six days with alternating chills and fever, distress and fullness in the chest and ribs (*Kyo Kyo Ku Man* 胸脅苦満—*Otsuka* abdomen #5), silence with loss of appetite, disturbance in the heart with a tendency to vomit or disturbances in the chest without vomiting, thirst, abdominal aching, obstruction and stiffness beneath the ribs (*Kyo Ka Hi Ko* 脅下痞硬—*Otsuka* abdomen #6); or palpitations beneath the heart (*Shin Ka Ki* 心下痞—*Otsuka* abdomen #10), dysuria, adypsia, mild generalized

fever, or cough, Minor Bupleurum Combination (*Sho Sai Ko To* 小柴胡湯 (Japanese), *Xiao Chai Hu Tang* (Chinese) is indicated.

The descriptive terminology used to identify specific abdominal patterns thus dates back to the *Shang Han Lun*; however, the text itself does not offer any theoretical model in respect to how the abdomen should be used in diagnosis, nor is there any systematic description of palpation techniques. Once again, it fell to the doctors in *Edo* period Japan to develop such protocols and interpretations for practical use in the clinic as we shall see later.

A final point to make in terms of the classical terminology used in defining abdominal patterns in the *Shang Han Lun* is that no clear differentiation is made in the text between subjective and objective findings nor whether they belong to Excess (*Jitsu* 實) or Deficiency (*Kyo* 虛) patterns (*Sho* 証). In other words, we cannot deduce from the text alone whether a particular abdominal description relates to a patient's reported sensation or if it rather describes a practitioner's tactile experience nor whether either is *Kyo* or *Jitsu*.

For example, the character usually translated as "Fullness" as in "Glomus" (Nigel Wiseman, *A Practical Dictionary of Chinese Medicine*, publ. Paradigm Publications, 2014), a sensation of obstruction (which can be in the throat, chest or abdomen), is 痞 *Hi* (*Pi* in Pinyin). This would seem to point to something experienced by the patient and was therefore treated as subjective by *Kampo* doctors. However, the character usually translated as "Hardness/ Tightness" as in an active resistance to the physician's palpatory pressure (with or without pain) is 硬 *Ko*. This, *Kampo* practitioners deduced, seemed to correspond to something felt by the physician and could therefore be considered a more "objective" finding. Such distinctions have obvious clinical significance in diagnosis.

So, for example, in the *Otsuka* system the two abdominal patterns, #3 *Shin Ka Hi Ko* 心下痞硬 and #4 *Shin Ka Hi* 心下痞 (see Figures 4.5 and 4.6), are differentiated from one another by just such a subjective and objective finding and notably each finding points to radically different formula applications even though they are apparently quite similar in nature in terms of the patient's subjective experience (i.e. fullness, bloating).

This process of differentiating the language of the *Shang Han Lun* used to describe the various *Fukusho* into subjective patient experiences (symptoms) and objective practitioner findings (signs) was one of the great achievements of *Edo* period Japanese *Kampo* doctors and accounts not only for the survival of *Fukushin* into contemporary practice but also its hierarchical importance in the *Kampo* dialectic.

Furthermore, the terms used to describe the abdominal patterns in the *Shang Han Lun*, whether subjective or objective, cannot on their own be determined as either Excess or Deficient in nature. A good example of this is the term Full Abdomen (*Fuku Man* 腹 滿). In the text there are numerous references to this term, but its interpretation is always left to context. Whereas for example in clause #119 (from the Sunlight *Yang/Yo Mei Byo* 陽明病 chapter) the term is used to describe a *Sho* 証 for which Major Rhubarb Combination (*Dai Joki To* 大承気湯) is prescribed (an obvious case of *Jitsu Sho* 實 証) in another clause, #134 (from the Greater *Yin/Tai In Byo* 太陰病 chapter), the same term is used to describe a very different *Sho* 証 for which Cinnamon and Peony Combination (*Keishi Ka Shaku Yaku To* 桂枝加芍薬湯) is prescribed (an obvious case of *Kyo Sho* 虛証).

Again, the ingenuity of *Edo Kampo* doctors in restructuring the language of the clinical narrative associated with each of the *Jing Fang* formulas included references to the patient constitution for which each formula is suited, expressed in terms of *Kyo* and *Jitsu*. Thus, in the examples given, the constitutional strength associated with *Daijokito* is described in *Kampo* as *Jitsu* whilst that of *Keishikashakuyakuto* is *Kyo*. So, even though the abdominal finding in both cases is described as *Fuku Man*, a *Kampo* practitioner would immediately be aware of the different tactile qualities associated with *Kyo Fuku Man* versus *Jitsu Fuku Man* in either case.

Thus, the language, methodology and techniques of the *Shang Han Lun* have undoubtedly influenced the development of *Kampo Yaku* in a profound way, and yet, as we shall see, the Japanese were not shy to reinterpret, modify and adapt classical Chinese teachings into their own style and culture of practice.

2. Early development (6th–13th centuries CE)

The earliest records of the transmission of medical texts and practices into Japan via what is now the Korean peninsula include references to the physician *Kim Moo* (金武) in the third year of the reign of Emperor *Ingyo* 允恭天皇 (412–453) and later the physician *De Lai* (徳来), both visiting the court of the *Yamato* period (*Yamato Jidai* 大和時代, 250–710). In the seventh year of the reign of Emperor *Keitai* 継体天皇 (513), various official Confucian teachers also visited Japan and from then on, the influx of medical, martial and philosophical teachings began in earnest.

The Chinese monk and physician *Zhicong* (智聡) arrived in Japan in the reign of the Emperor *Kinmei* 欽明天皇 (562), bringing with him 164 volumes of Chinese medical texts, and became a Japanese citizen. This period was marked by the introduction of Buddhism into Japan, bringing with it texts and teachings on Acupuncture and Moxibustion including the *Meidozu* 明堂図 (a chart of meridian points) and notably the *Yakusho* 薬書 (texts on medicines).

In 607, during the reign of the Empress *Suiko* 推古天皇, formal diplomatic relations were established with the *Sui* dynasty 隋朝 (581–618) court in China. This exchange continued through the *Tang* dynasty 唐朝 (618–907) and by 701, the *Yamato* court in Japan established first the *Taiho* code (大宝律令) then the *Yoro* code (養老律令), both of which included sections which governed the practice of medicine: *Ishitsuryo* (医疾令), which was regulated through the *Tenyakuryo* 典薬寮 ("Bureau of Medicine").

In 753 a Chinese Buddhist monk and renowned doctor named *Jianzhen* (鑒真, *Ganjin* in Japanese, 688–763), finally arrived in Japan after many attempts with 35 of his disciples, all doctors. Received by the Empress *Komyo* 孝謙天皇 (713–770), he initially presided over *Todaiji* temple 東大寺, which had just been finished in 752 along with its *Daibutsu* 大仏, the largest bronze Buddha statue in the world (now designated as a UNESCO World Heritage Site). He later set up his own temple, *Toshodaiji* (唐招提寺), also in Nara, where he died in 763. Along with his Buddhist teachings, the medical knowledge he and his many followers disseminated during *Nara* period Japan (710–794) consolidated that which had already been assimilated during the latter part of the *Kofun* period (*Kofun Jidai* 古墳時代, 250–538) and subsequently during the *Asuka* period (*Asuka Jidai* 飛鳥時代, 539–710) and paved the way for further exchange with China in the early part of the *Heian* period (*Heian Jidai* 平安時代, 794–1185).

However, with the decline of the *Tang* dynasty, Japan discontinued its missions to China by 894 and they were not destined to resume for more than 200 years (towards the end of the *Heian* period). Despite this extended period of "isolation," there were many advances in medical practice within Japan itself based on the many texts and teachings that had been imported from the Chinese mainland during the preceding 350 years.

The main source of textual evidence documenting all known references to Chinese medical and health practices in Japan dating from the *Han* dynasty to the time of its writing in 984, is the *Ishimpo* 醫心方 (*The Essentials of Medicine*). Compiled by Tamba Yasuyori 丹波康頼 in 30 volumes, this is the oldest surviving Japanese medical text, having been kept within generations of the Nakarai 半井 family for over a thousand years until, in 1984, it was designated as a National Treasure of Japan and is currently held in the Tokyo National Museum collection. This text, based on the *Zhubing Yuanhou Lun* 諸病源候論 ("General Treatise on Causes and Manifestations of All Diseases") by *Chao Yuanfang* 巢元方 of the *Sui* dynasty, is remarkable not only because it is the first known Japanese medical work but also because it has survived to the present day and includes more than 200 citations from classical Chinese texts, many of which have themselves been lost in the original. Amongst the 30 volumes which act as a veritable encyclopedia of medical knowledge of the time, there is one dedicated to Acupuncture and Moxibustion and the majority of others are on internal medicine including sub-specialties such as dermatology, OB/GYN, pediatrics and surgery. There are two volumes on pharmacology as well as others on dietary and preventive health practices as well as yet others on sexual practices, alchemy and magic. The role of the abdomen in diagnosis and treatment is alluded to repeatedly throughout the text.

As regards specifically the crude drugs referred to during the periods described above (from the 7th to the 10th centuries), up to and including those mentioned in the *Ishimpo*, medical historians have tended to rely on two main Japanese sources:

1. The 60 kinds of drugs preserved in the *Shosoin* 正倉院 (the "Treasure House") located within the *Todai-ji* temple complex in *Nara*. They formed part of 900 treasures originally dedicated by the Empress *Komyo* (Komyo-Kogo 光明皇后, 701–760) on the death of her husband, Emperor *Shomu* (*Shomu Tenno* 聖武天皇, 724–749). This group of medicinals were collectively studied by scholars in the late 1940s, the results of which were published as: Masutomi, K.: "The Shosoin Medicines" (*Shosoin Yakubutsu*正倉院薬物) (Ed. Asahina, Y. 1955), *Kodai Sekiyaki no Kenkyu* 1957, 39, 141, *Shokubutsu Bunken Kankokai*.

and:

2. The 209 crude drugs listed in the *Engishiki* 延喜式 ("Procedures of the *Engi* Era," completed in 927), which included 50 volumes on all aspects of political, religious and social (including medical) practices.

Following the *Ishimpo*, once Japan had re-established foreign exchange, this time with *Song* dynasty China (宋朝 960–1279) toward the end of the *Heian* period (794–1185) and into the *Kamakura* period (1185–1333), various significant Japanese medical texts were written such as: "Selected Therapies" (*Iryakusho* 医略抄, 1081) by *Tamba Masatada* 丹波雅忠 (1021–1088); "Treatise on Tea Drinking for Good Health" (*Kissa Yojoki* 喫茶養生記, 1193) by *Myoan Eisai* 明菴栄西, dedicated to Shogun *Minamoto no Sanetomo* 源実朝 (1192–1219) in 1214; and in particular two works by *Kajiwara Shozen* 梶原性全 (1266–1337), a monk from *Kamakura* with extensive medical knowledge, who wrote the *Tonisho* 頓医 抄 (1302–1304) in 50 volumes (in Japanese), a ground-breaking populist work aimed at interpreting Chinese medical literature of the time into a Japanese frame of reference, and the *Manampo* 万 安方 (begun in 1313) in 62 volumes, a much more scholarly work (written in Chinese characters) designed as a medical textbook. It was based on the *Seizai Soroku* 聖済総録 published in 1300 in *Yuan* dynasty China (1279–1368), which *Shozen* had come across several years after writing the *Tonisho*.

The *Kamakura* period saw a major shift in the medical patronage that had existed previously in Japan whereby the aristocracy, including the imperial court, had tended to provide the greatest influence and support in the development and dissemination of medical knowledge. From the late 13th century, such support transferred to Buddhist institutions where student monks, able to read classical Chinese, began to focus on the latest texts emanating from China at the time. This shift toward a more scholarly approach to the study and practice of medicine came to influence the development of TJM for the next 300 years.

Meanwhile in China during this period, a major medical reformation got under way in the early 12th century. After the fall of the Northern *Song* dynasty in 1127, two landmark texts were published, the "Commentary on the *Shang Han Lun*" *Zhu Jie Shang Han Lun* 註解傷寒論 (1172) and the "Logic of the *Shang Han Lun*" *Shang Han Ming Ni Lun* 傷寒明理論 (1157) both written by *Cheng Wuji* 成无己 (1063–1156) and published posthumously. They set out an entirely novel synthesis of the two classical *Han* dynasty texts, the *Nei Jing* and the *Shang Han Lun* (referenced above), which hitherto had been considered completely separate strands of medicine, the former setting out the philosophical logic and practical techniques of Acupuncture, the latter documenting a clinical handbook of herbal practice.

By this time in Japan, as mentioned previously, these two texts had been taken up separately, the former by the Acupuncture community, the latter by the herbalists and as such, these two professions had already set themselves on a divergent course. In China, however, this new movement to integrate Acupuncture and herbal theory began in earnest at this time and it had a resounding impact on the future of Chinese Medicine that can been seen right up to the present day in the TCM movement, which only began in the 1950s and which claims substantial integration between the practice of Acupuncture and herbs.

The earliest evidence of this attempted integration of different disciplines within the medicine is found in *Cheng Wuji's* two works. It was only after they were published, for example, that Acupuncture literature on individual point functions began to adopt similar language to that of the herbal materia medica. For example, Spleen 6 (*San Yin Jiao* 三阴交) began to be described for the very first time as a point with the potential to "drain Damp from the Lower *Jiao*," the kind of description that had hitherto been reserved exclusively for certain herbs considered to have such a pharmacological action. Similarly, these same works were the first to suggest in pharmacology that each herb might actually be thought to "enter" a specific meridian, a notion that had only ever been referred to until that point in the Acupuncture literature. Again, this thinking has survived into the present time—for example, Radix Bupleuri (*Chai Hu* 柴胡) "enters the Liver and Gall Bladder" (*Chinese Herbal Medicine: Materia Medica*, Bensky, D. and Gamble, A., publ. Eastland Press, 1986). Indeed, this revolutionary initiative to integrate the theories and practice of hitherto separate disciplines within the overall umbrella of East Asian Medicine has sometimes been referred to as the "Herbalization of Acupuncture" and vice versa.

The implications of this paradigm shift were profound, and in some ways mark the divergence of the new mainstream of Chinese Medicine at that time, not only from that of its own classical origins, but also from the future development of the medicine across the ocean in Japan. To appreciate this fact is to understand why, in essence, modern TJM resembles far more closely the style of medicine practiced from the *Han* to the *Song* dynasties in China than it does any of the styles that followed, including and especially TCM.

3. The influence of *Jin-Yuan* China (14th–16th centuries CE)

Cheng Wuji's legacy in 13th century China undoubtedly paved the way for the momentous reformational changes in medicine that occurred during the *Jin-Yuan* dynasty 金元 (1115–1368). This was a time of innovation during which many new medical theories flourished such as those of the "four great physicians" of the period: *Liu Wansu* 劉完素 (1110–1200)—"Cooling School"; *Zhang Zihe* 張子和 (1156–1228)—"Attack and Drain School"; *Li Dongyuan* 李東垣 (1180–1251)—"Center Tonifying School"; *Zhu Danxi* 朱丹溪 (1281–1358)—"Yin Nourishing School." Each of these schools represented not only remarkably novel and diverse approaches to treatment in their own right, but collectively marked a major departure from the classical teachings of the *Han–Song* dynasties that had preceded them for 1200 years and heralded the nature and content of medical philosophy and practice that was to follow in the *Ming* 明 (1368–1644) and *Qing* 清 (1644–1911) dynasties.

These same texts were all written during the time of the *Kamakura* period (1185–1333) in Japan. As has been mentioned, it was at this time that a shift in medical patronage occurred from the imperial court to the *Zen* monasteries, making the common people more of a primary target of medical practice than the aristocracy. Also, at this time, as mentioned, monks began to travel and pursue medical studies in China as well as read and translate contemporary Chinese texts such as *Kajiwara Shozen* (see above). This process was greatly facilitated by various serendipitous advances in printing techniques which made books more available to both scholars, physicians and the public at this time.

This trend continued into the *Muromachi* period 室町時代 (1336–1573) during which time many Japanese physicians and scholars spent protracted periods in (*Ming*) China, returning to influence medical circles of the time back home. The stage was set for a major shift in medical thinking and practice. Essentially, the increased availability of textual material, the social changes with regard to the patronage and dissemination of the medicine and the strong influence of the Neo-Confucionist teachings of the *Jin-Yuan* period, all combined to create a climate in Japan whereby scholarly medical knowledge was beginning to dictate therapeutic policy rather than the more pragmatic dialectic that had characterized the classical era. For a fascinating characterization of the Japanese adaptation of Confucian influences in the *Edo* period refer to Angurarohita, P. (1989) *Buddhist Influence on the Concept of the Neo-Confucian Sage*. Sino Platonic Papers 10. It was in this climate of rationalist philosophy in medicine that a new faction began to emerge in *Kampo*.

One such example of a Japanese *Zen* monk, who travelled to China at the age of 23 and remained there studying medicine for 12 years (1487–1498) was *Tashiro Sanki* 田代三喜 (1465–1537). He brought back with him two important texts—*Zenku Shu* 全九集 (1452) and *Saiin Ho* 済陰方 (1455)—which essentially reflected the teachings of the "four great physicians" from the *Jin-Yuan* era (mentioned above), in particular those of Li Dongyuan and Zhu Danxi, often referred to as *Li-Zhu* medicine in Japan, which focused on tonifying therapies. As such, Sanki is considered the pioneer of the *Gosei-Ha* 後世派 school of *Kampo*, literally meaning "Later Generation School" referring to *Jin-Yuan* medicine as having marked a move away from the earlier classical teachings of the *Han*, *Sui*, *Tang* and *Song* dynasties.

In the later *Muromachi* period and into the *Azuchi-Momoyama* period 安土桃山時代 (1573–1600), one of Sanki's most well-known students, *Manase Dosan* 曲直瀬道三 (1507–1594), came to prominence as perhaps the best-known proponent of *Gosei-Ha* philosophy, which essentially attempted to reintegrate the fundamental theories of *Yin/Yang* (*In/Yo* 陰陽) and the 5-Phases (*Go-Gyo* 五行) into *Kampo* practice, subjugating the classical teachings of the *Shang Han Lun* in the process. A monk, like his teacher before him, he also received his Confucianist/Buddhist education at the prestigious *Ashikaga* College 足利学校, founded in the *Kamakura* period, which dedicated its teaching to Chinese literature and science in the Neo-Confucianist tradition. He set up the "*Danxi* Society," which focused on the theory of the "four injuries by *qi*, blood, phlegm and stagnation," which was a precursor in fact to the *Qi*, Blood and Fluid theory developed much later in the *Koho-Ha* school by *Yoshimasu Todo*'s son, *Nangai* (more on them later).

The style of *Kampo* promoted by the *Gosei-Ha* therefore tended to be characterized by the use of a strict logical framework of diagnosis which sought to redefine the Pattern of Illness (*Byo Sho* 病証) using etiological and pathomechanistic language. This contrasted sharply with the classical method (from the *Shang Han Lun*) of identifying the Formula Pattern (*Yakusho* 薬証) that most closely matched the patient's presenting signs and symptoms, thus identifying the diagnosis and treatment by the same name.

In practical terms, the *Gosei-Ha* methodology of prescription began to employ the compounding of individual herbs into a formula that matched the theoretical logic of the diagnosis so that the use of *Jing Fang* formula units, hitherto favored in *Kampo* practice, began to lose currency.

Another Buddhist and Confucian scholar, *Nagata Tokuhon* 永田徳本 (1513–1630), also a student of *Tashiro Sanki*, continued the *Jin-Yuan* lineage into the *Edo* period and he, *Sanki* and *Manase* are collectively often known as the "three venerable physicians" of the *Gosei-Ha*. Their work and the influence of this faction impacted several generations of followers, including many who either translated or published original work based on prominent Chinese works of the *Ming* and *Qing* dynasties. These included *Manase Gensaku* 曲直瀬玄朔 (1549–1631), successor to *Manase Dosan* (see above) and his many students including *Okamoto Genya* 岡本玄治 (1587–1645), *Furubayashi Kengi* 古林見宜 (1579–1657) and *Nagasawa Doju* 長沢道寿 (year of birth unknown–1637). Later, *Kitayama Yushoshi* 北山友松子 (year of birth unknown–1701), *Nakayama Sanryu* 中山三柳 (1614–1684), *Katsuki Gyuzan* 香月牛山 (1655–1740), *Kato Kensai* 加藤謙斎 (1669–1724), *Tsuda Gensen* 津田玄仙 (1737–1809) and *Fukui Futei* 福井楓亭 (1725–1792) all published works significant to the *Gosei-Ha* faction during the middle of the *Edo* period.

Of particular relevance to the topic of this text, *Kitao Shunpo*

北尾春圃 (1658–1741), also from the *Gosei-Ha* school, developed a method of abdominal diagnosis based on the theory of the "Movement between the Kidneys" (腎間動氣), originally taken from the *Nan Jing* (難經), one of the classical *Han* dynasty texts (see above). What is significant here is that, though many of the *Gosei-Ha Kampo* practitioners were empirically orientated, they nonetheless, as in this case, tended to take a particular aspect of theory as their departure point in practical matters. This single feature, a focus on practical empiricism as opposed to philosophical theory, is what came to characterize yet another new faction that began emerging in the early *Edo* period, the *Koho-Ha* (see below).

4. "Return to the classics" in the *Edo* period (1603–1863)

The Classical School (*Koho-Ha* 古方派)

Just as the pendulum had swung away from the classical roots of Chinese Medicine, beginning in the *Kamakura* period, with the influence of *Jin-Yuan* teachings in Japan that had heralded *Sanki's* attempts to reconfigure the philosophy and practice of *Kampo* based on Neo-Confucianist doctrine (which itself resulted in the rise to prominence of the *Gosei-Ha* faction), so by the early *Edo* period, it was about to swing back in the opposite direction. By the mid 17th century, increasing dissatisfaction amongst many Japanese physicians at what they saw as the lack of concrete, practical dimensions to the practice of medicine began to confront and eventually oppose what was perceived as the overly abstract philosophical logic of the *Gosei-Ha*.

A movement began that took as its starting point the desire to "return to the classics" in terms of *Kampo* education and practice. This inevitably meant the re-emergence of the *Shang Han Lun* as the primary authority on medical doctrine in pharmacology and, by contrast, the abandonment of any reliance on overly abstract logic in the clinical setting. In time, as the *Gosei-Ha* continued its own trajectory through the *Edo* period and beyond, this new faction, known as the *Koho-Ha*, began to rely less and less on contemporary texts and teachings from China, preferring instead to develop its own interpretations of classical Chinese teachings and establishing many of its own, original adaptations of them.

In China, the *Shang Han Lun* had itself been subject to many revisions from the *Song* dynasty through the *Ming* into the *Qing*. Japanese *Kampo* physicians from the *Koho-Ha* were inspired by some of the more radical of these revisions and began to formulate their own practice based on them. The early proponents of this new brand of classicism included *Nagoya Gen'I* 名古屋玄医 (1628–1696), and his student *Goto Konzan* 後藤艮山 (1659–1733). They are credited as the "fathers" of the *Koho* style though in fact they each remained faithful to many of the theoretical concepts that had informed the work of the *Gosei-Ha* before them. They both made extensive use of *Yin/Yang* theory for example to explain aspects of disease and treatment and *Goto* in particular is well-known for his theory that:

> Most people today, regardless of whether they be old or young, depleted or plethoric, have congested vitality (*Shakki* 積気) knotted up (*Ketsu* 結) in the abdominal organs…the hundred diseases all arise from the stagnation (*Ryutai* 溜滞) of vitality (*Genki* 元気). (*Byoin Ko* ("Reflections on Etiology"), *Goto Konzan*, Yokoen, 1841)

In fact, this focus on a theoretical concept, in this case stagnant *Qi*, did not exactly resemble that of the *Gosei-Ha* whose interest was in diagnosing and treating deficiency in the Essence *Qi* (*Seiki* 生気) using tonic herbs (*Hozai* 補剤). In *Goto*'s theory by contrast, he advocated dispersing *Qi* Stasis using hot-spring baths, Moxibustion, bear gallbladder and such substances. This notion of removing the pathogenic *Qi* (*Jya Ki* 邪気) in order to allow the natural Defensive *Qi* (*Shoki* 正気) to flow was to become central to the *Koho-Ha* philosophy of practice.

Goto had three students who between them initiated the most radical of changes in the practice of *Kampo* in mid to late *Edo*. They were *Kagawa Shuan* 香川修庵 (1683–1755), *Yoshimasu Todo* 吉益東洞 (1702–1773) and *Yamawaki Toyo* 山脇東洋 (1705–1762). Their respective styles collectively established the *Koho-Ha* in clear and radical ways as completely distinct from, and in many ways opposed to, the *Gosei-Ha*. Kagawa, for example, refuted *Yin/Yang* theory, even daring to criticize the *Shang Han Lun* for its use of these terms. Later, *Yamawaki*, upon observing the dissection of the male body of a criminal in 1754, was to entirely disown the basis of traditional Chinese physiology by criticizing *Zang-Fu* organ theory as wholly inaccurate and unreliable. His famous text, "On the Viscera" (*Zoshi* 蔵志, 1759) included a detailed description of this experience deftly illustrated by one of his students *Asanuma Sukemitsu* 浅沼佐盈, and as the very first record of a human dissection in the *Tokugawa* (*Edo*) period, its implications for the medical world in Japan were to prove revolutionary and irreversible.

In many ways this single text cemented the orientation of the *Koho-Ha* away from *Gosei-Ha* in favor of the newly emerging medicine based on "Dutch Studies" (*Rangaku* 蘭学), which emanated from "Exit Island" (*Dejima* 出島), the Dutch trading post in the bay of *Nagasaki* through which *Tokugawa* period Japan (an era of sustained cultural isolation) retained contact with scientific and other developments from abroad. In fact this Dutch medicine had first been called *Komo Igaku* 薦菰医学 ("Medicine of the Red-Haired People") in rather the same way that the very first Western medical imports, which had originally been brought by the Portuguese (and later the Spanish) in the early 16th century long before the beginning of the *Edo* period, had been called *Nanban Igaku* 南蛮医学 ("Barbarian Medicine"), which had failed to flourish at that time.

Another landmark publication that filtered into *Edo* Japan was a Dutch anatomy text which formed the basis of "New Text on Anatomy" (*Kaitai Shinsho* 解体新書) by *Sugita Genpaku* 杉田玄白 published in 1774, possibly the single most pivotal text of the period and one which hastened the move towards Western medical thinking. This shift towards embracing modern textbook anatomy in the *Koho-Ha* and abandoning older abstract concepts of body structure and function naturally allowed for common ground between its own philosophy and practice of medicine and that of the emergent *Rampo* 蘭方 (Western Medicine), which may be one of the reasons for its survival into the 20th and 21st centuries alongside modern allopathic medicine.

Perhaps the best-known *Koho-Ha Kampo* physician, however, was *Yoshimasu*. Son of the surgeon and obstetrician *Hatakeyama Shigemune* 畠山重宗, he changed his name later on in honor of his birthplace, *Hiroshima* in *Yoshimasu*, and of his friend and patron, *Yamawaki Toyo* (see above), from whom he took *Todo*. Like Yamawaki, he also dismissed much of the logic and philosophy of the *Gosei-Ha* as purely speculative and is famous for his pragmatic pronouncements on the empirical nature of medical practice, "It is for me nonsense to discuss the pathogenesis of a disease, because pathogenesis is more or less a product of speculation…one depends upon what one has really seen and examined and nothing else" (from his *Yakucho*, 1771).

Most significantly, Yoshimasu recodified the *Shang Han Lun* and *Jin Gui Yao Lue* formulas according to the specific clinical evidence (*Sho* 証) which he believed identified them. His work in regard to attributing a specific pattern (*Yakusho* 薬証) for every *Jing Fang* formula (which of course included an abdominal pattern) became known as "Matching Pattern with Formula" (*Ho Sho Ichi* 方証一致) and is still very much used today in modern *Kampo* practice.

Of particular relevance to this book, *Yoshimasu* especially advocated the use of the abdomen in diagnosis. He regarded the pulse as too abstract and subjective (he would often admonish his students declaring, "Do not speak to me of things you cannot see or feel"), advocating instead the use of the abdomen as a more concrete and reliable assessment tool for establishing veracity in diagnosis by clearly identifying the "Toxin" (*Doku* 毒) or disease-causing agent, directly through *Fukushin*. It is perhaps this aspect of his legacy in particular that has survived into the modern era and, along with the *Shang Han Lun* itself, has most influenced the development of *Fukushin* into its present form within the modern *Koho-Ha*. Yoshimasu's most famous quote on this topic is still quite familiar to most *Kampo* physicians today and is lasting testimony to his profound belief in the importance of practical first-hand experience (*Shinshi Jikken* 親試実験) in distinguishing "fact" from "fiction" in medicine: "The abdomen is the origin of living. Thus, a hundred diseases root here. That is why we examine it without fail in order to diagnose a disease."

But perhaps the single most significant event following *Yoshimasu*'s death in relation to the importance placed on the abdomen within the *Koho-Ha* faction was the publication in 1800 of the *Extraordinary Views of Abdominal Patterns* (*Fukusho Ki Ran* 腹證奇覽), by *Inaba Katsubunrei* 稲葉克文禮 (date of birth unknown–1805). Compared with the erudite *Yoshimasu* who had been a prolific writer, *Inaba* was semi-illiterate and by his own account was introduced to the practice of *Fukushin* by his teacher, *Kaku Taiei* 鶴泰栄, who considered him unfit for more intellectual or scholarly pursuits and so agreed to teach him more practical skills in medicine. *Inaba*'s text documents the abdominal patterns (*Fukusho*) specific to most of the *Shang Han Lun* and *Jin Gui Yao Lue* formulas with detailed abdominal drawings accompanying each one (Figure 2.4).

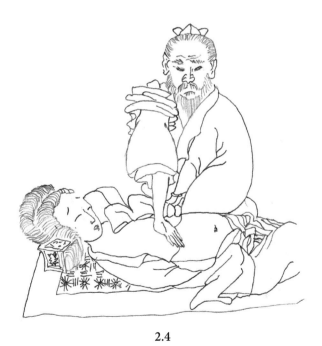

2.4

Since *Inaba* himself was either reluctant or incapable of writing down his lifetime experience concerning the abdomen, it was left to his students to pressure him to do so, subject to which he admits at the end of his author's preface, he finally succumbed: "I agreed…and subsequently recorded (my knowledge in) this book in order to provide instruction (to physicians concerning abdominal examination)."

This landmark text, together with that of one of his principal students *Wakuda Yoshitora* 和久田叔虎, who later wrote an addendum to the original—the *Fukusho Kiran Yoku* 腹證奇覽翼, contributed greatly to the survival of the practical art of *Fukushin* until today. Interestingly, *Inaba's* text is currently out of print in Japan though there are several Chinese translations circulating, especially in Taiwan, and we now have the first English language translation, *Extraordinary Views of Abdominal Patterns, Inaba Katsu Bunrei*, 1800, Transl. Kageyama, J., publ. The Chinese Medical Database, 2018.

A quote from the foreword to the English version by Arnaud Versluys, Ph.D., M.D. (China), L.Ac., serves as a summary of the significance of this text:

> Distilling detailed information on the ins and outs of abdominal diagnosis by reading the original writings of *Zhang Zhong Jing* is difficult to say the least. And we owe it to the wisdom and diligence of generations upon generations of formidable *Kampo* masters such as Todo Yoshimasu and…Inaba Katsubunrei, to have synthesized a clear and practical system for investigating a patient's abdomen as a guide for the selection of the exact canonical herbal formula.

The author of the English translation, Jay Kageyama, in his introductory remarks to the *Fukusho Kiran* makes a similar assessment of the significance of this text in the *Edo* period and its legacy in terms of the modern practice of *Kampo*:

> According to the Classification of Reference Books on Abdominal Diagnostics (*Fukushin Sho No Bun Ru*) by Otsuka Keisetsu (1900–1980), at least 50 works on abdominal examination from authors belonging to various schools of *Kampo* were published during the *Edo* (1603–1867) and *Meiji* (1868–1912) periods. Of these,

the works of Yoshimasu Todo 吉益東洞 (1702–1773), perhaps the most influential physician of the Ancient (Antiquity) School (*Koho-Ha* 古方派) of *Kampo*, and Inaba Bunrei 稲葉克文禮 (DOB unknown–1805) have been considered to be the most authoritative works on abdominal diagnosis in Japan.

The Eclectic School (*Secchu-Ha* 折衷派)

Inevitably there were those in late *Edo* Japan who found many of the *Koho-Ha* approaches extreme and in their view overly simplistic, preferring instead to attempt a kind of integration of *Jin-Yuan* medicine (*Gosei-Ha*) with *Koho* practice. Using the benefit of historical hindsight, they thus incorporated the more demonstrably successful theories and practices of both schools from the previous 400 years into a new faction, the "Eclectic" or "Compromise School," *Secchu-Ha* 折衷派. This school became well-known for its practical clinical innovations focused on "disease cure" rather than philosophical manifesto, such as those of *Wada Tokaku* 和田東郭 (1744–1803), whose use of formulas such as *Yokukansan* 抑肝散 (*Yi Gan San* in Chinese) for various psychiatric disorders is well-known and still used today. His approach embraced both the old (*Koho*) and new (*Gosei*) ways in a compromise that "looked at hardness and softness as the same" (*Tsuyoshi Ju So* 剛柔相摩). He famously considered the Liver and its pathologies (especially Qi Stagnation/*Ki Utsu* 気鬱) as the main culprit in emotional disorders. He reasoned that during times of peace and relative prosperity, such as those he lived in, that due to excessive spare time and "easy" living, the Liver became easily constrained: "We have been living in a peaceful era for a long time. This is why we commonly find all the people now have constraint in the liver and Gallbladder and suffer from ki constraint" (Wada, T. 和田東郭 "Idle Talk Under Palm Trees" 蕉窓雑話, 1821).

Others in this school wrote new formulations of their own synthesizing old and new such as *Hara Nanyo* 原南陽 (1752–1820) who created *Otsujito* 乙字湯 (*Yi Zi Tang* in Chinese), a formula for hemorrhoids and constipation. *Nakagami Kinkei* 中神琴渓 (1744–

1833), initially a student of *Yoshimasu*'s, famously converted to the *Secchu-Ha* faction arguing that the *Shang Han Lun* should be revered but also adapted to suit modern times adding, "It should only be used for its prescriptions and not its theories."

The *Secchu-Ha* survived into the *Meiji* period (*Meiji* 明治, 1868–1912), especially through such prominent doctors as *Asada Shohaku* (浅田宗伯, 1815–1894), a prolific writer of more than 80 books who in his later professional life claimed to have seen as many as 14,000 patients a year. Like *Nakagami* before him, he was also a student in the style of *Yoshimasu* but he nevertheless held that "the old theories are the main, and the new prescriptions are to be used." He wrote a number of original prescriptions including from his text "Experiential Prescriptions of *Asada Sohaku*" (*Asada Sohaku Keikenho* 浅田宗伯経験方) the gynecological formula Goddess Powder (*Nyo Shin San* 女神散, *Nu Shen San* in Chinese), still very much in use today in Japan.

Others in the *Sechu-Ha* tried to combine some of the new *Rangaku* teachings into *Kampo* practice including *Ogino Gengai* 荻野元凱 (1737–1806), a well-known court *Kampo* physician of his day (called to treat the Shogun in *Edo* in 1790) who reportedly spoke Dutch and was famous as a pioneer of bloodletting; and *Ishizaka Sōtetsu* 石坂 宗哲 (1770–1841), famous for his integration of modern anatomy into Acupuncture practice and his exchanges with Philipp Franz von Siebold (1796–1866), a German physician and botanist appointed resident physician in *Dejima* (see above) in 1823. Siebold, father of the first Japanese female Western doctor *Kusumoto Ine* 楠本イネ, brought many of *Ishikaza*'s teachings back to Holland in 1828.

Perhaps the most well-known of all the *Secchu-Ha* doctors to try to integrate *Kampo* and Western medicine was the surgeon *Hanaoka Seishu* 華岡青洲(1760–1846) whose several publications in late *Edo* Japan were mainly transcripts of his clinical experiences including that of his now famous surgery in 1804 to perform a partial mastectomy of breast cancer using an herbal anesthetic *Tsusen-san* (通仙散) which he had based on the one originally created by the *Han* dynasty surgeon *Hua To* 華佗, called *Ma Fei*

San 麻沸散. Performing over 150 surgeries in his life, he is also well-known for creating various herbal prescriptions including the topical first-aid ointment "Purple Cloud" *Shiun-ko* (紫雲膏) used also in Moxibustion therapy.

In popular Japanese culture, *Hanaoka*'s life has been well documented both in novel form—"The Doctor's Wife" 華岡青洲の妻 (1966), written by Sawako Ariyoshi—and on the screen as "The Wife of Seishu Hanaoka" (1967) directed by Masumura Yasuzo. *Seishu* trained several prominent students, among them *Honma Soken* 本間棗軒 (1804–1872), whose "Lectures on Skills of Doctors" was widely circulated amongst surgeons of the late *Edo*; and *Nakagawa Shutei* 中川修亭, who immortalized the doctrine of the *Secchu-Ha* by comparing it in a favorable light with the limitations of both the *Koho* and *Gosei* schools that had preceded it:

> If someone has diseases, just as there is a thief in the house, Koho school only seeks to drive the thief away without considering whether the house survives or perishes; whilst Gosei school holds to guard its house without daring to ask whether the thief is gone or not.

But the efforts of the *Secchu-Ha* to embrace the new while retaining the old in medicine were destined to stumble in the face of the momentous political, economic and cultural change that was about to sweep the nation. Even the serious academic pursuits of another faction, the "School of Textual Analyses" (*Kosho-Ha* 考証派) which, alongside the *Secchu-Ha*, dedicated itself to the commentary on and compilation and dissemination of scholarly works on *Kampo* as well as detailed analysis of specific aspects of the classical texts (such as the weights and measurements of *Jing Fang* prescriptions from the *Shang Han Lun*), was not enough to withstand the huge wave of change that was approaching with the end of the *Tokugawa* period. Nonetheless, the academic achievements of the *Kosho* faction, though appreciated more in China than in its homeland at the time, nonetheless laid some very important scholarly ground for the eventual resurgence of *Kampo* in the 20th century and in some ways set the standard for bench research in the field.

5. Introduction of modern medicine in the *Meiji* period (1868–1912)

The Meiji Restoration, *Meiji Ishin* 明治維新, saw a rapid decline in the popularity of *Kampo* as compared with the *Edo* period before it. Japan had emerged from its protracted period of relative isolation during the *Tokugawa* period and literally "opened its doors" to the world at the end of the 19th century starting with the arrival of Commodore Perry's "black ships" (*Kurofune* 黒船) into Tokyo harbor in 1853. The paradigm shift was exponential and exposed the Japanese culture to that of the modern industrialized world, initiating momentous change in philosophy, technology, politics, law, science and of course medicine.

Little by little the innovations of the *Rampo* school came to dominate what were increasingly seen as the antiquations of the *Kampo* system. Perhaps the final death-knell for *Kampo* was sounded with the introduction into Japan of Jennerian (heterologous) vaccination (especially for smallpox) in the early part of the 19th century (first administered by *Nakagawa Goroji* 中川五郎治 in 1824). By 1871 it was decided that the medical system should "modernize" in imitation of the German system and a series of legal changes followed, including in the "Medical Licensing Act" (*Isei* 医制) of 1875, introducing exams based on the natural sciences and Western medical knowledge. This led eventually to the revoking of the licenses of all existing TJM practitioners in 1883 (although well-known *Kampo* doctors such as *Asada Sohaku* [see above] continued to practice).

Various attempts were made by these remaining individuals to create organizations to preserve the practice of *Kampo* such as the *Teikoku Ikai* 帝国医会 (Imperial Medical Association) but by the end of the century, the *Kampo* movement was all but extinct.

Any attempt at rekindling the fire of the old traditional ideas and practice of medicine would have to be initiated by the newly trained Western physicians of the era, most of whom had little interest in looking to the past for their medical direction and training. Nonetheless, in 1910 *Wada Keijuro* 和田啓十郎 (1872–1916), a Western-trained doctor, wrote a text called "The Iron Hammer of the

Western World" (*Ikai No Tettsui* 医界之鉄椎) in which he compared the relative merits of *Kampo* and the new "Western" medicine. His summary was controversial at the time as he claimed traditional medicine to be far superior in most aspects to its modern rival. This text influenced a number of individuals who were dissatisfied with some of what they regarded as the limitations of modern medicine such as the side-effects of newly emerging pharmaceutical drugs. One amongst them was *Yumoto Kyushin* 湯本求真 (1876–1941), a graduate of *Kanazawa* Medical School who became a student of *Wada's* (and later the teacher of one of modern *Kampo's* most well-known doctors *Otsuka Keisetsu*—see below). His "Traditional Japanese and Chinese Medicine" *Kokan Igaku* 皇漢医学 (1927) as well as the publication in the same year of *A New Study of Chinese Medicine* (*Kampo Igaku no Shin Kenkyu*) by *Nakayama Tadanao* 中山忠直 (1895–1957) combined to initiate the beginnings of a *Kampo* "revival" which was to gather momentum as the new century began to unfold.

Kyushin was one of the more radical modern *Koho-Ha* practitioners who epitomized the divide, not only between his faction and the modern *Gosei-Ha* in Japan, but also in comparison to most traditional Chinese medical doctrine of that period. For example, an exchange between him and a Chinese colleague *Wu Hanxian* 吳漢僊 appeared in the publication *Authoritative Words about National Medicine* (*Kokui Seigan* 国医正言) in which *Kyushin* openly refused to accept any distinction between externally or internally caused disease in terms of the treatment strategy arguing that "*Shang Han Lun* formulas can be used to treat all disease." This was a clear rebuttal of the philosophical doctrines of *Li-Zhu* medicine in Japan (see above) and the Warm Disease (*Wen Bing* 温病) faction in China, both of which preferred the use of *Shi Fang* 时方 (Contemporary Formulas) and *Jin Fang* 今方 (Modern Formulas) for internally caused illness, something the *Koho* school scoffed at.

Interestingly, *Kyushin* had some sympathizers in China at the time who classed themselves (similar to the *Koho* tradition in Japan) as proponents of what they referred to as "evidential scholarship."

One such individual, *Zhang Taiyan* 章太炎 (1868–1936), a contemporary of *Kyushin*'s, was quite critical of the majority of commentaries on the *Shang Han Lun* (as were the *Koho* practitioners), pointing to Japan as the new heir to *Zhang Zhong Jing*'s legacy:

> With the spread of the Treatise to Japan, there have also been dozens of commentators. Their commentaries follow the text closely and are considerably more circumspect than ours. Their treatments demonstrate an ability to modify formula with virtuosity, unimpeded by past orthodoxies, and moreover with frequent clinical success. In terms of making *Zhongjing* [come to life in the] present, we must state: our Way has gone to the East.

> (Lu Yuanlei, 陆 渊雷, 1931)

Clearly the role of evidential scholarship that had marked the rise of the *Koho-Ha* in Japan also made its mark as a reaction to Neo-Confucianist doctrine in modern China. However, for multiple reasons, it was not destined to thrive in China whereas in Japan it was to drive the entire trajectory of the modern *Kampo* revival.

6. Renaissance of *Kampo* in modern Japan (1920–present)

Even though the practice of *Kampo* medicine had been suppressed and delegitimized by the end of the 19th century, the traditional medicines themselves were of great interest to botanists, pharmacognosists and pharmacologists. Their combined research into the crude drugs used in *Kampo* helped to legitimize their pharmacological potential and arouse the interest of the early pioneers of the pharmaceutical industry at the turn of the century.

In the 1920s, when *Kyushin* and others had already begun to initiate a *Kampo* renaissance, they were helped on a practical level in their endeavors by the founding of the first pharmaceutical companies to modernize the processing of crude drugs into a granular extract form. Nagakura Pharmaceutical Company in

Osaka was the first to develop this process closely followed by *Tsumura Juntendo* (the largest pharmaceutical company in Japan today), founded by *Tsumura Jusha* 津村重舎 (1871–1941), which established an institute to promote the standardization of *Kampo* manufacturing methods. This method of delivering the medicine in a high quality, easy-to-use, standardized format known as "Japanese–Chinese Formulas" *Wakan Yaku* 和漢薬 has become the most commonly used and accepted form of taking *Kampo* medicine today in Japan and is growing in acceptance throughout the world.

Thus, the seeds for the 20th century *Kampo* revival were sown before the Second World War, and in *Kyushin*'s footsteps there followed two giants of the modern *Kampo* era: one his student in the *Koho* style, *Otsuka Keisetsu* 大塚敬節 (1900–1980), the other from the *Gosei-Ha*, *Yakazu Domei* 矢数 道明 (1905–2002), who had studied *Kampo* at Tokyo Medical University under *Mori Dohaku* 森道白. Their professional lives, though enacted in different factions, unexpectedly came together when *Yakazu*'s younger brother *Yudo* was successfully treated by *Otsuka* for typhoid fever in 1933. There followed many years of collaborative activities between them, starting with the founding of the Japan *Kampo* Association (*Nihon Kampo Igakukai* 日本漢方医学会) in 1934 and in 1936 with both of them lecturing on *Kampo* at *Takushoku* University 拓殖 大学 in Tokyo. Later, at *Yakazu*'s initiation, the "Asia Medicine Association" (*Toa Igaku Kyokai* 東亜医学協会) was formed in 1938, a forerunner to the *Nippon Toyo Igakkai* 日本東洋医学会 (Japan Society of Oriental Medicine—JSOM) founded in 1950 (also by *Otsuka*, *Yakazu* and others) and which survives to this day with almost 9000 members.

Both *Otsuka* and *Yakazu* were involved in a landmark collaborative publication in 1941 entitled *The Actual Practice of Kampo Medicine* (*Kampo Shinryo no Jissai* 漢方新流の実際), which received a second edition in 1954 and was completely revised in 1969 under a new title "Medical Dictionary of *Kampo* Practice" (*Kampo Shinryo Iten* 漢方診療医典). This text has an English language version *Natural Healing with Chinese Herbs*, Ed. *Hsu Hong-Yen* 許鴻源, publ. Oriental Healing Arts, 1982, with a foreword by

Dr. *Yakazu*, by then the Director of Oriental Medical Research at the *Kitasato Kenkyujo* 北里研究所 (forerunner of *Kitasato* University, founded by the renowned bacteriologist *Kitasato Shibazaburo* 北里柴三郎—1853–1931) having taken over from its previous director, his colleague and friend, Dr. *Otsuka,* who had passed away in 1980.

Of note, Dr. *Hsu*, originally from Taiwan, had earned his pharmacy doctorate at Kyoto University, having graduated from *Meiji* University School of Pharmacy and also studied *Kampo* whilst in Japan, becoming well acquainted with Dr. *Otsuka*. He was an international scholar, publishing 24 books on *Kampo*, and held many prestigious posts in Asia including president of the Taiwan Pharmaceutical Association for 30 years. He went on to found the Sun Ten Pharmaceutical Company in 1946, based in Taipei, that manufactures and distributes Chinese Herbal formulas internationally using the same methodology as the Japanese to produce 5:1 ratio granulated extracts. Their inventory is strongly focused on *Jing Fang* formulas from the *Shang Han Lun* and *Jing Gui Yao Lue* and their publishing arm, the Oriental Healing Arts Institute (OHAI, founded in 1976), in its many publications includes a translation by *Hsu* and William Preacher of Dr. *Otsuka*'s own Japanese version of the *Shang Han Lun* (1981). One of Dr. *Hsu*'s many publications *Commonly Used Chinese Herbal Formulas with Illustrations*, publ. OHAI, 1980, became the first and one of the most influential English language texts on *Kampo* formulas in the West and includes many of the original *Edo* period abdominal illustrations from the *Fukusho Kiran* (see above).

The influence of *Otsuka, Yakazu* and others in legitimizing the practice of *Kampo* in the medical mainstream of modern Japan can hardly be overstated. The large percentage of physicians practicing some form of *Kampo* today (currently estimated at 90%) can in part be attributed to the influence of their flexible, open-minded approach to the integration of the traditional with the new and their willingness to disseminate knowledge through practice, teaching, research and publication.

As a result of its legitimization into mainstream medicine in Japan, the practice of *Kampo* today is highly regulated as are the formulas and individual herbs used in its practice. The Japanese Ministry of Health began approving *Kampo* medicines in 1967 for national health reimbursement and currently 148 formulas and 243 individual substances have been approved and licensed for use. They can be prescribed by licensed physicians and pharmacists and consequently basic *Kampo* education is now provided in all medical and pharmacy schools, though the unofficial title of "*Kampo* Specialist" is reserved for those who pursue much more detailed study, usually at postgraduate level.

7. The *Otsuka* lineage

Otsuka himself was perhaps the most influential *Kampo* practitioner of the last century. He was born in *Kochi* city on *Shikoku* island into a fourth generation medical family, his father having been a well-known OB/GYN doctor. He himself trained as a pediatrician and, after graduating *Kumamoto* medical college in *Kyushu* in 1923, returned home to practice. But a chance reading of the *Kokkan Igaku* (see above) was inspirational enough to uproot him from his family home and take him a thousand miles north to Tokyo where he pursued its author, *Yumoto Kyushin* (see above), and was accepted as his student for ten years. Also influenced by *Kimura Hiroaki* 木村 博昭 (1865–1931), a student of *Asada Sohaku* (see above), *Otsuka*, though he identified primarily with the *Koho* school, showed great flexibility and openness in his practice of *Kampo*, using old and new formulas alike and in many ways embodying more of the eclectic and diverse principles of the *Secchu-Ha* (see above).

His professional achievements were equally diverse, founding as mentioned the JSOM, directing the *Kampo* department at the *Kistasato* Institute (see above) as well as teaching, practicing and publishing—case studies, articles and books—including his seminal *Kampo* textbook, *Kanpo Igaku*, publ. *Sogensha Igakushinsho*, 1956. (An English translation of this text was published in 2010 by Churchill Livingstone as *Kampo: A Clinical Guide to Theory and Practice*, translated by Gretchen De Soriano and the author of this text, Nigel Dawes. A second edition was published by Singing Dragon in 2017.) Significantly this text has a section on abdominal diagnosis, and through his life, *Otsuka,* true to the *Koho* lineage, showed clear dedication to the practice and teaching of *Fukushin* and to him we owe a great deal for ensuring the survival of this practical art into the modern era.

What can be characterized as the "modern" *Koho-Ha* therefore owes a great deal to *Otsuka*, and while true to this school of thought— he did not pay much attention to either *Zang-Fu* organ theory nor to the meridians, for example—he nonetheless did not agree with, for example, the *Mengen* 瞑眩 ("Healing Crisis") theory of *Yoshimasu.* Neither did he dismiss out of hand the theory of "*Qi*," believing that to deny its existence, even if not fully understood, would be to deny the traditional foundation of the medicine itself. His focus was the traditional *Sho* (証), based on the Formula Patterns established by *Yoshimasu* and others though, as a medical doctor by training, he also believed the disease name could be seen as part of the "Pattern":

> The treatment of Oriental Medicine follows the *Sho* 証 and so it is described in the phrase: *Zui Sho Chi Ryo* 随証治療 (Treatment according to the proof). Another way of saying this is: The diagnosis is in itself the treatment plan. This method is not opposed to the way of treating in modern medicine, that is, treatment by the name of the illness. Sometimes, the determination of the name of the illness will facilitate the diagnosis of the proof. Even when a doctor depends only on the name of the illness to treat with *Kampo*, he or she can attain a certain effect with a somewhat high success rate.

Otsuka argued in fact that the two characters, 証 and 症, both pronounced as *Sho* (or *Zheng* in Chinese) in fact refer to radically different concepts. From his 1934 book "The Key to Classifying Clinical Presentations in Kampo Medicine" (*Rui Sho Kan Betsu Kani Yo Ketsu* 類證鑒別漢醫要訣):

> *Sho/Zheng* 證 presentation means evidence, verification, confirmation. It also means proof. It is completely different than

sho/zheng 症 symptoms… If you are examining a patient with pneumonia who has fever, chills, floating and tight pulse, absence of sweating, and panting, then this is called the Ephedra Decoction presentation (*sho/zheng* 證). If the patient has only a fever or wheezing, then this is a symptom, not a presentation.

This distinction is critical—for example, in distinguishing between what modern medicine might call a "syndrome" or TCM calls a "Pattern" as each of these terms refers to a broad category of symptoms that together summarize an overall clinical presentation. *Otsuka's* definition of *Sho* 證 is, however, far more precise, linking it to the signs and symptoms that characterize a specific formula, expressed in the concept of *Ho Sho* 方證 (*Fang Zheng* in Chinese) referring to the Formula (treatment) presentation. Additionally, *Otsuka* is differentiating the other use of *Sho* 症, which applies to a singular clinical symptom, insufficient on its own to guide treatment.

This hugely important semantic distinction had already been taken up by *Otsuka's* teacher, *Kyushin* in his "Sino–Japanese Medicine" (*Kokan Igaku* 皇漢医学) published in 1927:

> The symptomatic therapy 對症療法 of Western medicine and the "adjust the therapy to the presentation" 隨證治之 approach of *Kampo* medicine look similar but are different. The former focuses on the patient's uncertain self-reported symptoms 自覺症狀 and seeks to repress them. This approach is called treating the branch in *Kampo* medicine and is completely different than the "adjust the therapy to the presentation" approach. *Kampo* medicine combines the self-reported symptoms with the observed symptoms 他覺症狀 to discover the confirmed and unchanging symptoms 症狀 and treats that. For *Kampo* medicine, treating the presentation 證 is a causal therapy 原因療法 and a treatment of special efficacy 特効劑.

Otsuka was clearly a scholar who revered the classics but was equally pragmatic about the value of individual experience and was well-known for being brutally honest about his own failures and mistakes. As he often said to his students, "Read the classics. However, be aware that the ancient people could lie. Even what I have told you, you don't need to believe as I have told it. You try first, and if you like it, then use it" (Otsuka, 1956).

His legacy continues both in and outside Japan. His son, *Otsuka Yasuo* 大塚恭男 M.D., Ph.D. (1930–2009), in addition to practicing *Kampo* was also an accomplished academic and medical historian, teaching *Kampo* at the *Kitasato* Institute (北里研究所) after his father's death in 1980, and influencing many contemporary *Kampo* practitioners in his lifetime. One of his students is directly related to the *Otsuka* family by marriage—*Watanabe Kenji* 渡辺賢治, M.D., Ph.D., head of the Center for *Kampo* Medicine at Keio University School of Medicine in Tokyo, whose wife, *Noriko Watanabe*, M.D. is *Yasuo*'s daughter. They both studied *Kampo* under him and Dr. *Watanabe* was appointed director of the "*Otsuka* clinic" in Tokyo (founded by *Otsuka Keisetsu* in 1931) after *Yasuo*'s death in 2009. Thus, the legacy of the modern *Koho* tradition preserved through the *Otsuka* lineage continues including clinical work, research, publication and teaching.

Outside East Asia, the *Otsuka* legacy in modern *Kampo* is growing and has influenced generations including my own. Amongst *Otsuka Yasuo*'s foreign students at *Kitasato* Institute were two Westerners living in Tokyo in the 1980s: Peter Townsend, a pharmacist from New Zealand (who later taught *Kampo* and introduced Sun Ten products to Australia); and Gretchen De Soriano M.Sc., Bac.C., an American *Kampo* practitioner who now practices and teaches *Kampo* in London where she also introduced Sun Ten into the UK. Both studied *Kampo* at *Kitasato* with *Yasuo* and each became my teacher, Peter in Tokyo (in the mid 1980s) and later Gretchen in London (in the late 1980s.)

For his part, Dr. *Watanabe* has taught and collaborated with many foreign students at *Keio* University over the years, including visiting M.D.s, in particular from Germany such as Heidrun Reissenweber, M.D. from the Clinic for Japanese Medicine in Munich and Silke Cameron M.D. from the Gottingen University of Medicine as well as American doctors such as Gregory Plotnikoff

M.D. from the Minnesota Personalized Medicine Clinic, all of whom are very active in the *Kampo* field.

In addition to the many *Kampo* students taught by Gretchen in the UK and Peter in Australia (before his untimely death), I myself have set up the New York *Kampo* Institute and have been teaching *Kampo* throughout the US and internationally for the last 20 years. *Kampo* practice in many parts of Europe (with the notable exception of the UK) is open only to M.D.s, similar to Japan. However, in Australia, New Zealand and the US, licensed Acupuncturists are legally allowed to prescribe herbs in their practice. This affords great scope for developing continuing education at the graduate level in *Kampo* amongst the many thousands of licensed individuals in those countries.

International organizations that have sprung up in support of such a trend include the International Society for Japanese *Kampo* Medicine (ISJKM) based in Europe and the North American *Kampo* Consortium (NAKC), a collaboration between the NY *Kampo* Institute (my own); High Desert Hari Society in Santa Fe, NM; Dr. *Watanabe* at *Keio* University in Tokyo; and Sun Ten Pharmaceutical Company in Irvine, CA (headquarters Taipei, Taiwan).

The future internationally for *Kampo* looks therefore quite promising and in particular for the modern *Koho-Ha Otsuka* lineage, which always has and continues to espouse a very strong allegiance to the role of *Fukushin* in diagnosis and treatment.

3

METHODOLOGY

"The method to palpate abdominal patterns is to first ask the patient to lie supine and make his mind Qi (気) right. The physician must then also sit straight and correct his [own] breathing, while focusing his mind Qi on his subumbilical region. It is similar to a warrior who takes his sword and faces an enemy. [Such a physician] does not fear any major illnesses. He is not blinded by life and death. He does not yield to riches or nobility. He does not scorn the poor or those of low rank. The physician must perform examinations while keeping his mind focused on the goal of curing the disease and of removing suffering. This is the great method of physicians to examine patients."

From the introduction to *Extraordinary Views of Abdominal Patterns: Fukusho-Kiran, Inaba Katsu Bunrei*, 1800, Transl. Kageyama, J., publ. The Chinese Medicine Database, 2018.

THE ABDOMINAL EXAM—TECHNIQUE

"Skill comes before study, and lack of skill is just like a fading flower for it looks pitiful."

Otsuka Keisetsu (1900–1984) from the Preface to: Otsuka, K.: "30 Years of Kampo: Selected Case Studies of an Herbal Doctor", Oriental Healing Arts Institute, 1984, xxiii.

1. Preparation and materials

No equipment is necessary to perform the abdominal exam, which is typically done on a treatment table with the patient lying in the supine position. Adjust the table to a height at which the practitioner can comfortably "ground" their body weight yet still remain at the optimum height in relationship to the patient. If the table is too high, the practitioner will feel unable to properly "sink" into the *Hara* and their center of gravity will remain too elevated, giving rise to stiffness in the upper body, including the shoulders and hands, and an inability to properly relax. If too low, it may give rise to strain in the lower back and a tendency to lean too heavily on the patient, causing discomfort and potentially distorting the abdominal findings, leading to "false positives" in terms of the findings.

The only materials necessary will be a table cover and sheet and a low pillow and towels or equivalent for draping. The patient is not required to disrobe for the exam and may lie supine, fully clothed on the table, with their abdomen exposed from the lower border of the ribcage to the level of the pubic bone and anterior iliac spine. They should wear loose clothing and remove any belt or other constraints from the lower abdominal area. Initially, the patient should lie with their legs fully extended and may be asked to bring their knees up later during the exam (see below). Naturally, if an Acupuncture or other treatment is to follow then the patient should disrobe fully prior to the exam and should be draped in a similar manner as described above, leaving the abdominal area exposed.

The room should ideally be warm and conducive to relaxation as some patients may find exposing their abdomen, especially in a cool environment, may give rise to a mild sense of vulnerability and can lead to involuntary tension in the surface muscles of the areas to be palpated, thus distorting genuine findings. All sensory input should ideally be minimized—no perfumes, scents, music, bright light or other distracting influences—and the practitioner's movements and voice should remain smooth and rhythmic so as to induce an increased parasympathetic response in the patient that will enhance more positive receptivity to touch.

In short, any and all sources of stimuli that may potentially trigger a sympathetic response in the patient should be anticipated and avoided. In this way, abdominal palpation can be done with the least likelihood of subtle, involuntary tension being provoked in the surface musculature of the abdomen, which can cause distortions in the diagnostic findings leading to "false positives" in some instances (see below).

The practitioner should always ensure the hands are clean and warm, the nails short and that no intrusive jewelry or perfumes are worn.

2. Posture and positioning

In the section on "Form and function" in Chapter 1 ("Definition of *Fukushin*" section) I discussed at length the role of *Hara* and *Koshi* in regard to correct body posture and their corresponding relationship to power and efficacy in any given practice. Specifically, I noted that in Japanese culture (and I gave the example of the martial arts in particular), the *Shisei*, or outward form (posture), visibly betrays the inner strength or otherwise of the individual. Correct form indicates correct mind, intention and purpose, which, in diagnosis, are essentials for clarity and accuracy.

In the *Zen* tradition for example, the importance of correct form is linked directly to the right state of mind from which right action in any given practice will naturally and freely flow. But as *Suzuki Shunryu* (鈴木俊隆, 1904–1971) warns us in his *Zen Mind, Beginner's Mind*: "These forms are not the means of obtaining the right state of mind. To take this (right) posture is itself the right state of mind. There is no need to obtain some special state of mind."

Here, the term "correct" or "right," *Sei* 正 (*Zheng* in Chinese), is used in the sense of what is "upright" or "undistorted," i.e. true to its proper context and purpose. For example, in Japanese, *Genki* (元気) literally means "Healthy Energy" as in the exchange: "*Genki Desu Ka?*" ("How are you doing?"); "*Genki Desu*" ("I'm doing fine").

In *Kampo* terms we refer to this healthy energy as *Seiki* 正気

(*Zheng Qi* in Chinese), the "Upright" or "Correct" Energy related to the body's (anti-pathogenic) defenses, which stands in direct opposition to Pathological or "Evil Energy," *Jyaki* 邪気 (*Xie Qi* in Chinese), which can give rise to "Distorted Energy" *Byoki* 病気 (*Bing Qi* in Chinese), which means "Disease" in Japanese.

As such, "findings" in the context of abdominal palpation are sensory impressions, gained through touch, whose clarity will depend absolutely on correct form. Correct Form (*Koshi*) allows for the correct internal state (*Hara*) conducive to clear, concise and lucid perception of such tactile evidence and later, its accurate assessment and interpretation.

Thus, in preparing to perform the abdominal exam, critical attention must be paid to one's posture and positioning before attempting to make contact with and palpate the patient. Follow these steps:

1. Stand to the patient's right (if you are right-handed), or on the opposite side (if left-handed).

2. Place your feet shoulder width apart or slightly wider facing the patient (and table) at a 90-degree angle. You may brace your thighs against the side of the table, which helps stability. This position is referred to as "double weighted" meaning you are equally distributing your body weight on either foot.

3. Close your eyes and "ground" yourself by rooting your *Ki* 気 on exhalation. With your knees slightly bent, let the *Hara* sink and the *Koshi* establish itself. Take a few deep breaths in this position.

4. Relax and bring the mind/body into concentration or "single-mindedness" *Joriki* 定力. Now you are ready to begin the exam (see below).

5. Conduct the entire examination with confidence and skill, using smooth, flowing movements designed to cause the least discomfort to the patient.

3. Breathing

It can be said that the breath is none other than the source of life itself. Indeed, the character 気 (*Ki*), written as 氣 in classical Japanese, has multiple translations including that of breath, as in the "Breath of Life." It is made up of 气, the radical for "gas" or "air," and 米 meaning "rice" or "food," and according to the context, can mean air, gas, steam, smell, weather, atmosphere as well as several verbal connotations. In the context of East Asian Medicine, however, it is usually understood to indicate the Vital energy or Life Force permeating every living thing. It is the *Ki*, for example, that we seek to contact and manipulate in Acupuncture or any meridian-based healing modality, martial or fine art.

This term is clearly linked to the Sanskrit word *Prana* or "Breath," as in *Pranayama* or "breathing exercises" found in the Yogic tradition. In fact, some translators of East Asian Medical literature have preferred to use "breath" when translating the character 気, most notably the well-respected authors of the *Chinese Medicine from the Classics* series, Claude Larre and Elizabeth Rochat de la Vallee, publ. Monkey Press, 1989–1994.

So, since the language itself specifically links the concept of Vital energy with the breath, it follows naturally that we should pay careful attention to our own breathing and to that of the patient during the abdominal exam.

In Chapter 1 ("Language and terminology" section) I discussed the significance of the so-called "Elixir Field" (*Saika Tanden* 臍下 丹田) in relationship both to the specific Acupuncture point, "Sea of Qi" (*Kikai* 気海), located three finger widths on the midline below the navel, and also to the broader area of the *Hara* itself. This area of the lower abdomen forms the natural focus of breathing in all expressions of East Asian healing, martial and fine arts, giving a sense of concentrated intention and preparedness for action, something clearly implied in the Japanese phrase *Hara O Sueru* (literally "to set one's *Hara* in position") implying "to prepare oneself." In fixing your *Hara* (mind) on the task at hand, the quality of your focus becomes that of the task itself. Focusing your *Hara* is the same as preparedness. Again, a quote from *Suzuki Shunryu* (referenced above) comes to mind: "It is the readiness of the mind that is wisdom."

Typically, the ideal posture for the practice of this type of breathing is in the seated position. Whether in *Zen* Practice (*Zazen* 座禅), the Tea Ceremony (*Sa Do* 茶道), Acupressure (*Shiatsu* 指圧) or "The way of the sword" (*Iaido* 居合道), the practice of "Right Sitting" (*Seiza* 正座) includes "Right Breathing"—that is, breathing into and from the belly. This is done through the nose, with long, slow exhalations and shorter inhalations, such that the lower abdomen (*Hara*) and lower back (*Koshi*) literally "fill up" with the breath whilst the chest and upper body remain relaxed and still.

The abdominal exam in *Kampo* is typically rather done in the standing position (see above); however, attention is paid to all the same aspects of mind and body as discussed above and the manner of "belly-breathing" is the same as in the seated position.

The body's center of gravity will naturally rise slightly on inhalation and sink again on exhalation. Therefore, as we shall see below, pressure is always slightly released from the examining hand(s) during inhalation and applied during exhalation. It is this rhythmic application and release of pressure following the breath that comes to guide the form of the sequences that make up the exam. This form we call the *Kata* 型.

One word of caution in relationship to the patient's breath. It may be tempting, perhaps ideal, for the practitioner to coordinate the rhythm and rate of his or her breathing with that of their patient. Whilst this may naturally occur by itself, do not make this your fixed aim. To do so may distract from your own "right breath" and lead to loss of focus, ultimately distorting your findings. At the same time, encourage the patient to breathe in a natural, relaxed manner. They should not practice "belly-breathing" in the manner of the practitioner during the exam itself.

4. Pressure

In Chapter 2 I discussed the work of *Masunaga Shizuto*, the founder of the *Zen Shiatsu* style in respect to *Hara Shin* 腹診 (Abdominal Diagnosis). As previously noted, *Shi* 指 literally means "finger" and *Atsu* 圧 means "pressure" and *Masunaga* was well-known for his very particular approach to the application of pressure in diagnosis and treatment. His definition of "Correct Pressure" (*Seiatsu* 正圧), referring to the quality of pressure that will readily "penetrate", as in be able to connect deeply with the receiver, is based on three guiding universal principles which I have certainly found both profound and effective and apply equally in this case to the practice of *Fukushin*.

Perpendicular pressure

The angle of pressure applied to any given surface should be perpendicular to the angle of the surface itself.

In anatomical terms, this principle allows for pressure to penetrate the various levels of tissue (skin, fascia, muscles) without disturbing or causing stress to their integrity, allowing the practitioner to feel what is naturally present as opposed to sensing a potential "reaction" to the pressure itself.

In energetic terms, pressure that aims to penetrate to the depth of the main meridian or channel, the goal of any *Shiatsu* therapist or Acupuncturist, must pass through the more superficial layers of tissue without provoking any involuntary response such as tensing or tightening. Such responses could cause the body to "close up" and prevent access to the channels and their respective points. Perpendicular pressure avoids this in much the same way as a high diver, who when entering the water at a perfectly perpendicular angle, can "puncture" the water cleanly, avoiding even the smallest splash.

Continuous pressure

Pressure, once applied, should maintain an even, continuous depth and rhythm throughout any given *Kata* 型 or sequence of movements. The patient's experience of such pressure will feel as though there is no variation in the amount of overall pressure applied even though distinct locations are palpated successively and separately.

In order to achieve this "continuity" of pressure depth and flow, the practitioner must master the proper integration of what *Masunaga* referred to as the "Mother" or *In* 陰 (*Yin* in Chinese) and "Giving" or *Yo* 陽 (*Yang* in Chinese) hands. His concept of Continuous Pressure involved the effect of the static, supportive aspect of one with the dynamic, motive qualities of the other into a single, uniform, smooth and undifferentiated sensory experience for the patient. Such an experience is naturally conducive to a parasympathetic response and encourages relaxation and receptivity to the pressure itself, allowing it to penetrate more freely and without resistance.

In order to achieve this, the successful practitioner of *Fukushin* must fully appreciate how to differentiate between the respective qualities of *Yin* 陰 and *Yang* 陽 pressure, between the static and active, and how to harmonize the transition between these polarities in their posture, movement, breathing and of course in their hands— the point of actual contact with the patient.

To make an obvious analogy, those familiar with so-called "*Taiji* walking" in the practice of *Tai Kyoku Ken* 太极拳 (*Tai Ji Quan* in Chinese) or equally the style of walking meditation in Zen practice known as *Kinhin* 経行 will appreciate that the principle at work here is precisely the same. In both these examples, weight is fully absorbed into one leg/foot (*Yin*), thus supporting the potential for the other leg/foot (*Yang*) to move freely forward and into position at which point a natural shift of weight occurs reversing the *Yin/Yang* roles of each leg/foot, and so on. In this way, movement or "walking" involves the smooth maintenance of continuous pressure exerted (in this example on the earth) through the seamless transition of weight between the Full (*Jitsu* 実) and Empty (*Kyo* 虚) or the active and supportive.

So, in performing *Fukushin*, this same effortless and smooth transition must also characterize the movement of the "mother" and "giving" hands, rather like the stealthy and supremely coordinated "padding" of a tiger (or perhaps a cat!), if the exam is to render accurate and useful results.

Equal pressure

Palpatory pressure, in this case on the abdomen (or on any part of the body), when it includes more than one distinct source (both of the practitioner's hands in this case), must be applied in such a manner that neither giver nor receiver is able to consciously distinguish between the different points of contact.

Masunaga referred to this principle as "One-point pressure," giving rise to the subjective impression that, though multiple distinct tactile stimuli may be objectively applied at the same time, one's overall sensory experience can remain unified, whole and undifferentiated.

Technically, this principle is achieved in practice by literally equalizing the pressure applied through each hand during the *Fukushin* exam. In other words, in each of the specific locations to be palpated on the abdomen using both hands, each hand will register 50 percent of the total pressure applied by the practitioner at the moment of assessment. Such a moment will be very short lived, however, since in order to maintain the principle of Continuous Pressure (discussed above), the weight will then shift from one hand to the other in sequence allowing for the natural, smooth and uninterrupted flow of the weight transitions characteristic of the Form (*Kata*) of the exam.

Equal pressure in fact is less of a technical, objective principle, rather a subjective one, defined by the direct sensory experience of feeling two or more points of contact "as one." This sensation of "oneness" is not confined to the experience of the physical pressure applied on the abdomen; it also applies to the unified, non-discriminating mental state of both practitioner and patient during the exam. Such a state evolves naturally from the intense focus of bringing mind and body, posture and breath into alignment as described above in the "Posture and positioning" section, using what is referred to as "Power of Concentration" (*Joriki* 定力) in the Zen Buddhist lexicon.

In *Zen* seated meditation (*Zazen* 座禅) as well as in *Zen* walking meditation (*Kinhin* 経行), also mentioned above in the "Continuous pressure" section, the purpose of developing *Joriki* is to enter a state of "One-pointedness," *Ekagrata* in Sanskrit, the very state *Masunaga*, himself a lifelong devoted Buddhist, is advocating in respect to achieving his principle of "Equal Pressure."

As *Zen* Master *Dogen* (道元 1200–1253) reminds us, "In a snowfall that covers the winter grass a white heron uses his own whiteness to disappear."

For *Masunaga*, in the widest sense, achieving "Equal Pressure" is therefore none other than attaining "One-pointedness," itself the first step towards attaining the blissful state referred to in meditation practice by the Sanskrit word *Samadhi*. In turn, it is in this state that moments of insight or "enlightenment" may occur, either suddenly, in a flash, known as *Kensho Godo* (見性悟道) in *Zen*, or gradually, over time as in the practice of "Silent Illumination" (*Shinkantaza* 只管打坐).

Whilst such philosophical descriptions may appear quite abstract, it is important to mention that, for *Masunaga*, moments of sudden insight as described in the *Zen* literature were for him readily attainable in practice though developing *Joriki* through right posture, breath, attitude and technique as discussed above. Such moments were clearly equated by him with the art of "diagnosis" (in Latin, literally "seeing through") in the medical context. Concrete examples of *Kensho* for him not only were embodied in moments of insight in his meditation practice but were equated precisely with instances of clarity and understanding in his diagnostic work with patients.

In the practice of *Fukushin* then, the application of pressure to the abdomen is strictly defined by these three guiding principles, which, in practical terms, are not separate or distinct from one another, but rather characterize the overall quality and nature of the exam in its entirety:

1. Perpendicular

2. Continuous

3. Equal

The exam itself, in real time, takes only three minutes to perform. However, as we have seen above, there are a great many aspects to be aware of and to coordinate in order to conduct it successfully and discover its importance in diagnostic terms. From the external environment of the treatment space, to the internal environment of the practitioner including posture, movement, breath and intention, to the quality, depth and flow of the pressure itself, there are many things to be considered and practiced.

The basics of this technique are indeed simple; however, they are not easily mastered and in ten years of consistent practice you can expect only to begin to appreciate some of the more subtle aspects of this skill. Hopefully such a challenge will only excite the serious student and encourage them to embrace their mistakes and appreciate them as learning tools.

Repetition is the key. Between the expert and the beginner there is a natural gap but one's experience of this gap may either lead to a sense of despair or opportunity. It's up to you. Closing this gap requires patience, dedication and above all repetition since without repetition in practice, the goal will never be reached.

Paradoxically, it may indeed be the journey itself that holds more interest and satisfaction than the ultimate goal. Once again, as *Suzuki Shunryu* (see above) reminds us (talking of *Zazen* 座禅, but it could equally well be *Fukushin* 腹診), "If you continue this simple practice every day, you will attain some wonderful power (*Joriki* 定力). Before you attain it, it is something wonderful, but after you attain it, it is nothing special." In the meantime, he advises us to rejoice in our ignorance and take heart in the phrase, "In the beginner's mind there are many possibilities, in the expert's there are few."

5. Exam techniques and sequence (illustrated)

Refer to the final part of "Posture and positioning" above for a detailed description of how to prepare oneself to conduct the abdominal exam.

The exam sequence is described below in chronological order as illustrated by the photographs, which feature a right-handed practitioner standing on the patient's right side. Left/right references should therefore be reversed in the case of a left-handed practitioner who would in that case need to be standing on the patient's left side for the exam. In order to practice the exam correctly, follow these detailed descriptions carefully and refer to the illustrations as you go.

Whilst attempting to practice the following illustrated descriptions that make up the entire exam *Kata*, it will be important to make continued reference to the section on "Pressure" above as there are many aspects to keep in mind regarding the technique of applying pressure as well as shifting weight between the hands and between postural positions.

Key to terminology used in the exam

The following brief summary of key terms and concepts regarding the nature and depth of pressure will be a useful addition to those already discussed.

NATURE OF PRESSURE

- 触 (*Shoku*)—Light, non-penetrating touch used to make initial "contact" with the patient and help "ground" the practitioner

- 切 (*Setsu*)—Deeper, penetrating touch used in diagnosis,

achieved by the practitioner "sinking" the *Hara* on the out-breath and allowing natural body-weight pressure to "enter" without force or tension

DEPTH OF PRESSURE

The "Depth of pressure" 圧力深度 (*Atsuryoku Shindo*) refers to the three distinctly different depths of pressure used in this exam. They are as follows:

- 表面圧 (*Hyomen Atsu*)—"Superficial pressure" means the lightest of pressure applied by the fingertips to the very surface anatomy of the abdomen. This pressure only penetrates the level of the dermis and no deeper. This level applies *only* to Figures 3.7a–3.7e

- 深圧力 (*Shin Atsuryoku*)—"Deep pressure" refers to pressure that is aimed at reaching the level of the abdominal cavity, beyond the skin, fascia and muscle layers. This level applies only to Figures 3.10a and 3.10b

- 中圧 (*Chu Atsu*)—"Mid-level pressure," the most common level of pressure used throughout the exam, aims at reaching the fascia and muscle layers of the abdomen, in-between the superficial and deep levels. This level applies to all the illustrations except Figures 3.7 and 3.10

Exam sequence
FIRST TOUCH

Before making patient contact, the practitioner should adopt the correct posture and positioning (described above). Then, turning forward to face the patient's opposite shoulder, with the front leg bent at the knee and the rear leg straight but not locked (the "brush knee push" position in *Tai Ji Quan*), the practitioner should place the left (support) hand on the patient's right shoulder, spreading the fingers and palm as widely as possible to include the pectoral region so that weight is evenly and widely distributed over the contact surface. Avoid direct pressure on the acromion, which can be uncomfortable. At the same time, place the right (giving) hand, so that the fingertips rest comfortably in the epigastric area and the heel of the palm faces down towards (or over) the navel (Figures 3.1a and 3.1b).

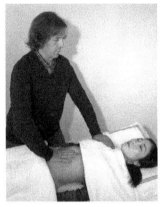
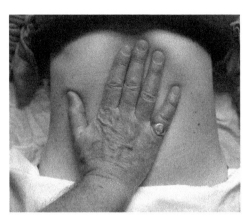

3.1a   3.1b

In this position, maintain even and equal pressure on both hands with a gentle touch that is neither invasive nor superficial. The practitioner should allow their right hand to rise and fall with the patient's breath and not actively apply pressure at this time. This is called "resting pressure." It is a kind of light, non-penetrating touch known in Japanese as 触 *Shoku* (see above) and will contrast quite clearly with the kind of penetrating, deeper touch employed in the exam itself, known as 切 *Setsu* (see above).

This "first touch" allows for initial contact between practitioner and patient and is used to establish mutual trust and confidence. It is a kind of initial tactile greeting that enables the practitioner to sense how easily or otherwise it might be to "enter" the patient's abdomen with the deeper pressure that will characterize the exam to follow. As such, depending on the relative state of relaxation/tension of the patient, the practitioner may choose to remain shorter or longer in this position in order to reach a mutual state of relaxation and receptivity.

Once this moment is reached, you are ready to begin the exam.

KNEADING THE ABDOMEN

After making "first touch" (Figures 3.1a and 3.1b), the practitioner returns to the double-weighted position, feet shoulder width apart with their weight equally distributed on each foot, facing at right angles to the patient in the direction of East, if the patient's head were North (Figure 3.2a).

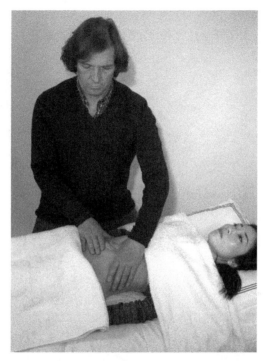

3.2a

With the knees slightly bent, the body and hands relaxed, the practitioner sinks their weight on the out-breath achieving correct alignment of *Koshi* and *Hara* (see above). It is this relaxed "sinking" of the weight that allows the practitioner's pressure to "go in" correctly, without resistance, thus avoiding the potential for "false positives" as described in detail in the section on "Pressure" above. This pressure is referred to as *Setsu* as opposed to the light touch of *Shoku* and is always used in the art of Touch Diagnosis known appropriately as *Setsu Shin*切診 in Japanese.

The technique illustrated in Figures 3.2b and 3.2c involves "kneading" the skin and fascia of the abdominal wall using a clockwise circular movement, alternately palpating the tissue with each hand using rhythmic, coordinated and smooth strokes. The pressure needs to be firm enough to sense the texture, resistance and thickness of the abdominal wall and the fascia and musculature of the abdomen as a whole without causing discomfort.

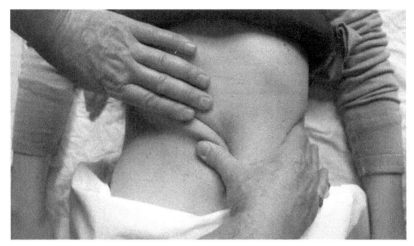

3.2b

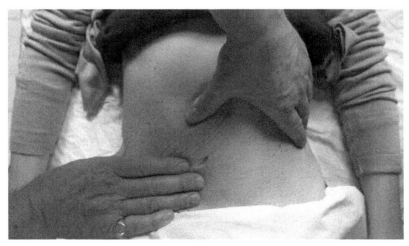

3.2c

The aim of this technique is to make an assessment of the patient's overall constitution, known in Japanese as 体質 *Taishitsu* (literally "the root of a person"), which in *Kampo* is used to determine a person's strength and thus their potential resistance toward disease, providing a useful determinate in the assessment and prognosis of any given illness.

Findings from this part of the exam will be defined in *Kampo* diagnostic terms as either:

1. *Kyo*

    a. Lax and Powerless (*Fuku Bu Nan Jyaku Mu Ryoku* 腹部軟弱無力) (see Figure 4.1)

    b. Tight and Powerless (*Fuku Bu Ko Ren Mu Ryoku* 腹部拘攣無力) (see Figure 4.2)

or:

2. *Jitsu*

    a. *Yang* Full Abdomen (*Yo Fuku Man* 陽腹滿) (see Figure 4.3)

    b. *Yin* Full Abdomen (*In Fuku Man* 陰腹滿) (see Figure 4.4)

The criteria for determining these findings and their clinical interpretations will be discussed in Chapter 4.

PALPATING THE EPIGASTRIUM

Returning to the "brush knee push" stance illustrated in Figure 3.1a, the practitioner should adopt the same hand positions as previously described with the left hand on the patient's right shoulder, weight well distributed, and the right hand, palm down, covering the mid abdomen from epigastrium to navel (Figure 3.1b). This time, unlike the *Shoku* (light touch) of Figures 3.1a and 3.1b, we will aim for the deeper *Setsu* (penetrating) pressure of Figure 3.2a, which is achieved by sinking the *Hara* on the out-breath (as described above) and allowing one's whole body weight to descend and settle without effort. This is done neither by leaning over and into the patient, nor by applying active pressure using the muscles of the fingers, hand or arm, any of which will tend to make the patient tense up and resist the practitioner's attempt to "enter."

Once 中圧 (*Chu Atsuryoku*) or "mid-level pressure" (described above) is achieved in this position, the practitioner will begin to absorb more of his/her weight into the left ("support") hand on the in-breath. In doing this, naturally and without effort, the right ("giving") hand will begin to release in proportion to the increased pressure of the left hand so that what was initially a 50:50 percent weight distribution between both hands now becomes closer to 75 percent in the left hand and 25 percent in the right. This technique is a classic example of the principle of "Continuous Pressure" discussed in the "Pressure" section above.

Once the 75:25 percent proportion is reached, the practitioner gently raises the heel of the right palm off the patient's abdomen so that the middle three fingers adopt a 45-degree angle to the abdominal surface (Figure 3.3). Then, on the out-breath, the left hand begins gradually to release pressure back toward the right hand until the point of "Equal Pressure" (discussed above) is reached.

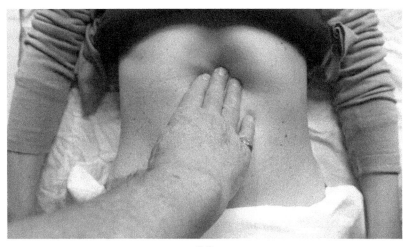

3.3

The aim of this technique is to make an assessment of the relative resistance or tightness of the epigastric region as well as to observe any patient adverse reaction to the pressure when applied.

Findings from this part of the exam will be defined in *Kampo* diagnostic terms as either:

- Abdomen #3 Epigastric Obstruction Resistance (*Shin Ka Hi Ko* 心下痞硬) (see Figure 4.5)

or:

- Abdomen #4 Epigastric Obstruction (*Shin Ka Hi* 心下痞) (see Figure 4.6)

The criteria for determining these findings and their clinical interpretations will be discussed in Chapter 4.

PALPATING THE HYPOCHONDRIUM

Maintaining the same posture and hand positioning from Figure 3.3, the practitioner, on the in-breath, again begins absorbing pressure into the left hand, thereby releasing the right hand to the same 75:25 percent proportions as before. At this point, the right hand moves from the central epigastric area to the right hypochondriac region at which point the hand is angled again at 45 degrees to the abdominal surface, this time with the lateral border of the index finger presenting in the direction of the patient's right shoulder, up and under the ribs on the patient's right side. On the out-breath, the practitioner begins slowly to release pressure from the supporting left hand, as before, into the active right hand until 50:50 percent proportional pressure is reached (Figure 3.4a).

Throughout the entirety of this movement, continuous pressure is maintained and the depth of pressure, as in Figure 3.3, is again *Chu Atsuryoku* 中圧力 or "middle-level," as described above.

On the next in-breath, the left hand again begins to absorb pressure so that the right hand is slowly released to a proportion of 75:25 percent once again. At this point the right hand smoothly slides over to the patient's left side as the left hand releases its position from the patient's right shoulder and again adopts a 45-degree angle to the skin surface, this time with the lateral border of the left little finger presenting downwards towards the patient's left floating rib. Once the left hand is in position, the right hand gently applies pressure on top of it up and under the ribs on the patient's left side in the mirror image of Figure 3.4a (see Figure 3.4b).

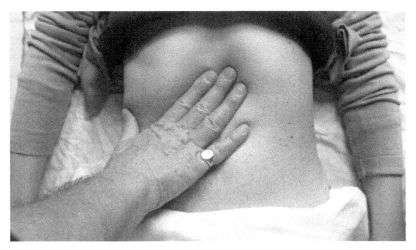

3.4a

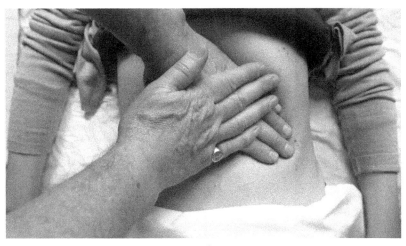

3.4b

The aim of this technique is to make an assessment of the relative resistance, tightness and possible reactive discomfort in the hypochondriac regions bilaterally.

Findings from this part of the exam will be defined in *Kampo* diagnostic terms as either:

- Abdomen #5 Hypochondriac Painful Fullness (*Kyo Kyo Ku Man* 胸脇苦満) (see Figure 4.7)

or:

- Abdomen #6 Hypochondriac Obstruction Resistance (*Kyo Ka Hi Ko* 脇下痞硬) (see Figure 4.8)

The criteria for determining these findings and their clinical interpretations will be discussed in Chapter 4.

PERCUSSING THE LEFT SUB-COSTAL AREA

The next sequence in the exam requires the practitioner to move back into the double-weighted position facing the patient at right angles (exactly the same as in Figure 3.2a). As this postural transition is made, the hand position, starting from that shown in Figure 3.4b, shifts at the same time and in a coordinated manner such that the right hand slides down away from the hypochondriac area gently stretching taut the skin of the abdomen on the patient's left side. This is done to create deliberate tension at the skin surface so that percussion of this area may be done much like the gentle beating of a drum.

As the right hand holds the skin taut, the practitioner uses a swift, staccato-like percussive technique with the three middle fingers of the left hand, "tapping" the sub-costal area on the left side (Figure 3.5). This technique is repeated several times in order to cover an area that corresponds to the entire upper left quadrant of the patient's abdomen, from the lateral border of the ribs to the midline and from directly under the ribs down as far as level with the umbilicus. The aim of this technique is to listen for tympanic gas sounds or the succussion sound associated with Fluid Accumulation in the stomach and upper intestines.

Findings from this part of the exam will be defined in *Kampo* diagnostic terms as:

- Abdomen #7 Epigastric Splash Sound (*Shin Ka Bu Shin Sui On* 心下部振水音) (see Figure 4.9)

The criteria for determining these findings and their clinical interpretations will be discussed in Chapter 4.

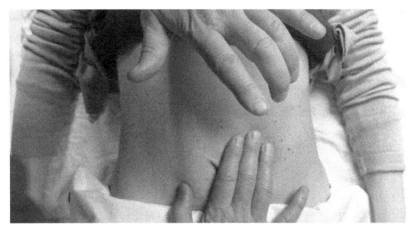

3.5

PALPATING THE RECTUS ABDOMINIS MUSCLE

For the next sequence the practitioner remains in the double-weighted position as for Figure 3.5. Bringing both hands alongside each other (Figure 3.6a), locate the lateral border of the rectus abdominis muscle with the tips of the fingers of both hands.

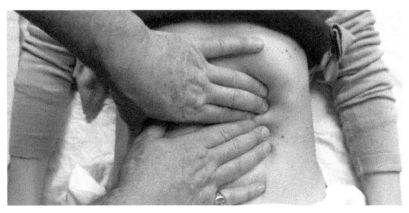

3.6a

Without actively pressing, on the out-breath sink into the *Hara* allowing both hands at the same time to sink into the patient's abdomen to the *Chu Atsuryoku* 中圧力 or mid-level pressure. Pay attention that you remain at this level—the level of the fascia and muscles—as to go deeper will undoubtedly cause discomfort and is not required in this part of the exam. Doing so may confuse your findings.

Start by placing both hands at the superior end of the rectus abdominis muscle, just inferior to the ribs on the left side (the far side of the patient's abdomen). Once the right depth of pressure has been achieved, begin by moving the hips back and drawing the hands gently with you so that the pressure of your fingers moves transversely through the muscle fibers from lateral to medial (i.e. towards you). Lean forward and return to your starting position and slide the hands a little further down in the direction of the navel. Repeat these steps several times so that you cover the entire trajectory of the muscle from superior to inferior, ending up down towards the inguinal area (Figure 3.6b).

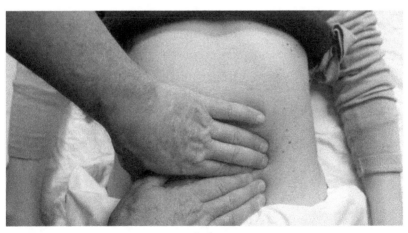

3.6b

When you have completed palpation of the patient's left (far) side, move your hips back a little, remaining in the double-weighted position, to bring your hands to the patient's right (near) side. Beginning as before at the superior portion of the rectus abdominis muscle, this time locating its medial border, repeat the steps previously described (as in Figures 3.6a and 3.6b). In this case, the practitioner's movements are the same, sinking into the muscle on the out-breath, moving the hips back and dragging the fingers of both hands transversely through the fibers of the muscle, only this time from medial to lateral as opposed to lateral to medial (Figures 3.6c and 3.6d).

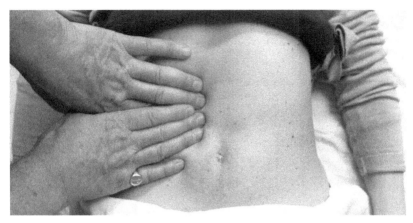

3.6c

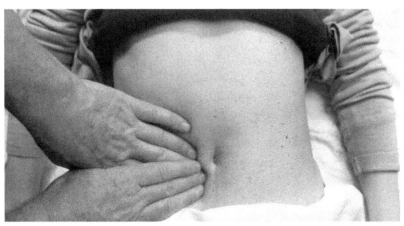

3.6d

In this technique it is essential that the fingers are very relaxed and that pressure is achieved by sinking the body weight in a relaxed fashion. The pressure itself, once the middle-level depth has been established, is actually applied laterally, moving across the muscle fibers and not perpendicularly downward. This is important, especially in the lower portions of the abdomen as perpendicular pressure applied too heavily there is likely to be confused with another part of the exam—Palpating for Blood Stasis (see Figures 3.10a and 3.10b). Thus, the findings can be confused with one another and errors in judgment made.

The aim of this technique is to assess the relative involuntary tension of the rectus abdominis and other muscles in this area of the abdomen. Since the patient is lying supine in a relaxed manner, these voluntary muscles are not engaged and thus should not feel involuntarily tight or spastic. If, in the upper abdomen, the practitioner can easily distinguish the muscle from the surrounding fascia and it feels chordal or like a rope, then this is taken as a positive finding. If, in the lower abdomen, not only the rectus abdominis muscle is spastic and chord-like, but in addition the entire lower abdominal surface is tight and reactive then this is what is called the "bowtie" (see Figure 4.13) and is also a positive finding.

Findings from this part of the exam will be defined in *Kampo* diagnostic terms as:

- Abdomen #8 Inside Spasm (*Ri Kyu* 裏急) (see Figures 4.11 and 4.12)

- Abdomen #9 Lower Abdominal Tight Spasm (*Sho Fuku Ko Kyu* 少腹拘急) (see Figure 4.13)

The criteria for determining these findings and their clinical interpretations will be discussed in Chapter 4.

PALPATING THE MIDLINE AND AROUND THE NAVEL
Again, the practitioner remains in the double-weighted position with both hands aligned alongside each other as in the sequences for Figures 3.6a–3.6d. After finishing the final sequence of palpating the

rectus abdominis muscle on the patient's right (near) side (Figure 3.6d) the practitioner should "float" his or her hands back up to the epigastric area, aligning the tips of the fingers of both hands along the midline of the abdomen beginning just inferior to the xiphoid process, taking care not to apply pressure directly onto this area of delicate cartilage (Figure 3.7a).

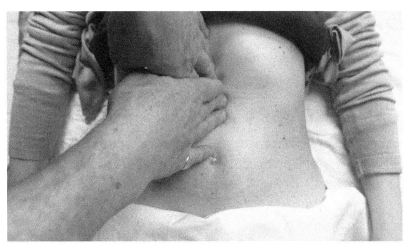

3.7a

On the out-breath, the practitioner sinks their weight allowing the fingers to gently make contact along the midline with the very lightest of pressure. This technique is the only one in the entire abdominal exam to use *Hyomen Atsu* 表面圧—"Superficial pressure" (see above for definition).

Releasing the pressure each time on the in-breath, and reapplying it on the out-breath, the practitioner gradually slides his or her fingers down the midline from superior to inferior towards the navel (Figure 3.7b).

Once at the level of the navel, using the same technique of releasing the pressure (on the in-breath), sliding and then applying the pressure (on the out-breath), gently palpate on either side of the navel itself (Figures 3.7c and 3.7d).

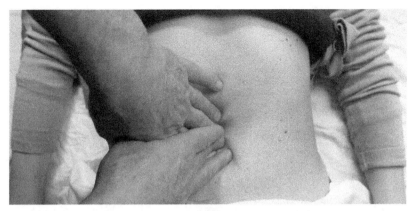

3.7b

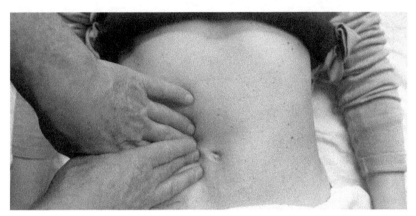

3.7c

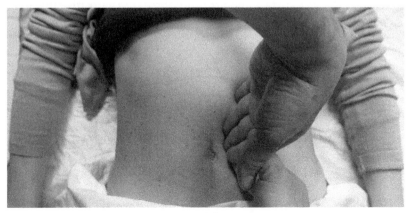

3.7d

Finally, slide down to the lower abdomen and, using the same technique as before, gently palpate the area along the midline from the umbilicus to the pubic bone (Figure 3.7e).

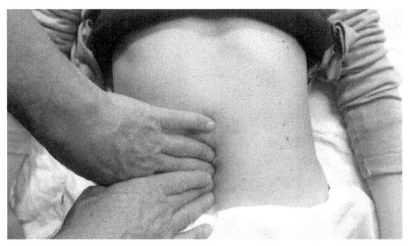

3.7e

The aim of this technique is to feel for any pulsations along the trajectory of the abdominal aorta from the upper to the lower abdomen and including the bifurcation of the aorta at the level of the umbilicus. Naturally, with moderate or deep pressure it should easily be possible to feel these pulsations. However, with the very light pressure used in this part of the exam, if pulsations can still be felt (or seen) at the surface then this is considered a positive finding.

Findings from this part of the exam will be defined in *Kampo* diagnostic terms as:

- Abdomen #10 (see Figure 4.14)

  - Cardiac Pulsations (*Shin Ki* 心悸)

  - Epigastric Pulsations (*Shin Ka Ki* 心下悸)

  - Pulsations around the Navel (*Sei Ka Ki* 臍下悸)

The criteria for determining these findings and their clinical interpretations will be discussed in Chapter 4.

PALPATING THE LOWER ABDOMEN
ALONG THE MIDLINE

Once completing the sequence illustrated in Figure 3.7e, the practitioner, maintaining the same position with both posture and hand position, now moves both hands to the patient's left (far) side lower abdomen, similar to the illustration in Figure 3.6b.

As in that description, on the out-breath, the practitioner sinks his or her pressure, using the *Hara*, so that the fingers of both hands contact the lateral border of the rectus abdominis muscle at the middle level of pressure depth. Leaning the hips back slightly, the hands are drawn transversely through the muscle fibers as in the technique for Figure 3.6b. But this time, on reaching the medial (near) border of the muscle, the practitioner continues to slide the fingers of both hands towards the patient's midline until they finally sink into the area between the navel and pubic bone (Figure 3.8).

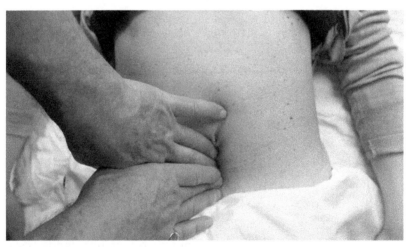

3.8

It is important for purposes of comparison to maintain the same amount of pressure on the far side of the patient's lower abdomen as when reaching the midline, both of which should be done with *Chu Atsu* 中圧—"Mid-level pressure."

The aim of this technique is to compare the tonus of the skin, fascia and musculature on the (left) side of the lower abdomen with that of the abdominal midline between the navel and pubic bone. Whilst normal anatomy will assume a moderate degree of difference in tonus between these two areas, if such a difference is marked, either with the midline feeling unusually tight or full or with the same area feeling extremely empty, then each of these would be considered positive findings.

Findings from this part of the exam will be defined in *Kampo* diagnostic terms as:

- Abdomen #11 (see Figures 4.15–4.18)

    – Lower Abdomen Lacking Benevolence (*Sho Fuku Fu Jin* 小腹不仁) (Figure 4.15)

    – Lower Abdomen Pencil Line (*Sho Fuku Ko Ren* 小腹拘攣) (Figure 4.16)

    – Lower Abdominal Resistance and Fullness (*Sho Fuku Ko Man* 小腹硬満) (Figure 4.17)

    – Lower Abdominal Fullness (*Sho Fuku Man* 小腹満) (Figure 4.18)

The criteria for determining these findings and their clinical interpretations will be discussed in Chapter 4.

PALPATING BESIDE AND BELOW THE NAVEL
Following the sequence in Figure 3.8, the practitioner, maintaining the same body positioning, now moves his or her hands back up to the left (far) side of the patient's navel in much the same manner illustrated in Figure 3.7d, this time using *Chu Atsuryoku* 中圧力—"Mid-level pressure" instead of 表面圧 (*Hyomen Atsu*)— "Superficial pressure" (Figure 3.9a).

After releasing pressure on the in-breath, the practitioner's hands move to the right (near) side of the navel, again applying mid-level pressure (Figure 3.9b).

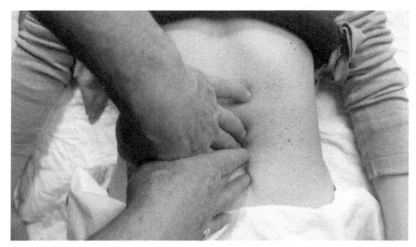

3.9a

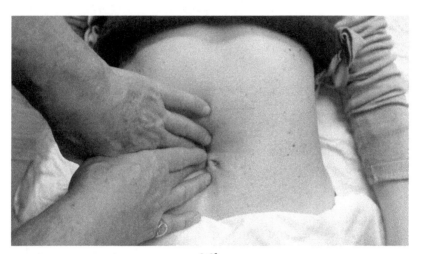

3.9b

The aim of this technique is to assess any resistance to pressure that may be detected in the peri-umbilical areas. This will often feel like a hard, flat surface at the mid-level pressure depth, which resists further penetration of pressure and seems to be almost "mass-like" in form. There may or may not be patient reaction to such a finding when pressed and unlike in the following sequence (Figures 3.10a and 3.10b), the patient's response to this pressure does not constitute part of the finding.

Findings from this part of the exam will be defined in *Kampo* diagnostic terms as:

- Abdomen #13 Navel Spastic Knot Point (*Sai Bu Kyu Ketsu* 臍部急結) (see Figure 4.19)

The criteria for determining these findings and their clinical interpretations will be discussed in Chapter 4.

PALPATING THE LOWER LEFT/RIGHT QUADRANTS

We are now reaching the final sequence of the abdominal exam. It should have been noted that, up to this point, the majority of sequences have been conducted using what we have termed *Chu Atsuryoku* 中圧力—"Mid-level pressure." Only one sequence, described in Figures 3.7a–3.7e, "Palpating along the midline and around the navel" was conducted using—*Hyomen Atsu* 表面圧—"Superficial pressure."

This final sequence of the exam will require the use of *Shin Atsuryoku* 深圧力—"Deep pressure," details of which have been already discussed above. This technique is the most likely of all to provoke reactive discomfort in the patient and, though short-lived, is always best left till the end for this reason.

The practitioner, still maintaining the same double-weighted position, places both hands together, the palm of one on top of the dorsum of the other, and with perpendicular pressure, uses the *Hara* to allow the fingers of both hands to sink deeply into a point on the patient's left (far) side lower abdomen (Figure 3.10a).

The precise location of the area is measured as midway on an imaginary line drawn between the navel and the anterior superior iliac spine. This point equates roughly with the location of the Acupuncture point *Daiko* 大巨 (S.27). Deep pressure must be applied so as to reach the level of the abdominal cavity, beyond skin, fascia and muscle layers.

The equivalent bilateral area is then palpated on the patient's right (near) side in exactly the same manner (Figure 3.10b).

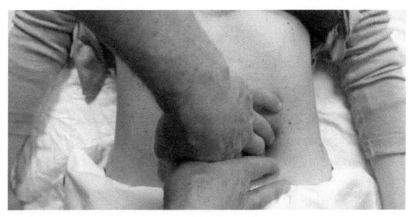

3.10a

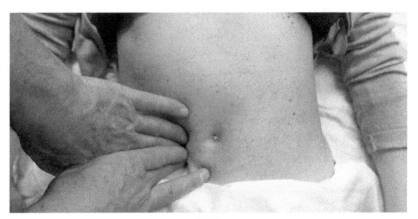

3.10b

The aim of this technique is to assess any resistance to pressure that may be detected either unilaterally or bilaterally. This will often feel like a discrete, nodular mass, as small as a pea though potentially a lot larger. At the "deep" level, if such a point of resistance is detected, the practitioner must then deliberately agitate or laterally displace the nodule or obstruction to test whether there is reactive discomfort on the part of the patient. This may be sudden and severe at times and may even cause the patient to cry out and draw the knees up toward the chest in an involuntary protective reaction. It is the simultaneous confirmation of nodular resistance by the practitioner along with reactive discomfort on the part of the patient that establishes a positive finding in this case. If findings are noted, have the patient bend the knees and place a support underneath in order to recheck the findings. It is possible that the *Oketsu* point might be misdiagnosed as muscular tension in one of the smooth muscles deep in the lower abdomen. With the knees bent these muscles will relax, reducing the possibility for this error.

Findings from this part of the exam will be defined in *Kampo* diagnostic terms as:

- Abdomen #14 Lower Abdomen Spastic Knot Point (*Sho Fuku Kyu Ketsu* 小腹急結) (see Figure 4.20)

The criteria for determining these findings and their clinical interpretations will be discussed in Chapter 4.

Completing the exam

After palpating for the *Oketsu* point bilaterally (Figures 3.10a and 3.10b), release the deep pressure from the patient's abdomen and begin the "Finishing strokes," which are as follows:

1. Make large clockwise circular strokes around the patient's entire abdomen with both palms with the intention of "smoothing out" your work.

2. Reach around both sides of the patient's waist and draw both hands together reaching from behind the patient's back round to their navel with the intention of "gathering up" and "pulling" everything together.

3. Return to the original "brush knee push" position in which you began the very first part of the exam—"First touch" (Figure 3.1). Hold this position for several moments, allowing your palm pressure to slowly float off your patient's abdomen, one breath at a time.

This completes the entire abdominal exam sequence.

4

INTERPRETATION

"Sensations from the outside rule the pulse. Internal damages govern the abdomen."

> Quoted by *Otsuka Keisetsu* in *Kampo: A Clinical Guide to Theory and Practice*, Transl. De Soriano, G. and Dawes, N., 1st edn. publ. Churchill Livingstone, 2010; 2nd edn. publ. Singing Dragon, 2017

The author goes on to explain:

> *"This means that the diagnosis of exogenous-induced disease (Gai Sho 外傷) such as an acute febrile disease depends upon the pulse, while the progress of chronic illness is taken to be endogenous-induced (Nai Sho 内傷) and so should be made according to the abdominal pattern (Fukusho 腹証). In this way Deficiency (Kyo 虚) and Excess (Jitsu 実) can be determined."*

CLINICAL FINDINGS IN THE ABDOMINAL EXAM

"The aim of 腹診 *(Fuku Shin) in Kampo is to determine the* 虚 *(Kyo) or* 実 *(Jitsu) of the patient. However, making this judgment based solely on Fuku Shin could lead to a misdiagnosis. Without fail, make a comprehensive diagnosis by referring to the pulse* 脈証 *(Myaku Sho) and individual complaints as well as other symptoms."*

From "The Aim of the Abdominal Examination 腹診の目的
Fuku shin no moku teki" in *Kampo: A Clinical Guide to Theory
and Practice*, Transl. De Soriano, G. and Dawes, N., 1st edn. publ.
Churchill Livingstone, 2010; 2nd edn. publ. Singing Dragon, 2017

In Chapter 3 the precise methodology of the abdominal exam was discussed and clearly illustrated. Critical aspects of technique such as body posture and positioning, breathing, pressure and the actual step-by-step sequences (*Kata*) of the exam were thoroughly explained and documented. The exam should be practiced countless times over a long period in order to attain basic proficiency and be ready for the next step.

Once the practitioner has gained confidence and skill in these basic techniques, they will be ready to chart the specific findings of the exam and to begin the challenging process of interpretation. This chapter will identify the nature and quality of these individual findings, obtained through the exam, and how to interpret them in the clinical context.

The descriptive narratives (clinical evidence) that accompany each of the specific abdominal patterns (known as the *Sho* 証) are detailed below in the same sequence as in Chapter 3 and follow a concise and consistent rubric including subheadings described below.

Morphology

The source for the material in the "Morphology" section is based on the text *Kampo: A Clinical Guide to Theory and Practice*, Otsuka, K.; Transl. De Soriano, G. and Dawes, N., 1st edn. publ. Churchill Livingstone, 2010; 2nd edn. publ. Singing Dragon, 2017.

This section provides a description of the exact palpatory qualities associated with each specific abdominal pattern in both anatomical and energetic terms. At times it makes reference to associated diagnostic signs including the pulse as well as specific symptoms related to the pattern.

- *Comment*: Additional comments on the morphology of each abdominal pattern provided by Dr. *Otsuka* and with additions from the author

- *Notes*: These are provided based on the author's own clinical experience and attempt to offer more detailed qualitative analysis of the findings and their implications in pathology

- *Charting*: An illustration of each abdominal finding is provided with the precise method of charting shown in each case. The system of charting in *Kampo* is standardized and is usually consistent throughout the literature

- *Clinical interpretation*: In this section specific formulas or formula "families" are identified in regard to each of the abdominal patterns shown. This is the section where formula matching in relation to specific abdominal patterns is systematically discussed

The following 14 Abdominal Conformations will be presented in the same order as in the sequences of the practical exam set out in Chapter 3. The first 4 Conformations relate to Constitutional findings, the remaining 10 belong to Disease findings.

MORPHOLOGY, CHARTING AND INTERPRETATION
A. Constitutional Findings

Refer to Figures 3.2a–3.2c for the technique involved in palpating the two following possible findings.

1. Empty Abdomen 腹力弱(虚)
(*Fuku Ryoku Jyaku [Kyo]*)

- Lax and Powerless Abdomen (*Fuku Bu Nan Jyaku Mu Ryoku* 腹部軟弱無力)

- Tight and Powerless Abdomen (*Fuku Bu Ko Ren Mu Ryoku* 腹部拘攣無力)

Morphology

According to Dr. *Otsuka*:

> The term *Fuku* means abdomen and *Bu* means place. *Mu* means "lack of" and *Ryoku* is strength or power. Due to this lack of strength, the abdomen can be described as flaccid, soft or non-elastic; we shall call it lax and powerless.
>
> The lax abdomen (flaccid, powerless, non-elastic): this speaks of the abdomen as a single unit, as a plane or plate; the muscles are limp, weak and powerless.
>
> When at the same time the abdomen is non-elastic, with a weak 弱 *Jyaku*, and deep 沈 *Chin* pulse, and the hands and feet are cold, then this is the Inside Empty Pattern *Ri Kyo Sho*, 裏虚証.

Comment

The abdominal wall is either thin, weak and without tonus or there may be excessive layers of fatty tissue which are flaccid and atonic upon palpation. It is often cool to the touch and there is a marked decrease in abdominal pressure. The patient often likes the pressure applied by the practitioner.

This abdomen is often referred to as *Yin* within *Yin* (*In Chu No In* 陰中の陰), that is to say, cold, lax, flaccid, empty and wet—all *Yin* qualities.

Notes

This technique is done with Mid-level Pressure (*Chu Atsuryoku* 中圧力) so that the practitioner can assess the tonus and vitality not only of the skin but also of the fascia and muscles of the abdomen.

In addition to the Lax and Powerless Abdomen described above, there is also within the same category the Tight and Powerless (*Kyo* Tight) Abdomen (*Fuku Bu Ko Ren Mu Ryoku* 腹部拘攣無力). This is known as the *Yang* within *Yin* Abdomen (*In Chu No Yo* 陰中の陽), and is still considered an Empty (*Kyo* 虚) Abdomen, but with some apparent "*Yang*" qualities nonetheless. For example, in this case, the abdominal wall is thin and malnourished (*Yin*) but its surface may be tight, resistant and drum-like (*Yang*) where all the superficial musculature is involuntarily tense and strained (*Ko Kyu* 拘急). However, below this surface resistance there is an emptiness and lack of power or strength (*Mu Ryoku* 無力), a *Yin* quality, which can be sensed by the practitioner as a kind of last line of defense in a weak (*Kyo* 虚) individual.

In *Kampo*, the *Yin* within *Yin* type abdomen is often associated constitutionally with Water Types who tend to be damp.

The *Yang* within *Yin* type abdomen is rather associated constitutionally with Blood Types who tend to be dry.

Charting

This abdominal finding is charted as follows according to whether the finding is:

- #1a Lax and Powerless (*Fuku Bu Nan Jyaku Mu Ryoku* 腹部軟弱無力) (Figure 4.1) or:

- #1b Tight and Powerless (*Fuku Bu Ko Ren Mu Ryoku* 腹部拘攣無力) (Figure 4.2)

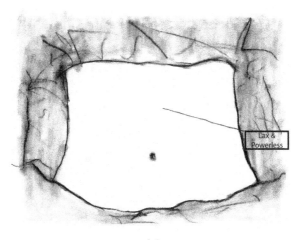

4.1

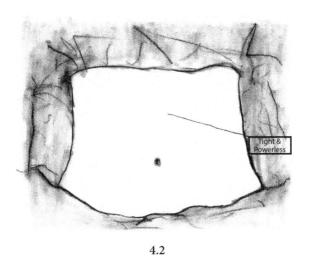

4.2

Clinical interpretation

The interpretation of the findings derived from the very first part of the abdominal exam, "Kneading the abdomen" (see Figures 3.2a,

3.2b and 3.2c), has to do exclusively with the patient constitution (*Taishitsu Sho* 体質証). When we perform this part of the exam our intention is to get an overall sense of "who this person is" and "what they are made of," meaning what type of constitutional strength they possess. This helps in prognosis with regard to assessing their potential susceptibility to illness as well as their response timeframe to any given treatment. It also helps determine the kind of formulas that the person will be able to tolerate, regardless of the pattern of disease (*Byo Sho* 病証) that they are being treated for.

Examples of the language of constitutional typing in *Kampo* include:

- Strong (*Jitsu Taishitsu Sho* 実体質証)

- Weak (*Kyo Taishitsu Sho* 虚体質証)

- *Qi* (*Ki Taishitsu Sho* 気体質証)

- Blood (*Ketsu Taishitsu Sho* 血体質証)

- Water (*Sui Taishitsu Sho* 水体質証)

- Cold (*Hie Taishitsu Sho* 冷え体質証)

- Weak Digestion (*I Cho Kyo Jyaku Taishitsu Sho* 胃腸虚弱体質証)

- Sensitive (*Shin Kei Shitsu Taishitsu Sho* 神経質体質証)

When the abdomen is Weak (*Fuku Ryoku Jyaku* [*Kyo*] 腹力弱[虚]), whether it is Lax (*Nan Jyaku* 軟弱)—*Yin* within *Yin*, or Tight (*Ko Ren* 拘攣)—*Yang* within *Yin*, this is always interpreted as a sign of a Weak Constitution (*Kyo Taishitsu Sho* 虚体質証) in *Kampo*.

Lax and Powerless Abdomen (*Fuku Bu Nan Jyaku Mu Ryoku* 腹部軟弱無力)

When the abdomen is Lax and Powerless (Figure 4.1) this indicates exclusively *Yin* interpretations involving a constitution of *Yang Qi*

Deficiency (*Yo Ki Kyo Sho* 陽気虚証), Coldness (*Hie Sho* 冷え症) and Dampness (*Shitsu Sho* 濕証) along with a tendency for weak Gastro-Intestinal Function (*I Cho Kyo Jyaku* 胃腸虚弱).

This abdomen (*Yin* within *Yin*) suggests a constitution that will require formulas to Warm the *Yang* (*Un Yo* 溫陽), Activate the *Qi* (*Gyo Ki* 行氣) and Resolve Dampness to Activate *Qi* (*Ka Shitsu Gyo Ki* 化濕行氣) such as those found in the *Taiyin* (*Tai In Byo* 太陰病) and *Shaoyin* (*Sho In Byo* 少陰病) Stages of the "Treatise on Damaging Cold" (*Shang Han Lun* 傷寒論).

According to *Yin-Yang* Theory (*In Yo Setsu* 陰陽説), both *Taiyin* and *Shaoyin* Stages indicate Interior Deficiency Cold Patterns (*Ri Kyo Kan Sho* 裏虚寒証) and according to *Zang-Fu* Organ theory (*Zo Fu Setsu* 臟腑説) they would conform with Patterns of Spleen and/or Kidney *Yang* Deficiency (*Hi/Jin Yo Kyo Sho* 脾／腎陽虚証) respectively, although these references are used here to describe a constitutional state (*Taishitsu Sho* 体質証) as opposed to a Disease Pattern (*Byo Sho* 病証).

In the example of what might be called a "*Taiyin* Constitutional Type," in whom the primary Cold and Deficient symptoms will occur in the gut (such as abdominal distention, poor appetite, loose stool) the warming, activating and fluid regulating actions are provided by Dry Ginger (*Kan Kyo* 乾姜), Ginseng (*Ninjin* 人参) and Atractylodes (*Byaku Jutsu* 白朮) respectively exemplified in the Formula Pattern:

- Ginseng and Ginger Combination (*Ninjin To* 人参湯—also known as *Ri Chu To* 理中湯)

In this case, in addition to being Lax and Powerless (*Fuku Bu Nan Jyaku Mu Ryoku* 腹部軟弱無力) (Figure 4.1), the abdomen will also evidence abdomen #4 Epigastric Obstruction (*Shin Ka Hi* 心下痞) (Figure 4.6), which matches the subjective symptoms of abdominal fullness, distention and bloating and is a finding (in Deficiency patterns) calling for formulas containing Ginseng.

This abdomen will also evidence the finding of abdomen #7 Epigastric Splash Sound (*Shin Ka Bu Shin Sui On* 心下部振水音)

(Figure 4.9), along with abdomen #10 Epigastric Pulsations (*Shin Ka Ki* 心下悸) (Figure 4.14), which together match the symptoms of nausea and heavy, foggy head in this Formula Pattern—both Counterflow Water (*Sui Nobose* 水のぼせ) signs. Naturally, as fluid (Damp) accumulates in the stomach and intestines due to lack of Middle Jiao *Yang Qi* (*Chu Sho Yo Ki* 中焦湯気) it will give rise to counterflow, which is addressed not only by the Ginseng and Dry Ginger in this formula (both considered *Qi* herbs in *Kampo*), but also by the White Atractylodes (*Byaku Jutsu* 白朮)—a Water herb—which regulates fluid and in this case removes Toxic Water (*Sui Doku* 水毒) due to Deficiency.

Other formulas that could match this so-called *Taiyin* type (*Yang* Deficient) Lax and Powerless Abdomen as described above, including the other abdominal findings already mentioned, each according to its individual Formula Pattern (*Yakusho* 薬証), include:

More *Yang* Deficiency and Cold:

- Aconite Ginseng and Ginger Combination (*Bu Shi Ri Chu To* 附子理中湯)—with the additional abdominal finding of abdomen #11 Lower Abdomen Lacking Benevolence (*Sho Fuku Fu Jin* 小腹不仁) (see Figure 4.15)

- Cardamom and Fennel Combination (*An Chu San* 安中散)

More *Qi* Deficiency:

- Four Major Herb Combination (*Shi Kun Shi To* 四君子湯)

- Six Major Herb Combination (*Rikkun Shi To* 六君子湯)

- Cardamom and Saussurea Combination (*Ko Sha Rikkun Shi To* 香砂六君子湯)—with the additional abdominal finding of #3 Epigastric Obstruction Resistance (*Shin Ka Hi Ko* 心下痞硬) (Figure 4.5), or possibly #4 Epigastric Obstruction (*Shin Ka Hi* 心下痞) (Figure 4.6)

- Ginseng and Astragalus Combination (*Ho Chu Ekki To* 補中益気湯)

- Stephania and Astragalus Combination (*Boi Ogi To* 防已黄耆湯)

More (deficiency) Fluid Accumulation:

- Hoelen Combination (*Buku Ryo In* 茯苓飲)

- Alisma and Hoelen Combination (*Bukuryo Takusha To* 茯苓沢瀉湯)

- Atractylodes and Hoelen Combination (*Ryo Kei Jyutsu Kan To* 苓桂朮甘湯)

- Inula and Hematite Combination (*Sen Puku Ka Tai Sha Seki To* 旋覆花代赭石湯)

- Pinellia and Gastrodia Combination (*Hange Byakujutsu Tenma To* 半夏白朮天麻湯)

In the example of what we might call a "*Shaoyin* Constitutional Type," in whom the cold has penetrated deeper into the body slowing down the entire metabolic processes (*Yang*) of the body, warming and activating in this case is provided by Aconite (*Bushi* 附子) exemplified in the formula:

- Aconite, Ginger and Licorice Combination (*Shi Gyaku To* 四逆湯)

As in the above *Taiyin* type, all the same kinds of symptom will be present, and the abdomen findings will include:

- #1a Lax and Powerless (*Fuku Bu Nan Jyaku Mu Ryoku* 腹部軟弱無力) (Figure 4.1)

- #4 Epigastric Obstruction (*Shin Ka Hi* 心下痞) (Figure 4.6)

- #7 Epigastric Splash Sound (*Shin Ka Bu Shin Sui On* 心下部振水音) (Figure 4.9)

- #10 Epigastric Pulsations (*Shin Ka Ki* 心下悸) (Figure 4.14)

Additionally, due to the extreme deficiency of body *Yang* in *Shaoyin* types, there will be more pronounced fatigue of the kind that renders the person dysfunctional ("the need to curl up and lie down" as it states in the *Shang Han Lun*). This "curling up" is the person's attempt to stay warm and indicates a level of cold that results in frigidity of the extremities as well as a tendency for watery diarrhea. This degree of cold and the metabolic hypo-functioning of the entire body system is what distinguishes the *Shaoyin* from the *Taiyin* types. An additional abdominal finding that can help identify the *Shaoyin* Constitutional Type and the need for Aconite (*Bushi* 附子) in the formula is:

- #11 Lower Abdomen Lacking Benevolence (*Sho Fuku Fu Jin* 少腹不仁) (Figure 4.15)

Other formulas that could match this so-called *Shaoyin* type (*Yang Deficient*) Lax and Powerless Abdomen as described above, each according to its individual Formula Pattern (*Yakusho* 薬証), include:

- Vitality Combination (*Shinbu To* 真武湯)

- Aconite Combination (*Bushi To* 附子湯)

- Mahuang and Asarum Combination (*Mao Bushi Sai Shin To* 麻黄附子細辛湯)

- Mahuang, Aconite and Licorice Combination (*Mao Bushi Kanzo To* 麻黄附子甘草湯)

- Ginger, Licorice and Aconite Combination (*Shi Gyaku Ka Ninjin To* 四逆加人参湯)

Tight and Powerless Abdomen (*Fuku Bu Ko Ren Mu Ryoku* 腹部拘攣無力)

When the abdomen is Tight and Powerless (Figure 4.2) this indicates that within a *Yin* or Weak constitution (*Kyo Taishitsu Sho* 虚体質証) which is also Cold, there tends to be *Ying* (Nutrient *Qi*) Deficiency (*Ei Ki Kyo Sho* 栄気虚証) and Dryness (*Kan Sho* 乾証) along with a tendency for Weak Gastro-Intestinal Function (*I Cho Kyo Jyaku* 胃腸虚弱). In addition, due to the lack of *Ying* at the center of the body, the *Qi* will be weak, lack root and easily rise or counterflow (*Ki Nobose* 気のぼせ or *Ki Gyaku* 気逆) so that these constitutions tend easily to be sensitive and vulnerable to both their physical and emotional environment.

This abdomen (*Yang* within *Yin*) suggests a constitution that will require formulas to warm and circulate the *Yang* (*Un Yo* 温陽) and moisten the *Ying* (*Jun Ei* 潤栄) and/or the Blood (*Jun Ketsu* 潤血) but also to subdue or stabilize counterflow (*Ko Gyaku Ka Ki* 降逆下氣).

According to *Yin-Yang* Theory (*In Yo Setsu* 陰陽説), this abdomen reflects both *Taiyin*, *Shaoyin* and in this case *Jueyin* (*Ketsu In Byo* 厥陰病) Constitutional Types, who tend to suffer from Interior *Yin* Deficiency Patterns (*Ri In Kyo Sho* 裏陰虚証) and according to *Zang-Fu* Organ theory (*Zo Fu Setsu* 臓腑説) they would present with Patterns of Spleen and/or Liver and Kidney *Yin* Deficiency (*Hi Jin/Kan In Kyo Sho* 脾腎／肝陰虚証) respectively. Again, this is a constitutional not a disease reference.

In the example of what might be called a "*Taiyin* Constitutional Type" who is dry, there will be deficiency in the Nutrient or *Ying Qi* (*Ei Ki* 栄気) causing the surface muscles on the abdomen to be dry, tight and cold leading to abdominal cramps and pain as well as loose stools. Such cases require gentle warming, circulating and softening with formulas containing Cinnamon (*Keishi* 桂枝) and Peony (*Shaku Yaku* 芍薬) in example formulas such as:

- Cinnamon and Peony Combination (*Keishi Ka Shakuyaku To* 桂枝加芍薬湯)

In this case, in addition to being abdomen #1b Tight and Powerless (*Fuku Bu Ko Ren Mu Ryoku* 腹部拘攣無力) (Figure 4.2), this abdomen will also evidence #8 Inside Spasm (*Ri Kyu* 裡急) (Figure 4.11), reflecting surface muscular tension due to deficient Dryness and Cold. There will be no splash sound as this is a dry pattern but there will likely be gas accumulation in the upper left quadrant (part of the #7 finding—Figure 4.10). Additionally, there will be #10

Epigastric Pulsations (*Shin Ka Ki* 心下悸—Figure 4.14) due to the tendency for Counterflow *Qi* (*Ki Nobose* 気のぼせ) caused by deficiency (inability of the *Qi* to root itself in the middle).

In this constitutional type when these pulsations are strong and there is clinical evidence of *Nobose* (such as anxiety, palpitations, insomnia), the use of Cinnamon (*Keishi* 桂枝) to treat Counterflow *Qi* is common in such formulas as:

- Cinnamon Combination (*Keishi To* 桂枝湯)

In more extreme cases there may be the need for formulas that also sedate (or "calm the spirit" *An Shin* 安神) such as:

- Cinnamon and Dragon Bone Combination (*Keishi Ka Ryukotsu Borei To* 桂枝加竜骨牡蠣湯)

If, in addition, the abdominal wall is thin and lacking adipose tissue and the person is underweight then along with the above actions, moistening and building the *Ying Qi* (*Ei Ki* 栄気) with sweet substances like Maltose (*Ko I* 膠飴) will also be necessary in example formulas such as:

- Minor Cinnamon and Peony Combination (*Sho Kenchu To* 小建中湯)

- Astragalus Combination (*Ogi Kenchu To* 黄耆建中湯)

- Major Zanthoxylum Combination (*Dai Kenchu To* 大建中湯)

or there may be the need to moisten the Lungs (an aspect of *Tai In*) with substances such as Ophiopogon (*Bakkumundo* 麦門冬) in example formulas such as:

- Ophiopogon Combination (*Bakumondoto* 麦門冬湯)

- Bamboo Leaves and Gypsum Combination (*Chikuyo Sekko To* 竹葉石膏湯)

In such cases, within this #1b Tight and Powerless (*Fuku Bu Ko Ren Mu Ryoku* 腹部拘攣無力) Abdomen (Figure 4.2), there will likely be abdomen #8 Inside Spasm (*Ri Kyu* 裡急) (Figure 4.11), which involves involuntary tension of the rectus abdominis muscle and/or there may be the "Jumping Fishes" finding (Figure 4.12).

In the example of what might be called "*Shaoyin* or *Jueyin* Constitutional Types" there will be deficiency (Dryness) in the *Ying* and Blood levels (*Ei Ketsu Kan* 栄血乾). On the one hand, therefore, the surface muscles and skin on the abdomen (and the whole body) will be dry and tight. This will give rise to the same tendency for the abdominal finding #8 Inside Spasm (*Ri Kyu* 裡急) (Figure 4.11) as in the *Taiyin* types (above). In this case, however, there will be the additional finding of #9 Lower Abdominal Tight Spasm (*Sho Fuku Ko Kyu* 少腹拘急) (Figure 4.13) confirming the *Shaoyin* aspect of this abdomen pattern.

In addition, due to Dryness at the Blood level, there will be evidence of Blood Stasis (*Oketsu* 瘀血) in the abdominal exam, confirmed by the finding #13 Navel Spastic Knot Point (*Sai Bu Kyu Ketsu* 臍部急結) (Figure 4.19). The location of this Blood Stasis finding beside and/or below the navel is always linked to deficiency patterns (*Kyo Sho* 虚証), where through lack of fluids, the blood has become dry and stuck. Therefore, blood moistening and invigoration is required.

Note: This finding must always be differentiated from #14 Lower Abdomen Spastic Knot (*Sho Fuku Kyu Ketsu* 少腹急結) (Figure 4.20), which is palpated in a different location and is linked to the *Oketsu* found in patterns of Excess (*Jitsu Sho* 実証), requiring Blood cracking (sometimes cooling) and invigorating formulas.

In addition, as in the *Taiyin* types, the abdomen exam will reveal #10 Pulsations (*Shin Ki* 心悸) (Figure 4.14), but these will occur lower down the abdomen surrounding the navel: *Sei Ka Ki* 臍下悸, in the same areas in fact that the *Oketsu* points in #13 Navel Spastic Knot Point (*Sai Bu Kyu Ketsu* 臍部急結) (Figure 4.19) are found.

Such constitutions require *Yin* tonifying and Blood moistening and invigorating as well as gentle warming, circulating and softening with formulas containing Rehmannia (*Ji O* 地黄), *Dang Gui* (*Toki* 当帰), Cnidium (*Sen Kyu* 川芎), Cinnamon (*Keishi* 桂枝) and Peony (*Shaku Yaku* 芍薬) in example formulas such as:

For the *Shaoyin* Type:

- Rehmannia Eight Combination (*Hachi Mi Jio Gan* 八味地黄丸腎気丸)
- Baked Licorice Combination (*Sha Kanzo To* 炙甘草湯)

For the *Jueyin* Type:

- *Dang Gui* Four Combination (*Shi Motsu To* 四物湯)
- *Dang Gui* and Jujube Combination (*Toki Shi Gyaku To* 当帰四逆湯)
- *Dang Gui* Evodia and Ginger Combination (*Toki Shi Gyaku Ka Goshuyu Shokyo To* 当帰四逆加呉茱萸生姜湯)

2. Full Abdomen 腹満 (*Fuku Man*)

- *Yang* Full Abdomen (*Yo Fuku Man* 陽腹満)
- *Yin* Full Abdomen (*In Fuku Man* 陰腹満)

Morphology
According to Dr. *Otsuka*:

The word *Fuku* 腹 means abdomen, while *Man* 満 is used to mean fullness. The full abdomen: in the full abdomen there exist both the *Jitsu* 実証 and *Kyo Sho* 虚証. Full with constipation is usually *Jitsu Sho*, but there are exceptions. Examples of constipation with *Kyo Sho* are: peritonitis, ileus (bowel obstruction) and such illnesses. Diarrhea and a swollen abdomen together, which seems like an unlikely complaint, exist in the *Kyo Sho*. Likewise, when the full abdomen occurs as a result of ascites it is the *Kyo Sho*. Where there is a full abdomen, strength in the depths and constipation, then if the pulse has strength, 力のある *Chikara no aru*, this is the *Jitsu Sho*. With a full abdomen, tight on the surface, and powerless in the depths, *Chikara Naku*, if the pulse is Faint, 微 *Bi* and Weak, 弱 *Jyaku*, then this is *Kyo Sho*.

Comment

Caused by occlusion of gas or feces. This sensation of fullness on the part of the patient can occur in the chest and/or abdomen and causes discomfort and pressure. There may be breathing difficulties (from restricted movement of the diaphragm), gas pain and generalized aching as well as indigestion and constipation. The entire abdomen will feel distended and resistant to the practitioner and the patient often dislikes pressure being applied. This abdomen is often referred to as *Yang* within *Yang* 陽中の陽 (*Yo Chu No Yo*), that is to say, tight, resistant, warm and full—all *Yang* qualities.

Notes

This technique is done with Mid-level Pressure 中圧 (*Chu Atsu*) in exactly the same manner as when palpating for abdomen #1 described above. In addition to the Full and Resistant finding in this category, there is also the *Yin* within *Yang* abdomen 陽中の陰 (*Yo Chu No In*), still considered a Full 実 (*Jitsu*) abdomen, but with some apparent *Yin* qualities to it. For example, in this case, though visibly swollen and full (*Yang*), to the touch it may feel somewhat soft though still warm and well nourished. Thus, there is a certain *Yin* quality to the touch so that this may be called a *Yin* within *Yang* abdomen in *Kampo*. The *Yang* within *Yang* abdomen type is usually associated with Blood Constitutions (*Ketsu Tasishitsu Sho* 血体質証) whereas the *Yin* within *Yang* abdomen is more likely a Water Constitutional Type (*Sui Taishitsu Sho* 水体質証).

Charting

This abdominal finding is charted as follows according to whether the finding is *Jitsu* Tight (*Yang* within *Yang*) or *Jitsu* Soft (*Yin* within *Yang*). These are referred to as *Yang* Fullness (*Yo Fuku Man* 実腹満) (Figure 4.3) and *Yin* Fullness (*In Fuku Man* 陰腹満) (Figure 4.4) respectively.

Note: The Full Abdomen 腹満 (*Fuku Man*) can also be differentiated into Excess Fullness (*Jitsu Fuku Man* 実腹満), or Empty Fullness (*Kyo Fuku Man* 虚腹満) as described in the "Morphology" section above. But this description has a markedly different meaning. It refers to Disease Patterns (*Byo Sho* 病証), not Constitutional Patterns (*Taishitsu Sho* 体質証), and therefore distinguishes between the Fullness (*Man* 満) that is found in Excess Patterns (*Jitsu Sho* 実証) as opposed to the Fullness found in Deficiency Patterns (*Kyo Sho* 虚証). As always, this distinction between references to constitution as opposed to disease is crucial to the *Kampo* diagnostic process.

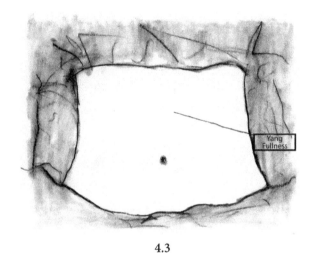

4.3

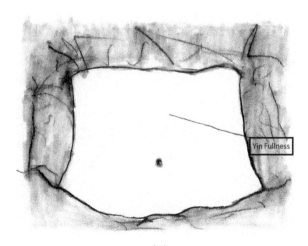

4.4

Clinical interpretation

Again, it is important to stress, as above, that the interpretation of the findings derived from this very first part of the abdominal exam, "Kneading the abdomen" (see Figures 3.2a, 3.2b and 3.2c), have to do exclusively with the patient constitution (*Taishitsu Sho* 体質証).

Thus, when the abdomen is Strong (*Fuku Ryoku Jitsu* 腹力実), whether it is a *Yang* Full Adomen (*Yo Fuku Man* 陽腹滿) or a *Yin* Full Abdomen (*In Fuku Man* 陰腹滿), this is always interpreted as a sign of a Strong Constitution (*Jitsu Taishitsu Sho* 実体質証) in *Kampo*.

Yang Full (*Yo Fuku Man* 陽腹滿)

When the abdomen is Full and Tight (Figure 4.3) this indicates exclusively *Yang* interpretations involving a constitution of Strong *Yang Qi* (*Yo Ki Jitsu Sho* 陽気実証), Heat (*Netsu Sho* 熱症) and Dryness (*Kan Sho* 乾証), all qualities of *Yang*. These are usually Blood Constitutional Types (*Ketsu Taishitsu Sho* 血体質証).

This abdomen (*Yang* within *Yang*) suggests a constitution that will require formulas to Move and Regulate *Qi* (*Gyo Ri Ki* 行理氣), Harmonize *Qi* (Wa Ki 和気, Direct *Qi* Downward (*Fu Gyaku Ka Ki* 降逆下氣, Clear Heat (*Sei Netsu* 清熱) and sometimes Purge (*Tsu Ka* 通下) such as those found in the *Shaoyang* (*Sho Yo Byo* 少陽病) and *Yangming* (*Yomei Byo* 陽明病) Stages of the "Treatise on Damaging Cold" (*Shang Han Lun* 傷寒論).

According to *Yin-Yang* Theory (*In Yo Setsu* 陰陽説), both *Shaoyang* and *Yangming* Stages indicate Interior Excess Heat Patterns (*Ri Jitsu Nestu Sho* 裏実熱証) and according to *Zang-Fu* Organ theory (*Zo Fu Setsu* 臟腑説), they would conform with Patterns of Liver, Gall Bladder, Stomach and Large Intestine *Yang* Excess (*Kan/Tan/I/Daicho Yo Jitsu Sho* 肝 / 胆 /胃/大腸 陽実証) respectively, although these references are used here to describe a constitutional state (*Taishitsu Sho* 体質証)as opposed to a Disease Pattern (*Byo Sho* 病証).

In the example of what might be called a "*Shaoyang* Constitutional Type," in whom the primary *Qi* Constraint, Heat and Excess symptoms will occur in the Middle *Jiao* (such as abdominal and chest fullness, distention, pain, reflux and so on), the *Qi* moving, regulating, harmonizing and downward directing actions are provided by Bupleurum (*Saiko* 柴胡) and/or Pinellia (*Hange* 半夏); while the cooling action is provided by Coptis (*Oren* 黄連), Scute (*Ogon* 黄芩) or Gardenia (*Shi Shi* 梔子) in such example formulas as:

- Minor Bupleurum Combination (*Sho Saiko To* 小柴胡湯)

- Coptis Combination (*Oren To* 黄連湯)

- Pinellia Combination (*Hange Sha Shin To* 半夏瀉心湯)

In cases where a purgative action is required (with constipation) formulas that also contain Rhubarb (*Daio* 大黄) can be used such as:

- Major Bupleurum Combination (*Dai Saiko To* 大柴胡湯)

- Coptis and Rhubarb Combination (*San O Shashin To* 三黄瀉心湯)

- Capillaris Combination (*In Chin Ko To* 茵蔯蒿湯)

The abdomen of this *Shaoyang* Constitutional Type, in addition to being Full (*Fuku Man* 腹滿), will either tend to show #5 Hypochondriac Painful Fullness (*Kyo Kyo Ku Man* 胸脅苦滿) (Figure 4.7) or #6 Hypochondriac Obstruction Resistance (*Kyo Ka Hi Ko* 脅下痞硬) (Figure 4.8),which in *Kampo* indicates the need for a Bupleurum-based formula (amongst the above examples).

Alternatively, the *Qi* constraint may be more located in the epigastrium rather than the hypochondrium as in finding #3 Epigastric Obstruction Resistance (*Shin Ka Hi Ko* 心下痞硬) (Figure 4.5), which calls for the use of a Pinellia-based formula (amongst the above examples).

If in the abdomen exam, there is also the finding #14 Lower Abdomen Spastic Knot (*Sho Fuku Kyu Ketsu* 少腹急結) (Figure 4.20), aka the *Otsuka* Blood Stasis (*Oketsu* 瘀血) Point, then Rhubarb is called for in the formula (amongst the above examples).

In the example of what might be called a "*Yangming* Constitutional Type," in whom the primary *Qi* Constraint, Heat and Excess symptoms will occur in the Lower *Jiao* (such as abdominal fullness, distention, pain, constipation, and so on), the *Qi* moving, regulating, harmonizing and downward directing actions are provided by Magnolia Bark (*Koboku* 厚朴) and/or Chi Shi (*Ki Jitsu* 枳実), while the cooling and purgative action is provided by Rhubarb (*Daio* 大黄) and/or Mirabilitum (*Bo Sho* 芒硝) in such example formulas as:

- Major Rhubarb Combination (*Dai Joki To* 大承気湯)

- Minor Rhubarb Combination (*Sho Joki To* 小承気湯)

The abdomen of this *Yangming* Constitutional Type, in addition to being Full (*Fuku Man* 腹満), will tend to manifest either #12 Lower Abdomen Resistant Fullness (*Sho Fuku Ko Man* 少腹硬満) (Figure 4.17) or #14 Lower Abdomen Spastic Knot (*Sho Fuku Kyu Ketsu* 少腹急結) (Figure 4.20), the so-called *Otsuka* Blood Stasis (*Oketsu* 瘀血) Point for which the above-mentioned Rhubarb formulas are indicated.

There are also cases in this Abdominal Conformation where the Excess Heat for the *Yangming* moves more toward the surface and causes it to "vent" through the skin rather than to get stuck in the bowel. This is sometimes referred to as *Yangming* channel disease (*Yomei Kei Byo* 陽明経病) and is often treated with:

- Gypsum Combination (*Byaku Ko To* 白虎湯)

Yin Full Abdomen (*In Fuku Man* 陰腹満)

When the abdomen is Full and Soft (Figure 4.4) this indicates a *Yin* within *Yang* interpretation involving a constitution of Strong *Yang Qi* (*Yo Ki Jitsu Sho* 陽気実証) and Heat (*Netsu Sho* 熱症) (*Yang* qualities) and Dampness (*Shitsu Sho* 湿証) (a *Yin* quality). These are usually Water Constitutional Types (*Sui Taishitsu Sho* 水体質証).

This abdomen, in addition to being #2 Full (*Fuku Man* 腹満), is often so distended that individual areas of constraint such as #5

Hypochondriac Painful Fullness (*Kyo Kyo Ku Man* 胸脅苦滿) (Figure 4.7), #6 Hypochondriac Obstruction Resistance (*Kyo Ka Hi Ko* 脅下痞硬) (Figure 4.8), or #3 Epigastric Obstruction Resistance (*Shin Ka Hi Ko* 心下痞硬) (Figure 4.5) cannot clearly be distinguished.

Rather, the whole abdomen as a unit is Full (滿) and the only additional abdominal finding that was not necessarily seen in the *Yang* Full Abdomen (*Yo Fuku Man* 陽腹滿) above is #7 Epigastric Splash Sound (*Shin Ka Bu Shin Sui On* 心下部振水音) (Figure 4.9), indicating the presence of Toxic Water (*Suidoku* 水毒).

This abdomen (*Yin* within *Yang*) suggests a constitution that will require herbs to Regulate/Drain Dampness (*Ri Shitsu* 利濕) like Atractylodes (*Jutsu* 朮), Hoelen (*Buku Ryo* 茯苓), Polyporus (*Cho Rei* 猪苓) or Alisma (*Taku Sha* 沢瀉) in formulas such as:

- Hoelen 5 Formula (*Go Rei San* 五苓散)

- Capillaris and Hoelen Combination (*Inchin Go Rei San* 茵蔯五苓散)

- Bupleurum and Hoelen Combination (*Sai Rei To* 柴苓湯)

- Hoelen and Alisma Combination (*Bun Sho To* 分消湯)

- Atractylodes Combination (*Eppi Ka Jutsu To* 越婢加朮湯)

When, in addition to Dampness, there is the need to Clear Heat (*Sei Netsu* 清熱, minerals like Gypsum (*Sekko* 石膏) or Talc (*Kasseki* 滑石) and additionally purgative actions (*Shita Ho* 下法) with Rhubarb (*Daio* 大黄) and Mirabilitum (*Bo Sho* 芒硝) may be required in formulas like:

- Siler and Platycodon Formula (*Bofutsu Sho San* 防風通聖散)

In summary, the #2 Full Abdomen (*Fuku Man* 腹滿) finding, whether *Yang* or *Yin* in nature, suggests a Strong Constitutional Type that will likely suffer from patterns of Excess. They can tolerate strong approaches to treatment whereby sudorifics, diuretics and purgatives may be used.

The interpretation of the findings derived from the remaining parts of the abdominal exam (Figures 4.5–4.20) relates to specific Herbs or Formula Patterns (*Yakusho* 薬証) and therefore facilitates the diagnosis of Disease Patterns (*Byo Sho* 病証) as opposed to those of patient Constitution (*Taishitsu Sho* 体質証) described above.

In each case, the individual findings listed below will tend to fall into one or other of the four types of Constitutional abdomens that have been identified above. That is:

1. *Yang* within *Yang* 陽中の陽 (*Yo Chu No Yo*)—Strong Dry Types.

2. *Yin* within *Yang* 陽中の陰 (*Yo Chu No In*)—Strong Wet Types.

3. *Yang* within *Yin* 陰中の陽 (*In Chu No Yo*)—Weak Dry Types.

4. *Yin* within *Yin* 陰中の陰 (*In Chu No In*)—Weak Wet Types.

B. Disease Findings

Refer to Figure 3.3 for the technique involved in palpating the two following possible findings.

3. Epigastric Obstruction Resistance
心下痞硬 (*Shin Ka Hi Ko*)
Morphology
According to Dr. *Otsuka*:

> *Shin Ka* 心下 refers to the epigastrium, and the *Hi* 痞 refers to a subjective feeling of obstruction, while the *Ko* 硬 is an objective resistance. This means that there is a resistance, which the physician can feel with the hand, as well as the patient's complaints of a feeling of obstruction in the epigastrium. Resistance (and obstruction): patients report that their epigastrium feels "stuffed," and upon palpation by the physician, tightness and resistance are detected. This is the meaning of this term.

Comment

Palpable resistance in the epigastric area generally accompanies neither tension of the abdominal muscles such as the rectus abdominis, nor tenderness. The patient sometimes feels pressure pain, however, or may report spontaneous subjective discomfort in that area. The key finding in this case is the objective sense of hardness in the area felt by the practitioner which, when pressed, will elicit reactive discomfort from the patient.

Notes

This technique is done with Mid-level Pressure 中圧力 (*Chu Atsuryoku*) and indicates a true Excess 実 (*Jistu*) finding, otherwise thought of as *Yang* within *Yang* 陰中の陽 (*Yo Chu No Yo*).

Charting

This abdominal finding (Figure 4.5) is charted as follows and must be clearly differentiated from Figure 4.6, which is also located in the epigastric region but has a different clinical interpretation.

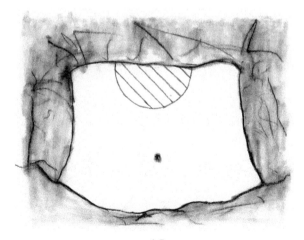

4.5

Clinical interpretation

This finding has two major clinical interpretations depending on the Constitutional strength of the patient as indicated by the overall strength of the abdomen itself. For example:

1. If the overall abdomen is #2 Full Abdomen (*Fuku Man* 腹滿) (Figures 4.3 and 4.4), indicating a Strong Constitution (*Jitsu Taishitsu Sho* 実体質証), then this finding is an indication for the use of formulas containing Pinellia (*Hange* 半夏).

2. If the overall abdomen is #1b Tight and Powerless (*Fuku Bu Ko Ren Mu Ryoku* 腹部拘攣無力) (Figure 4.2), indicating a Weak Constitution (*Kyo Taishitsu Sho* 体質証), then this finding is an indication for formulas containing Cinnamon (*Keishi* 桂枝).

In the case of point 1 above, in an Average to Strong Type, the abdomen may be either #2a *Yang* Full Abdomen (*Yo Fuku Man* 陽腹滿)—*Yang* within *Yang* or #2b *Yin* Full Abdomen (*In Fuku Man* 陰腹滿)—*Yin* within *Yang* (Figures 4.3 and 4.4), and other typical findings that accompany this #3 Epigastric Obstruction Resistance (*Shin Ka Hi Ko* 心下痞硬) will include:

- #7 Epigastric Splash Sound (*Shin Ka Bu Shin Sui On* 心下部振水音) (Figure 4.9)

- #10 Epigastric Pulsations (*Shin Ka Ki* 心下悸) (Figure 4.14)

This is a pattern of Excess (*Jitsu Sho* 実証) where there is true stasis in the epigastric area and example formulas used in this case to drain downwards, according to their *Sho* (証) include:

- Coptis Combination (*Oren To* 黃連湯)

- Pinellia Combination (*Hange Shashinto* 半夏瀉心湯)

- Pinellia and Licorice Combination (*Kanzo Shashin To* 甘草瀉心湯)

- Pinellia and Ginger Combination (*Sho Kyo Shashin To* 生姜瀉心湯)

In the case of point 2 above, in a Weak, Dry Type, the abdomen is #1b Tight and Powerless (*Fuku Bu Ko Ren Mu Ryoku* 腹部拘攣無力) (Figure 4.2) (*Yang* within *Yin*) and other typical findings that accompany #3 Epigastric Obstruction Resistance (*Shin Ka Hi Ko* 心下痞硬) may include:

- #8 Inside Spasm (*Ri Kyu* 裡急) (Figure 4.11)

- #10 Epigastric Pulsations (*Shin Ka Ki* 心下悸) (Figure 4.14)

This is a pattern of Deficiency (*Kyo Sho* 実証) where the epigastric obstruction is related to anxiety creating tightening in the solar plexus and example formulas used in this case to warm, circulate and treat Counterflow *Qi*, according to their *Sho* (証) include:

- Cinnamon Combination (*Keishi To* 桂枝湯)

- Cinnamon and Peony Combination (*Keishi Ka Shakuyaku To* 桂枝加芍薬湯)

- Cinnamon and Dragon Bone Combination (*Keishi Ka Ryukotsu Borei To* 桂枝加竜骨牡蠣湯)

There is also this pattern in Moderate to Strong Types where the epigastric obstruction is also related to anxiety creating tightening in the solar plexus but in this case generating heat in the pattern in example formulas such as:

- Coptis and Scute Combination (*Oren Ge Doku To* 黄連解毒湯)

4. Epigastric Obstruction 心下痞 (*Shin Ka Hi*)
Morphology
According to Dr. *Otsuka*:

This is the above-mentioned *Shin Ka Hi Ko* 心下痞硬 conformation when the patient complains of obstruction with only subjective symptoms. Upon palpation by the physician there is no objective resistance. Obstruction in the epigastrium: this heading refers to complaints of a stuffed feeling in the pit of the stomach, when, upon examination of the area, there is no resistance, obstruction or tightness, or pain with pressure there. This subjective fullness is often accompanied by the epigastric splash sound, and is usually *Kyo Sho* 虚証.

Comment

There is a subjective feeling of obstruction in the pit of the stomach (epigastrium), often accompanied by heaviness and distention. This likely occurs more obviously after eating and when the stomach is full. The practitioner may also notice the area from the navel up to the xiphoid process may be visibly distended though soft and non-resistant to the touch.

Notes

This technique is done with Mid-level Pressure 中圧 (*Chu Atsu*) and indicates by itself a Full 実証 (*Jistu Sho*) finding, yet usually occurs within a pattern of Emptiness 虚証 (*Kyo Sho*). This would be thought of as an example of *Yang* within *Yin* 陰中の陽 (*In Chu No Yo*) in *Kampo*.

Charting

This abdominal finding (Figure 4.6) is charted as follows and must be clearly differentiated from Figure 4.5, which is also located in the epigastric region but has a different clinical interpretation.

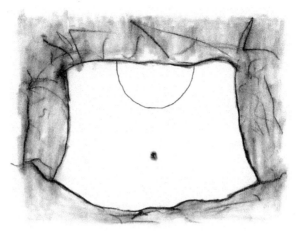

4.6

Clinical interpretation

This finding is associated with the use of formulas containing Ginseng (*Ninjin* 人参).

This abdominal finding belongs to the weak, wet type constitution which belongs to the #1 Lax and Powerless (*Fuku Bu Nan Jyaku Mu Ryoku* 腹部軟弱無力) (Figure 4.1) (*Yin* within *Yin*), and will have the following findings that accompany this subjective #4 Epigastric Obstruction (*Shin Ka Hi* 心下痞) such as:

- #7 Epigastric Splash Sound (*Shin Ka Bu Shin Sui On* 心下部 振水音) (Figure 4.9)

- #10 Epigastric Pulsations (*Shin Ka Ki* 心下悸) (Figure 4.14)

This is a pattern of Deficiency (*Kyo Sho* 虚証) where the feeling of obstruction (Branch Excess—*Hyo Jitsu* 標実) is due to poor transformation and transportation by the Spleen and Stomach (Root Deficiency—*Hon Kyo* 本虚) and example formulas used in this case to tonify and warm as well as regulate fluids, according to their *Sho* (証) include:

- Ginseng and Ginger Combination (*Ninjin To* 人参湯, also known as *Ri Chu To* 理中湯)

- Four Major Herb Combination (*Shi Kun Shi To* 四君子湯)

- Six Major Herb Combination (*Rikkun Shi To* 六君子湯)

- Cardamom and Saussurea Combination (*Ko Sha Rikkun Shi To* 香砂六君子湯)

- Ginseng and Astragalus Combination (*Ho Chu Ekki To* 補中益気湯)

If in the same abdominal pattern, Toxic Water (*Sui Doku* 水毒) and Water Counterflow (*Sui Nobose* 水のぼせ) symptoms predominate then use formulas according to their *Sho* (証) such as:

- Hoelen Formula (*Buku Ryo In* 茯苓飲)

- Alisma and Hoelen Combination (*Bukuryo Takusha To* 茯苓沢瀉湯)

- Atractylodes and Hoelen Combination (*Ryo Kei Jyutsu Kan To* 苓桂朮甘湯)

- Inula and Hematite Combination (*Sen Puku Ka Tai Sha Seki To* 旋覆花代赭石湯)

- Pinellia and Gastrodia Combination (*Hange Byakujutsu Tenma To* 半夏白朮天麻湯)

- Evodia Combination (*Go Shuyu To* 呉茱萸湯)

If in the same pattern, Cold (*Kan* 寒) and *Yang* Deficient (*Yo Kyo* 陽虚) symptoms predominate, where in addition to the #1a Lax and Powerless Abdomen (*Fuku Bu Nan Jyaku Mu Ryoku* 腹部軟弱無力) (Figure 4.1) and other findings mentioned above there is also:

- #11 Lower Abdomen Lacking Benevolence (*Sho Fuku Fu Jin* 少腹不仁) (Figure 4.15)

then use formulas such as:

- Aconite, Ginseng and Ginger Combination (*Bu Shi Ri Chu To* 附子理中湯)

- Aconite, Ginger and Licorice Combination (*Shi Gyaku To* 四逆湯)

- Vitality Combination (*Shinbu To* 真武湯)

- Aconite Combination (*Bushi To* 附子湯)

- Mahuang and Asarum Combination (*Mao Bushi Saishin To* 麻黄附子細辛湯)

- Mahuang, Aconite and Licorice Combination (*Mao Bushi Kanzo To* 麻黄附子甘草湯)

- Ginger, Licorice and Aconite Combination (*Shi Gyaku Ka Ninjin To* 四逆加人参湯)

Refer to Figures 3.4a and 3.4b for the technique involved in palpating the two following possible findings.

5. Hypochondriac Painful Fullness
胸脅苦滿 (*Kyo Kyo Ku Man*)
Morphology
According to Dr. *Otsuka*:

> This first *Kyo* 胸 means the chest, and the second *Kyo* 脅 the flanks. This refers to fullness and resistance in the hypochondrium, including the area under the arch of the ribs. The *Ku* 苦 is "suffering", a subjective pain or discomfort. The *Man* 滿 again means fullness (as in Full Abdomen, *Fuku Man* 腹滿 #2 above). Pain and resistance: there is a feeling of fullness in the hypochondrium, as well as distress and pain there. It can be verified objectively as resistance and pressure pain. It may appear on both sides at the same time or on either side separately. Enlargement of the liver and spleen may well be regarded as *Kyo Kyo Ku Man*…

Comment

Tenderness and the feeling of fullness (*Ku* 苦 and *Man* 滿) in the hypochondriac area can occur in the subcutaneous structures outside the peritoneum, such as the muscles and fascia of the diaphragm, the greater pectoral muscles, and the upper portions of the rectus abdominis muscle. There have been reports on the relationship of 胸脅苦滿 (*Kyo Kyo ku Man*) with the morbid states of splenoma, pleurisy, chronic hepatitis and hepatomegaly. It must be related to those organs in the thorax or below the diaphragm, such as the liver, stomach, spleen and pancreas. It can occur also when lymphocyte functions accelerate and can also be found in certain lung diseases such as bronchitis.

Notes

This technique is done with Mid-level Pressure 中圧力 (*Chu Atsuryoku*), indicating a Full 実証 (*Jistu Sho*) finding, and would be thought of as an example of *Yang* within *Yang* 陽中陽 (*Yo Chu Yo*) in *Kampo*. It is usually indicative of acute patterns.

Charting

This abdominal finding is charted as follows (Figure 4.7) and must be clearly differentiated from Figure 4.8, which is also located in the hypochondriac region. Note that this finding *always* occurs bilaterally.

Clinical interpretation

This finding is associated with the use of formulas containing:

- Bupleurum (*Saiko* 柴胡)

Within the category of Strong (*Fuku Ryoku Jitsu* 腹力実), this #5 Hypochondriac Painful Fullness (*Kyo Kyo Ku Man* 胸脅苦滿) (Figure 4.7) is usually found within a #2a *Yang* Full Abdomen (*Yo*

Fuku Man 陽腹滿) (Figure 4.3) and will usually have the following findings that accompany it:

- #3 Epigastric Obstruction Resistance (*Shin Ka Hi Ko* 心下痞硬) (Figure 4.5)

- #8 Inside Spasm (*Ri Kyu* 裡急) (Figure 4.11)

- #10 Epigastric Pulsations (*Shin Ka Ki* 心下悸) (Figure 4.14)

- #14 Lower Abdomen Spastic Knot (*Sho Fuku Kyu Ketsu* 少腹急結) (Figure 4.20)

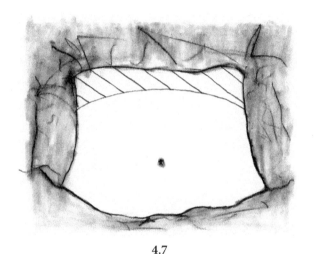

4.7

This is a pattern of Excess (*Jitsu Sho* 実証) where *Qi* constraint (*Ki Tai* 気滞) has occurred in the hypochondriac area, which must be dispersed using Bupleurum (*Saiko* 柴胡) and which often gives rise to Excess Heat (*Jitsu Netsu* 実熱), which must be purged through the bowels using Rhubarb (*Daio* 大黄). This Heat may either move down in the body (causing constipation) or it may counterflow upwards (*Netsu Nobose* 熱ののぼせ), disturbing the mind (*Shin* 神) so that the following example formulas can be used in each case according to their *Sho* (証):

- Major Bupleurum Combination (*Dai Saiko To* 大柴胡湯)

- Bupleurum and Dragon Bone Combination (*Saiko Ka Ryu Kotsu Borei To* 柴胡加竜骨牡蠣湯)

#5 Hypochondriac Painful Fullness (*Kyo Kyo Ku Man* 胸脅苦満) (Figure 4.7) is also found in certain respiratory conditions when the diaphragm is tight and the Lung *Qi* cannot descend properly (bronchitis, asthma, etc.). In such cases the following Bupleurum (*Saiko* 柴胡)-based formulas can be considered according to their *Sho* (証):

- Bupleurum and Scute Combination (*Sai Kan To* 柴陥湯)

- Bupleurum and Magnolia Combination (*Sai Boku To* 柴朴湯)

The main feature of this abdominal finding #5 Hypochondriac Painful Fullness (*Kyo Kyo Ku Man* 胸脅苦満) (Figure 4.7) is that it is found only in very Strong individuals who are suffering from acute patterns of Excess (*Jitsu Sho* 実証) where in addition to *Qi* stagnation (*Ki Tai* 気滞) that needs to be dispersed, there is likely a lot of Heat that needs to be cooled or drained out of the body. Formulas in these cases are used for relatively short periods of time.

6. Hypochondriac Obstruction Resistance 脅下痞硬 (*Kyo Ka Hi Ko*)
Morphology
According to Dr. *Otsuka*:

> This *Kyo* 脅 is the second *Kyo* from #5 above (Hypochondriac Painful Fullness, *Kyo Kyo Ku Man* 胸脅苦満), here referring to the flanks. This refers to a (*Hi Ko* 痞硬) obstruction resistance (as in #3 Epigastric Obstructive Resistance 心下痞硬, *Shin Ka Hi Ko*), both subjective and objective at the lower border of the ribcage. It may occur at the same time as *Kyo Kyo Ku Man* 胸脅苦満.

Comment

This finding exhibits palpable resistance in the hypochondriac area very similar in quality to abdomen #3 Epigastric Obstruction Resistance (*Shin Ka Hi Ko* 心下痞硬) (Figure 4.5). Enlargement of the Liver and Spleen may well be regarded as *Kyo Kyo Ku Man*.

Notes

This technique is done with Mid-level Pressure 中圧 (*Chu Atsu*) and, as with Abdomen #5 above, this indicates a Full 実証 (*Jistu Sho*) finding. However, on palpation, though the patient will likely notice there is resistance, the practitioner's pressure does not elicit pain or discomfort as in abdomen #5 Hypochondriac Painful Fullness (*Kyo Kyo Ku Man* (胸脅苦満). It can be argued that this finding is more commonly found in chronic patterns of Stasis and therefore belongs to a pattern of *Yin* within *Yang* 陽中の陰 (*Yo Chu No In*).

Charting

This abdominal finding (Figure 4.8) is charted as follows and must be clearly differentiated from Figure 4.7, which is also located in the hypochondriac region. Note that this finding may occur unilaterally or bilaterally and must be charted accordingly. Additionally, the relative strength of the resistance palpated is reflected by the number of lines used to chart it—one line being mild, two moderate and three lines indicating strong resistance to pressure.

Clinical interpretation

This finding is also associated with the use of formulas containing:

- Bupleurum (*Saiko* 柴胡)

However, unlike abdomen #5 Hypochondriac Painful Fullness (*Kyo Kyo Ku Man* 胸脅苦満) (Figure 4.7), this finding can be palpated in both Full (*Jitsu Sho* 実証) and Empty (*Kyo Sho* 虚証) Abdomens.

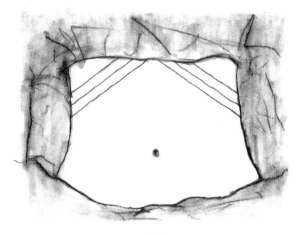

4.8

Full Patterns (*Jitsu Sho* 実証)

Within the category of Strong and Full (*Fuku Ryoku Jitsu* 腹力実), this #6 Hypochondriac Obstruction Resistance (*Kyo Ka Hi Ko* 脅下痞硬) (Figure 4.8) is usually found within either the #2a *Yang* Full Abdomen (*Yo Fuku Man* 陽腹滿) or the #2b *Yin* Full Abdomen (*In Fuku Man* 陰腹滿) (Figures 4.3 and 4.4 respectively).

In the case that the *Qi* has become stagnant (*Ki Tai* 気滞) in the hypochondriac area, calling for a dispersing action using Bupleurum (*Saiko* 柴胡), the following abdominal findings will also be apparent:

- #3 Epigastric Obstruction Resistance (*Shin Ka Hi Ko* 心下痞硬) (Figure 4.5)

- #8 Inside Spasm (*Ri Kyu* 裡急) (Figure 4.11)

Example formulas that may be considered in this case according to their *Sho* (証) include:

- Minor Bupleurum Combination (*Sho Saiko To* 小柴胡湯)

- Bupleurum and Chi Shi Formula (*Shi Gyaku San* 四逆散)

In the case that there is evidence of Counterflow *Qi* (*Ki Nobose* 気の

ぼせ), due to *Qi* Stasis (*Ki Tai* 気滞), the abdomen will clearly reflect this in the additional finding of:

- #10 Cardiac Pulsations (*Shin Ki* 心悸) and Epigastric Pulsations (*Shin Ka Ki* 心下悸) (Figure 4.14)

Example formulas that may be considered in this case according to their *Sho* (証) include:

- Bupleurum and Cyperus Formula (*Saiko Sokan San* 柴胡疎肝散)

- Bupleurum Formula (*Yoku Kan San* 抑肝散)

- Bupleurum and Magnolia Combination (*Sai Boku To* 柴朴湯)

In the case that there is evidence of Toxic Water (*Sui Doku* 水毒), the abdomen will clearly reflect this in the additional finding of:

- #7 Epigastric Splash Sound (*Shin Ka Bu Shin Sui On* 心下部振水音) (Figure 4.9)

Example formulas that may be considered in this case according to their *Sho* (証) include:

- Bupleurum and Hoelen Combination (*Sai Rei To* 柴苓湯)

- Bupleurum, Citrus and Pinellia Formula (*Yoku Kan San Ka Chin Pi Hange* 抑肝散加陳皮半夏)

- Evodia and Pinellia Combination (*En-Nen Hange To* 延年半夏湯)

In the case that there is evidence of Blood Stasis (*Oketsu* 瘀血), the abdomen will clearly reflect this in the additional finding of:

- #14 Lower Abdomen Spastic Knot (*Sho Fuku Kyu Ketsu* 少腹急結) (Figure 4.20)

Example formulas that may be considered in this case according to their *Sho* (証) include:

- Bupleurum and Evodia Combination (*So Kan To* 疎肝湯)

- Bupleurum and Peony Formula (*Kami Shoyo San* 加味逍遥散)

In the case that there is evidence of what *Kampo* calls Toxic Blood (*Ketsu Doku* 血毒) where there is a need to detoxify and dispel heat from the surface (in dermatological disorders) then use:

- Bupleurum and Schizonepeta (*Ju Mi Bai Doku To* 十味敗毒湯)

Empty Patterns (*Kyo Sho* 虚証)

Within the category of a Weak and Empty Abdomen (*Fuku Ryoku Kyo* 腹力虚), this #6 Hypochondriac Obstruction Resistance (*Kyo Ka Hi Ko* 脅下痞硬) (Figure 4.8) is usually found within the #1b Tight and Powerless (*Fuku Bu Ko Ren Mu Ryoku* 腹部拘攣無力) abdomen (Figure 4.2)

In the case that additional abdominal findings include:

- #3 Epigastric Obstruction Resistance (*Shin Ka Hi Ko* 心下痞硬) (Figure 4.5)

or:

- #8 Inside Spasm (*Ri Kyu* 裡急) (Figure 4.11)

then this would likely call for the use of Cinnamon (*Keishi* 桂枝) in addition to Bupleurum (*Saiko* 柴胡) in such example formulas according to their *Sho* (証) as:

- Bupleurum and Cinnamon Combination (*Saiko Keishi To* 柴胡桂枝湯)

In the case that there is evidence of Toxic Water (*Sui Doku* 水毒), the abdomen will clearly reflect this in the additional finding of:

- #7 Epigastric Splash Sound (*Shin Ka Bu Shin Sui On* 心下部振水音) (Figure 4.9)

Example formulas that may be considered in this case according to their *Sho* (証) include:

- Bupleurum, Cinnamon and Ginger Combination (*Saiko Keishi Kankyo To* 柴胡桂枝乾姜湯)

In the case that there is evidence of Blood Stasis (*Oketsu* 瘀血) related to Blood deficiency (*Ketsu Kyo* 血虚) and Dryness, the abdomen will clearly reflect this in the additional finding of:

- #13 Navel Spastic Knot Point (*Sai Bu Kyu Ketsu* 臍部急結) (Figure 4.19)

Example formulas that may be considered in this case according to their *Sho* (証) include:

- Bupleurum and Rehmannia Combination (*Saiko Seikan To* 柴胡清肝湯)

The main feature of this abdominal finding, #6 Hypochondriac Obstruction Resistance (*Kyo Ka Hi Ko* 脅下痞硬) (Figure 4.8), is that it is found in moderately Strong but also sometimes Weaker individuals who are suffering from mixed patterns of Excess (*Jitsu Sho* 実証) and Deficiency (*Kyo Sho* 虚証). In such cases, in addition to *Qi* stagnation (*Ki Tai* 気滞) that needs to be dispersed using formulas containing Bupleurum (*Saiko* 柴胡), there is likely more complicated pathology that may include Dampness (*Shitsu* 湿) or Dryness (*Kan* 乾), Heat (*Netsu* 熱) or Cold (*Kan* 寒), Counterflow *Qi* (*Ki Nobose* 気のぼせ) and in some cases Blood Stasis (*Oketsu* 瘀血). These complex patterns more likely reflect chronic disease and formulas used in such cases are often prescribed for longer periods of time.

Refer to Figure 3.5 for the technique involved in palpating the two following possible findings.

7. Epigastric "Splash" Sound 心下部 振水音 (*Shin Ka Bu Shin Sui On*)

Morphology

According to Dr. *Otsuka*:

> *Shin Ka Bu* 心下部 means the place below the heart, referring here to the epigastrium; *Shin Sui On* 振水音 refers to a sound like splashing water. The splash sound: in patients with gastric ptosis, gastric atony and such like, this sound is often easily detectable. The author often uses a closed hand, the back of the fist or the second joint of the middle finger lightly tapping, or percusses lightly with the tips of the middle and fourth fingers together. Most often patients with the splash sound are Empty 虚証 *Kyo Sho*.

Comment

When the stomach wall is relaxed and there is a certain amount of stagnant gastric juices and air, sloshing sounds come from inside the stomach and intestines. The cause of this sound is thought to occur in conditions where the smooth muscles of the stomach are weak and atonic, as in the case of gastroptosis. Under such circumstances, intestinal peristalsis is decreased, and gastric secretions and air cannot properly be excreted, accumulating instead in the stomach lumen (lower portion). These signs point to a functional deterioration of the vagus nerve, and they usually accompany other signs of autonomic nervous system disorders. The sounds may occur not only in the stomach but also in the transverse section of the duodenum, and in the jejunum, when intestinal secretions have accumulated there.

Notes

This technique is done with Mid-level Pressure 中圧 (*Chu Atsu*) and the exam technique is critical here. As explained in Chapter 3, it is important to cover the entire upper left quadrant of the abdomen with the percussion technique described. Failing to do this comprehensively may mean you will miss this important finding.

The sounds themselves are distinctive: gas accumulations will sound tympanic or drum-like when percussed while the water splash literally sounds like a glass jar half full of liquid being shaken. Whilst considered a Full 実証 (*Jistu Sho*) finding in itself, it typically occurs within a pattern of Emptiness 虚証 (*Kyo Sho*) although there are patterns of Fullness 実証 (*Jistu Sho*) in which it can also be found.

Charting

These abdominal findings (Figures 4.9 and 4.10) are charted as follows and whether gas or water or both are detected must clearly be indicated as shown:

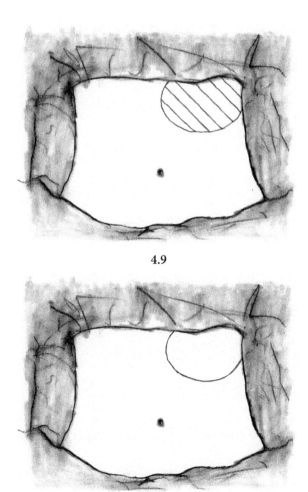

4.9

4.10

Clinical interpretation

This finding is interpreted in two different ways, using the same palpatory technique, according to whether there is:

1. Water (Figure 4.9)—associated with Damp Patterns which are more commonly Empty (*Kyo Sho* 虚証) though can also be Full (*Jitsu Sho* 実証)

or:

2. Gas (Figure 4.10)—associated with Dry Patterns which may be either Empty (*Kyo Sho* 虚証) or Full (*Jitsu Sho* 実証).

Figure 4.9 Epigastric Splash Sound (*Shin Ka Bu Shin Sui On* 心下部振水音)

This finding is associated with the use of formulas containing Hoelen (*Bukuryo* 茯苓) and Atractylodes (*Jyutsu* 朮).

Empty Patterns (*Kyo Sho* 虚証)

Within the category of Weak and Empty (*Fuku Ryoku Kyo* 腹力虚), this #7 Epigastric Splash Sound (*Shin Ka Bu Shin Sui On* 心下部振水音) (Figure 4.9) is usually found within abdomen #1a Lax and Powerless Abdomen (*Fuku Bu Nan Jyaku Mu Ryoku* 腹部軟弱無力) (Figure 4.1). This Toxic Water accumulation (*Sui Doku* 水毒) has itself been caused by weakness of the Spleen/Stomach transformation confirmed by the abdominal finding:

- #4 Epigastric Obstruction (*Shin Ka Hi* 心下痞) (Figure 4.6)

In turn, this Fluid Accumulation will tend to obstruct the natural downward movement of *Qi* giving rise to Water Counterflow (*Sui Nobose*) symptoms (such as nausea) which will be confirmed on the abdomen as:

- #10 Epigastric Pulsations (*Shin Ka Ki* 心下悸) (Figure 4.14)

Thus, this abdominal interpretation resembles that of both #1a Lax and Powerless abdomen (*Fuku Bu Nan Jyaku Mu Ryoku* 腹部軟弱無力) (Figure 4.1) and #4 Epigastric Obstruction (*Shin Ka Hi* 心下痞) (Figure 4.6).

This is a pattern of Deficiency (*Kyo Sho* 虚証) where the feeling of obstruction (Branch Excess—*Hyo Jitsu* 標実) is due to poor transformation and transportation by the Spleen and Stomach (Root Deficiency—*Hon Kyo* 本虚) and example formulas used in this case to tonify and warm as well as regulate fluids, according to their *Sho* (証) include:

- Ginseng and Ginger Combination (*Ninjin To* 人参湯—also known as *Ri Chu To* 理中湯)

- Four Major Herb Combination (*Shi Kun Shi To* 四君子湯)

- Six Major Herb Combination (*Rikkun Shi To* 六君子湯)

- Cardamom and Saussurea Combination (*Ko Sha Rikkun Shi To* 香砂六君子湯)

- Ginseng and Astragalus Combination (*Ho Chu Ekki To* 補中益気湯)

If in the same abdominal pattern, Toxic Water (*Sui Doku* 水毒) and Water Counterflow (*Sui Nobose* 水のぼせ) symptoms predominate then use formulas such as:

- Hoelen Combination (*Buku Ryo In* 茯苓飲)

- Alisma and Hoelen Combination (*Bukuryo Takusha To* 茯苓沢瀉湯)

- Atractylodes and Hoelen Combination (*Ryo Kei Jyutsu Kan To* 苓桂朮甘湯)

- Inula and Hematite Combination (*Sen Puku Ka Tai Sha Seki To* 旋覆花代赭石湯)

- Pinellia and Gastrodia Combination (*Hange Byakujutsu Tenma To* 半夏白朮天麻湯)

- Bamboo and Hoelen Combination (*Untan To* 温胆汤)

If, in the same pattern, Cold (*Kan* 寒) and *Yang* Deficient (*Yo Kyo* 陽虚) symptoms predominate, where in addition to the #7 Epigastric Splash Sound (*Shin Ka Bu Shin Sui On* 心下部振水音) (Figure 4.9) and other findings mentioned above there is also:

- #11 Lower Abdomen Lacking Benevolence (*Sho Fuku Fu Jin* 少腹不仁) (Figure 4.15)

then use formulas that again contain Water herbs such as such as Hoelen (*Bukuryo* 茯苓) and/or Atractylodes (*Jyutsu* 朮) but also Aconite (*Bushi* 附子) such as:

- Aconite, Ginseng and Ginger Combination (*Bu Shi Ri Chu To* 附子理中湯)

- Vitality Combination (*Shinbu To* 真武湯)

- Aconite Combination (*Bushi To* 附子湯)

Full Patterns (*Jitsu Sho* 実証)

Within the category of Strong and Full (*Fuku Ryoku Jitsu* 腹力実), this #7 Epigastric Splash Sound (*Shin Ka Bu Shin Sui On* 心下部振水音) (Figure 4.9), though less common than in Empty Patterns (*Kyo Sho* 虚証), is usually found within the #2b *Yin* Full Abdomen (*In Fuku Man* 陰腹満) (Figure 4.4) and will include the additional abdominal findings of:

- #6 Hypochondriac Obstruction Resistance (*Kyo Ka Hi Ko* 脅下痞硬) (Figure 4.8)

and/or:

- #3 Epigastric Obstruction Resistance (*Shin Ka Hi Ko* 心下痞硬) (Figure 4.5)

Formulas that may be relevant to these Full Pattern (*Jitsu Sho* 実証) abdominal findings can be reviewed under the heading #2b *Yin* Full Abdomen (*In Fuku Man* 陰腹満) (Figure 4.4).

Figure 4.10 Epigastric "Drumming" Sound
(*Shin Ka Bu "Don Don"* 心下部どんどん)

This finding is associated with the use of formulas already discussed under one of the following:

- #2a *Yang* Full Abdomen (*Yo Fuku Man* 陽腹滿) (Figure 4.3)

or:

- #1b Tight and Powerless Abdomen (*Fuku Bu Ko Ren Mu Ryoku* 腹部拘攣無力) (Figure 4.2)

These formulas for treating this tympanic sound in the epigastrium tend to have *Qi* moving and regulating qualities—see above for details of example formulas.

The main significance of this finding is to be able to distinguish between Dry Patterns (where there is gas) and Damp Patterns (where there will be water). As a finding on their own, each belongs to Excess (*Jitsu Sho* 実証) since they involve accumulation. However, more often than not, these findings will be present in Patterns of Deficiency (*Kyo Sho* 虚証). In the case of Toxic Water (*Sui Doku* 水毒), sometimes referred to as Rheum (thin watery fluid), the finding is significant as treating it at this stage is usually far more straightforward than if these thin watery substances transform into Phlegm, which is then notoriously difficult to treat. Thus, this finding might be said to have very useful prognostic significance in all manner of disease.

Refer to Figures 3.6a–3.6d for the technique involved in palpating the two following possible findings.

8. Inside Spasm 裡急 (*Ri Kyu*)
Morphology
According to Dr. *Otsuka*:

> The *Ri* 裡 refers to the inside and this *Kyu* 急 means acute or sudden. The acuteness referred to here is a cramp inside the stomach wall.

Jumpy, ropy abdomen: the *Ri Kyu* can be detected as a spasm which feels like a sudden jerk or contraction beneath the surface of the abdomen. This spasm may occur along the rectus abdominis muscle or elsewhere. Even without the spasm, when there is peritonitis or such diseases, prodding an abdomen swollen with gas gives rise to that sensation inside the abdominal wall. The term *Ri Kyu* includes both the spasm of the rectus abdominis and any stiffening, contraction or tension in that area. *Ri Kyu* is seen only in the *Kyo Sho*, so that even if there is constipation, purgatives should not be used.

Comment

Figure 4.11 Rectus abdominis tension: As neither pain on palpation nor deep pain are generally found, this strain is not related to muscle contraction such as in the reflection of an organ's movement. Rather, *Ri Kyu* 裡急 is a result of overly strained rectus abdominis compensating for low abdominal pressure. Again, the muscle fibers, which with the patient in this relaxed supine position should not be engaged or tense, nonetheless feel cord-like or tight and often respond with an involuntary spasm or twitch.

Figure 4.12 "Jumping Fishes": Due to the cold, digestive functions have deteriorated, and gas and intestinal fluids are occluded or flow in the intestines causing them to expand. These fasciculations are sporadic and they do not succeed in excreting the contents of the intestines. The palpatory experience is defined by an involuntary spasm that occurs immediately in response to the light pressure of the practitioner and can sometimes be seen directly with the eye.

Notes

This technique is done using either Superficial Pressure 表面圧 (*Hyomen Atsu*) or Mid-level Pressure 中圧力 (*Chu Atsuryoku*). Figure 4.12 findings may be detected using a specific shallow, transverse pressure technique described in Chapter 3, whilst Figure 4.11 findings are detected using a slightly deeper transverse pressure that follows the trajectory of the rectus abdominis muscle from superior to inferior, also described in Chapter 3. Pay attention to the different techniques in each case.

Whilst considered an Empty (*Kyo Sho* 虚証) finding in itself, as Dr. *Otsuka* points out (above), nevertheless this finding (Figure 4.11) can occur also in Full Patterns (*Jistu Sho* 実証) whilst the finding in Figure 4.12 only ever occurs in Empty Patterns (Kyo Sho 虚証).

Charting

These abdominal findings (Figures.4.11 and 4.12) are charted as follows according to whether the surface fasciculations, sometimes called "Jumping Fishes" (Figure 4.12), or the rectus abdominis tension (Figure 4.11) is detected. Rectus tension can occur unilaterally or bilaterally and must be charted accordingly. Additionally, the length of the charted finding indicates how far down the rectus abdominis muscle tension was detected, whilst the width of the charting itself indicates the intensity of the tension (thin being mild and thick being strong).

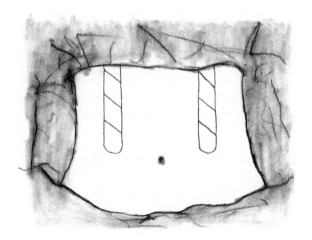

4.11

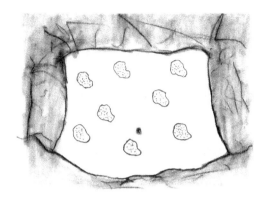

4.12

Clinical interpretation

This finding is most commonly associated with Empty Patterns (*Kyo Sho* 虚証) since it indicates an insufficiency of *Qi* and Blood (*Ki Ketsu Kyo* 気血虚) flow to the surface. In the case of Figure 4.11 this refers to the rectus abdominis muscle on either side of the midline, which feels involuntarily tight and rope-like. In the case of Figure 4.12 it means the skin and adipose tissue at the very surface of the abdomen are lacking nourishment and are tight, giving rise to the "Jumping Fishes."

These findings usually occur within the category of Weak and Empty (*Fuku Ryoku Kyo* 腹力虚), and are associated with the following abdomen:

- #1b Tight and Powerless Abdomen (*Fuku Bu Ko Ren Mu Ryoku* 腹部拘攣無力) (Figure 4.2)

and there will also be a tendency for:

- #10 Cardiac Pulsations (*Shin Ki* 心悸) and Epigastric Pulsations (*Shin Ka Ki* 心下悸) (Figure 4.14)

There will be no splash sound as this is a Dry pattern but there will likely be gas accumulation in the upper left quadrant (part of the #7 finding, Figure 4.10).

In Figure 4.11 the involuntary tension in the rectus abdominis muscle reveals a deficiency in the Nutrient or *Ying Qi* (*Ei Ki* 栄気) and Blood (*Kekkyo* 血虚) causing the surface muscles on the abdomen to be dry, tight and cold leading to abdominal cramps and pain as well as loose stools. Additionally, the #10 Epigastric Pulsations (*Shin Ka Ki* 心下悸) (Figure 4.14) are due to the tendency for Counterflow *Qi* (*Ki Nobose* 気のぼせ) caused by deficiency (inability of the *Qi* to root itself in the middle). Such cases require gentle warming, circulating and softening with formulas containing Cinnamon (*Keishi* 桂枝) and Peony (*Shaku Yaku* 芍薬) in example formulas such as:

- Cinnamon Combination (*Keishi To* 桂枝湯)

- Cinnamon and Peony Combination (*Keishi Ka Shakuyaku To* 桂枝加芍薬湯)

If these pulsations are strong and there is clinical evidence of more substantial *Nobose* (such as anxiety, palpitations, insomnia) the use of Cinnamon (*Keishi* 桂枝) to treat Counterflow *Qi* is common along with minerals that "sedate" (or "calm the spirit" *An Shin* 安神) such as Dragon Bone (*Ryu Kotsu* 竜骨) and Oyster Shell (*Bo Rei* 牡蠣) in such formulas as:

- Cinnamon and Dragon Bone Combination (*Keishi Ka Ryukotsu Borei To* 桂枝加竜骨牡蠣湯)

In Figure 4.12, the abdominal wall is thin and lacking adipose tissue and the person is underweight so that building the *Ying Qi* (*Ei Ki* 栄気) with sweet substances like Maltose (*Ko I* 膠飴) will be necessary in example formulas such as:

- Minor Cinnamon and Peony Combination (*Sho Kenchu To* 小建中湯)

- Astragalus Combination (*Ogi Kenchu To* 黄耆建中湯)

- Major Zanthoxylum Combination (*Dai Kenchu To* 大建中湯)

In Full Patterns (*Jitsu Sho* 実証) where this #8 Inside Spasm (*Ri Kyu* 裡急) (Figure 4.11) is palpated, though much less common than in Patterns of Deficiency (*Kyo Sho* 虚証), it is usually accompanied by the #2 Full Abdomen (*Fuku Man* 腹満) (Figures 4.3 and 4.4) in which there will either be:

- #3 Epigastric Obstruction Resistance (*Shin Ka Hi Ko* 心下痞硬) (Figure 4.5)

or:

- #4 Hypochondriac Obstruction Resistance (*Kyo Ka Hi Ko* 脇下痞硬) (Figure 4.8)

For details of example formulas that might match these findings see above under these two sections.

The main significance of this finding is that it only *ever* occurs in Patterns of Dryness, whether Deficient (*Kyo Sho* 虚証) or Excess (*Jitsu Sho* 実証). This will therefore always call for herbs that combine a *Qi* action (activating) with a Blood action (moistening) so that both *Qi* and Blood can be brought to the surface muscle layer to "soften" the tension of this #8 Inside Spasm (*Ri Kyu* 裡急).

In Excess Patterns of *Qi* Stasis (*Ki Tai* 気滞) this effect might be achieved, for example, by the combination of Bupleurum (*Saiko* 柴胡) and Peony (*Shaku Yaku* 芍薬) within formulas such as:

- Major Bupleurum Combination (*Dai Saiko To* 大柴胡湯)

In Deficiency Patterns where either the *Ying Qi* (*Ei Ki* 栄気) or the Blood (*Ketsu* 血) itself are not reaching the surface muscle layers this effect might rather be achieved by the combination of Cinnamon (*Keishi* 桂枝) and Peony (*Shaku Yaku* 芍薬) within such formulas as:

- Cinnamon Combination (*Keishi To* 桂枝湯)

In patterns of mixed *Jitsu* and *Kyo* consider:

- Bupleurum and Cinnamon Combination (*Saiko Keishi To* 柴胡桂枝湯)

9. Lower Abdomen Tight Spasm
少腹拘急 (*Sho Fuku Ko Kyu*)
Morphology
According to Dr. *Otsuka*:

> *Sho* 少 means small, and *Fuku* 腹 means abdomen, hence the "lower abdomen." The *Ko* 拘 means restricted, seized-up or arrested, and as in the above (inside spasm, *Ri Kyu*), *kyu* 急 means acute or sudden. Lower-abdomen spasm: here the spasms of the rectus abdominis muscle are in the zone between the navel and the pelvic bone. This is referred to as lower burner *In Kyo* 陰虚. It is the Abdominal *Pattern* 腹証 (*Fukusho*) belonging to a kidney *pattern* 腎虚 (*Jin Sho*).

Comment
This is a very similar finding to abdomen #8 Inside Spasm (*Ri Kyu* 裡急) (Figure 4.11). In this case the location of the spasms or contractions is along the rectus abdominis muscle of the lower abdomen and they may extend across the whole of the lower abdominal surface. As previously stated, *Ri Kyu* is a result of overly strained rectus abdominis compensating for low abdominal pressure.

Notes
The technique for palpating this part of the exam is discussed in Chapter 3 (Figures 3.6b and 3.6d) and care must be taken to identify *only* the muscle layer in this sequence. This is done by applying pressure at the 中圧力 (*Chu Atsuryoku*)—"Mid-level pressure" already described, as opposed to, for example, at a deeper level—深圧力 (*Shin Atsuryoku*) where, later in the exam, we will be palpating for the #14 Lower Abdomen Spastic Knot 少腹急結 (*Sho Fuku Kyu Ketsu*) (Figure 4.20) otherwise known as the *Yu Xue* (瘀血) or *Oketsu* point. Care must be taken not to confuse these two findings with one another as their clinical interpretations are distinctly different.

Charting

This abdominal finding (Figure 4.13) is charted as follows and is often nicknamed the "bowtie" or "butterfly" abdomen.

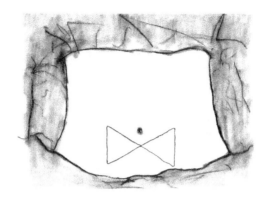

4.13

Clinical interpretation

This finding is very closely allied with that of the previous #8 Inside Spasm (*Ri Kyu* 裡急) (Figure 4.11) and indeed is palpated as part of the same sequence in the exam itself (Figures 3.6a–3.6d). In the same manner, it is most commonly associated with Empty Patterns (*Kyo Sho* 虚証) since it indicates an insufficiency of *Qi* and Blood (*Ki Ketsu Kyo* 気血虚) flow to the surface. In this case, however, instead of calling for Cinnamon (*Keishi* 桂枝), Peony (*Shaku Yaku* 芍薬) or Maltose (*Ko I* 膠飴) to nourish the *Ying* (*Ei* 栄) as in the previous abdomen, this finding suggests the need to nourish the *Yin* and Blood with Rehmannia (*Jio* 地黄).

This finding usually occurs within the category of Weak and Empty (*Fuku Ryoku Kyo* 腹力虚), and is associated with the following abdomen:

- #1b Tight and Powerless Abdomen (*Fuku Bu Ko Ren Mu Ryoku* 腹部拘攣無力) (Figure 4.2)

There may also be:

- #8 Inside Spasm (*Ri Kyu* 裡急) (Figure 4.11)

and:

- #10 Lower Abdominal Pulsations (*Sei Ka Ki* 臍下悸) (Figure 4.14)

The location of these abdominal pulsations in the lower abdomen, beside and below the navel, is related to the presence of the (deficiency) Blood Stasis (*Oketsu* 瘀血) that occurs there also and is reflected in the finding:

- #13 Navel Spastic Knot Point (*Sai Bu Kyu Ketsu* 臍部急結) (Figure 4.19)

Such Patterns (*Sho* 証) require *Yin* tonifying and Blood moistening and invigorating as well as gentle warming, circulating and softening with formulas containing Rehmannia (*Ji O* 地黄), *Dang Gui* (*Toki* 当帰), Cnidium (*Sen Kyu* 川芎), Cinnamon (*Keishi* 桂枝) and Peony (*Shaku Yaku* 芍薬) in example formulas such as:

- Rehmannia Eight Combination (*Hachi Mi Jio Gan* 八味地黄丸腎気丸)

- Achyranthes and Plantago Formula (*Go Sha Jin Ki Gan* 牛車腎気丸)

- Baked Licorice Combination (*Sha Kanzo To* 炙甘草湯)

- Phellodendron Combination (*Ji In Ko Ka To* 滋陰降火湯)

- *Dang Gui* Four Combination (*Shi Motsu To* 四物湯)

- *Dang Gui* Cinnamon and Peony Combination (*Toki Kenchu To* 当帰建中湯)

- *Dang Gui* and Evodia Combination (*Un Kei To* 温経湯)

- *Dang Gui* and Rehmannia Combination (*Ho In To* 補陰湯)

- Eucommia and Achyranthes Combination (*Isho Ho* 痿証方)

As with #8 Inside Spasm (*Ri Kyu* 裡急) (Figure 4.11) the main significance of this #9 Lower Abdominal Tight Spasm (*Sho Fuku Ko Kyu* 少腹拘急) (Figure 4.13) finding is that it only *ever* occurs in Patterns of Dryness. Additionally, in this case, it also only *ever* occurs in Patterns of Deficiency (*Kyo Sho* 虚証). This finding will therefore always call for tonifying herbs and formulas of the kind discussed above.

Refer to Figures 3.7a–3.7e for the technique involved in palpating the two following possible findings.

10. Cardiac/Epigastric/Lower Abdominal Pulsations 心悸 / 心下悸 / 臍下悸 (*Shin Ki/Shin Ka Ki/Sei Ka Ki*)
Morphology
According to Dr. *Otsuka*:

> The *Shin* 心 refers to the heart, and this *Ki* 悸 means pulsation. *Shin Ka Ki* 心下悸: this *Ka* means below, hence pulsations below the heart (in the epigastrium). *Sei Ka Ki* 臍下悸: this *Sei* is the navel, so here the pulsations are beside or below the navel. Cardiac pulsations: these are known as pulsations of the cardiac area. If the area known in Acupuncture as the point *Kyo Ri*, 虚里 (apex of the heart), is swollen, it points clearly to this cardiac *Sho*. Pulsations below the heart (epigastric), pulsations below the navel, and pulsations in the area called *Sui Bun*, 水分 (Ren.9 Acupuncture point), where the abdominal aorta encircles the navel, or the area *Jin Mon*, 腎間 ("kidney gate"), where the kidneys lie under the abdominal wall, show an obvious influence of these abdominal aorta pulsations. This can be identified objectively by observation, or by a light touch of the hand. Generally these passages refer to instances where the pulsations are progressing, soon to be Empty 虚証 (*Kyo Sho*), so that diuretics, sudorifics, purgatives or emetics are forbidden.

Comment

These are pulsations of the aorta abdominalis. This is divided into the left and right common iliac arteries at the level of the umbilicus. *Shin Ki* 心悸 is the pulsation of the aorta abdominalis itself. *Shin Ka Ki* 心下悸 could be the pulsation of the furcation of the aorta abdominalis, above the umbilicus. *Sai Ka Ki* 臍下悸 could be the pulsation of a furcation below the umbilicus. In a healthy individual, the artery is situated on the floor of the abdomen and is impossible to palpate with light touch. But in the case of a patient with Deficiency (*Kyo Sho* 虚証) where the abdominal wall is thin and lax, it can be felt. Also, in a patient with Excess (*Jitsu Sho* 実証) who has sympathetic nervous system strain, the pulsation of the abdominal aorta will become strong and refers to the abdominal wall where it can be felt at the surface.

Notes

This technique employs Superficial Pressure (*Hyomen Atsu* 表面圧) and is the lightest pressure used in the entire abdominal exam as has been noted in Chapter 3 (Figures 3.7a–3.7c). Care must be taken not to press too deeply since this finding will then tend to be over-diagnosed. Whilst considered an Empty (*Kyo Sho* 虚証) finding in itself, as has been mentioned (above), nevertheless this finding can occur also in Full Patterns (*Jistu Sho* 実証).

Charting

This abdominal finding (Figure 4.14) is charted as follows and care should be taken to reflect on the chart both the exact location *and* the relative strength of the pulsations. One cross indicates mild (strength), two crosses moderate and three strong.

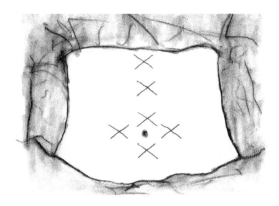

4.14

Clinical interpretation

This finding is one of the most common abdominal patterns (*Fukusho* 腹証) and is always a sign of Counterflow (*Nobose* のぼせ). In *Kampo* Counterflow symptomology is divided into three types:

1. *Qi* Counterflow (*Ki Nobose* 気のぼせ), which includes symptoms of a neurological and psycho-emotional nature such as headache, light-headedness, anxiety, panic attack, nervous arrythmia, insomnia and what is called in *Kampo* "Troublesome Heart" or "Heart Vexation" (*Shin Pan* 心煩), which describes a restless feeling in the chest.

2. Blood Counterflow (*Ketsu Nobose* 血のぼせ), which includes symptoms of a vascular nature such as headache (vasomotor—throbbing), rosacea, bloodshot eyes, racing heart and feeling hot sensations such as flushing.

3. Water Counterflow (*Sui Nobose* 水のぼせ), which includes symptoms of a neurological or inflammatory nature such as headache (dull heavy feeling), heavy head, dizziness, tinnitus, palpitations, facial edema.

In the abdominal exam, when these pulsations are felt by the practitioner (or the patient), their location on the abdomen and their strength is significant. For example, they fall into the categories of *Qi*, Blood and Fluid pulsations according to the following criteria:

- Cardiac Pulsations (*Shin Ki* 心悸) are located typically above the navel, usually from about the acupoint Ren.12 (*Chukan* 中脘) and above, often around the acupoint Ren.14 (*Koketsu* 巨闕, the Front-Mu point of the Heart) or around the apex of the heart itself (located in the 5th intercostal space below the left nipple)

- Epigastric Pulsations (*Shin Ka Ki* 心下悸) occur along the midline from around Ren.12 down to the navel and often especially around the acupoint Ren.9 (*Sui Bun* 水分)

- Lower Abdominal Pulsations (*Sei Ka Ki* 臍下悸) are found clustered around the navel, to either side and below it as far down as the acupoint Ren.6 (*Kikai* 気海)

Cardiac Pulsations (*Shin Ki* 心悸) occur in patterns of Counterflow *Qi* (*Ki Nobose* 気のぼせ), both Excess (*Jitsu Sho* 実証) and Deficiency (*Kyo Sho* 虚証), and thus are associated with the types of symptoms mentioned above that can be found in *Qi* Formulas (*Ki Yakusho* 気薬証) in which *Nobose* is found such as in the following examples:

Jitsu:

- Bupleurum and Dragon Bone Combination (*Saiko Ka Ryukotsu Borei To* 柴胡加竜骨牡蠣湯)

- Bupleurum Formula (*Yokukansan* 抑肝散)

- Bupleurum and Cyperus Formula (*Saiko Sokan San* 柴胡疎肝散)

- Gambir Formula (*Cho to San* 釣藤散)

- Pinellia and Magnolia Combination (*Hange Ko Boku To* 半夏厚朴湯)

- Inula and Hematite Combination (*Senpuku Ka Taisha Seki To* 旋覆花代赭石湯)

Kyo:

- Cinnamon and Dragon Bone Combination (*Keishi Ka Ryukotsu Borei To* 桂枝加竜骨牡蠣湯)

- Hoelen, Licorice and Jujube Combination (*Ryo Kei Kan So To* 苓桂甘棗湯)

- Licorice and Jujube Combination (*Kan Baku Tai So To* 甘麦大棗湯)

- Pinellia and Gastrodia Combination (*Hange Byaku Jutsu Ten Ma To* 半夏白朮天麻湯)

- Cardamom and Fennel Combination (*An Chu San* 安中散)

Epigastric Pulsations (*Shin Ka Ki* 心下悸) occur in patterns in which Toxic Water (*Sui Doku* 水毒) is also a finding (confirmed by abdomen #7 Epigastric Splash Sound (*Shin Ka Bu Shin Sui On* 心下部振水音 (Figure 4.9) and they are associated with the types of Water Counterflow (*Sui Nobose* 水のぼせ) symptoms mentioned above. Again, these patterns can be either *Jitsu* or *Kyo* in nature and include example Water Formulas (*Sui Yakusho* 水薬証) such as:

Jitsu:

- Hoelen Five Formula (*Go Rei San* 五苓散)

- Bupleurum and Hoelen Combination (*Sai Rei To* 柴苓湯)

- Magnolia and Hoelen Combination (*I Rei To* 胃苓湯)

Kyo:

- Atractylodes and Hoelen Combination (*Ryo Kei Jutsu Kan To* 苓桂朮甘湯)

- Hoelen Combination (*Buku Ryo In* 茯苓飲)

- Alisma and Hoelen Combination (*Bukuryo Takusha To* 茯苓 沢瀉湯)

- *Dang Gui* and Peony Combination (*Toki Shaku Yaku San* 当 帰芍薬散)

Lower Abdominal Pulsations (*Sei Ka Ki* 臍下悸) are found mostly in patterns of Blood Stasis (*Oketsu* 瘀血). They involve the kind of Blood Counterflow (*Ketsu Nobose* 血のぼせ) symptoms mentioned above and can also be either:

- Excess Patterns (*Jitsu Sho* 実証) of *Oketsu* including Blood Heat (*Ketsu Netsu* 血熱) and Toxic Blood (*Ketsu Doku* 血 毒), which will require such example Blood Formulas (*Ketsu Yakusho* 血薬証) as:

  - Rhubarb and Moutan Combination (*Daio Botanpi To* 大 黄牡丹皮湯)

  - Persica and Rhubarb Combination (*Tokaku Joki To* 桃核 承気湯)

  - Cinnamon and Persica Combination (*Sessho In* 折衝飲)

  - Cinnamon and Hoelen Formula (*Keishi Bukuryo Gan* 桂 枝茯苓丸)

or:

- Deficient Patterns (*Kyo Sho* 虚証) of *Oketsu* related to Dryness (*Kan Sho* 乾証), which require moistening and tonifying formulas such as:

  - *Dang Gui* and Gardenia Combination (*Unsei In* 温清飲)

  - Rehmannia Eight Formula (*Hachi Mi Gan* 八味丸)

  - Rehmannia Six Formula (*Roku Mi Jio Gan* 六味地黄丸)

- Anemmarhena, Phellodendron and Rehmannia Combination (*Chi Baku Hachi Mi Gan* 知柏八味丸)

- Ginseng Nutritive Combination (*Ninjin Yoei To* 人参養栄湯)

- Ginseng, Longan and Bupleurum Combination (*Kami Kihi To* 加味帰脾湯)

- Baked Licorice Combination (*Sha Kanzo To* 炙甘草湯)

As mentioned, this finding can occur within almost any pattern which can be either *Jitsu* or *Kyo* in nature. This means that they are found in abdomens that are Strong and Full (*Fuku Ryoku Jitsu* 腹力実, and Weak and Empty (*Fuku Ryoku Jyaku [Kyo]* 腹力弱[虚]) alike. They can therefore be associated with any of the other findings mentioned in this book but the most helpful clinical interpretation they offer is whether they belong to *Qi*, Blood or Fluid Patterns (*Ki Ketsu Sui Sho* 気血水証).

Refer to Figure 3.8 for the technique involved in palpating the two following possible findings:

11. Lower Abdomen Lacking Benevolence
少腹不仁 (*Sho Fuku Fu Jin*)
Morphology
According to Dr. *Otsuka*:

> *Sho* 少 means small, and *Fuku* 腹 means abdomen, hence the "lower abdomen." *Fu* 不 means without or lacking while *Jin* 仁 is the character associated with the virtue of the Liver, standing for benevolence or human kindness. So, the meaning here is that this area along the midline of the lower abdomen is empty or hollow to the touch, as if it has "nothing to give" or lacks the ability to emanate strength or abundance.

Comment

Figure 4.15—this Abdominal Pattern (*Fukusho* 腹証) is characterized by decreased tension of the linea alba in the lower abdomen below the navel and relatively exacerbated tension of the rectus abdominis muscle on either side, backed by a decline in overall abdominal pressure.

Figure 4.16—the anatomical structure of the median plane core (*Seichu Shin* 正中心) below the level of the umbilicus is plica umbilicalis mediana (the medial umbilical fold), which here can be palpated on the median plane. On the other hand, the structure above the umbilicus is ligamentum reres hepatis (the round ligament of the liver), the debris of the umbilical artery and the vein. Under normal circumstances, these structures cannot be palpated from the surface of the body due to the "padding" of the surrounding adipose tissue. But when this tissue atrophies or reduces in density and tonus, the normal tension of the linea alba (the white line) is reduced, in turn causing a decrease in abdominal pressure, and these findings may then be detected.

Notes

This technique is done with Mid-level Pressure 中圧 (*Chu Atsu*), and a positive finding should be charted if the differential in tonus between the rectus abdominis muscle and the linea alba below the navel is significantly great. Naturally, the midline below the navel will feel less firm to the touch than on either side, but in this case the fingers will literally "fall into" this area almost like falling into a hollow pit (Figure 4.15) and in some cases, at the bottom, a thin, taught line of tissue may be felt, often called the "Pencil Line" (Figure 4.16). Either of these findings always belongs to an Empty Pattern (*Kyo Sho* 虚証).

Charting

These abdominal findings are charted as follows and may include either Figure 4.15 or Figure 4.16 or both.

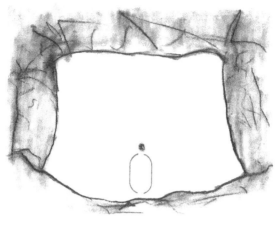

4.15

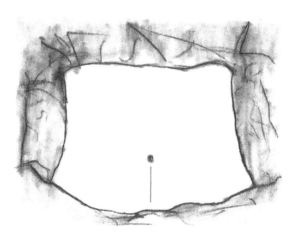

4.16

Clinical interpretation

This #11 Lower Abdomen Lacking Benevolence (*Sho Fuku Fu Jin* 少腹不仁) (Figure 4.15) can be palpated as two distinct findings which can also be found together. Both belong to Deficiency (*Kyo Sho* 虚証) though it could be said that the "Pencil Line" (*Sho Fuku Ko Ren* 小腹拘攣) (Figure 4.16) suggests an even more chronic, empty state than Figure 4.15.

Typically, either of these findings is related to Kidney Deficiency (*Jin Kyo Sho* 腎虚証) and more specifically Kidney *Yang* Deficiency (*Jin Yo Kyo Sho* 腎陽虚証) which can be thought of as a Shaoyin Pattern (*Sho In Byo* 少陰病) in *Kampo*, calling for the use of the herb Aconite (*Bushi*).

This #11 *Sho Fuku Fu Jin* 少腹不仁 finding only ever occurs within:

- #1a Lax and Powerless Abdomen (*Fuku Bu Nan Jyaku Mu Ryoku* 腹部軟弱無力) (Figure 4.1)

We have already seen that this indicates exclusively *Yin* interpretations involving a constitution of *Yang Qi* Deficiency (*Yo Ki Kyo Sho* 陽気虚証), Coldness (*Hie Sho* 冷え症) and Pathological Fluids (*Tan In* 痰飲).

Other findings in this kind of Deficient (*Kyo* 虚), Cold (*Kan* 寒) and Damp (*Shitsu* 湿) abdomen will include:

- #7 Epigastric Splash Sound (*Shin Ka Bu Shin Sui On* 心下部振水音) (Figure 4.9)

- #10 Epigastric Pulsations (*Shin Ka Ki* 心下悸) (Figure 4.14)

Example formulas used to treat this kind of *Shaoyin* Abdominal Pattern (*Sho In Fukusho*) include:

- Aconite Ginseng and Ginger Combination (*Bushi Richu To* 附子理中湯)

- Aconite, Ginger and Licorice Combination (*Shi Gyaku To* 四逆湯)

- Vitality Combination (*Shinbu To* 真武湯)

- Aconite Combination (*Bushi To* 附子湯)

- Rehmannia Eight Formula (*Hachi Mi Gan* 八味丸)

- Licorice and Aconite Combination (*Kanzo Bushi To* 甘草附子湯)

- Cinnamon and Aconite Combination (*Keishi Ka Bushi To* 桂枝加附子湯)

However, patients with this kind of abdomen will often manifest the constitutional finding of weak gastro-intestinal function (*I Cho Kyo Jyaku* 胃腸虚弱) and in such cases there will likely be the additional abdominal finding of:

- #4 Epigastric Obstruction (*Shin Ka Hi* 心下痞) (Figure 4.6)

In such cases, *Qi* tonics may also be used such as Ginseng (*Ninjin* 人参), in formulas that address the *Taiyin* (*Tai In Byo* 太陰病) in the overall abdominal pattern such as:

- Ginseng and Ginger Combination (*Ninjin To* 人参湯—also known as *Ri Chu To* 理中湯)

- Four Major Herb Combination (*Shi Kun Shi To* 四君子湯)

- Six Major Herb Combination (*Rikkun Shi To* 六君子湯)

- Cardamom and Saussurea Combination (*Ko Sha Rikkun Shi To* 香砂六君子湯)

- Ginseng and Astragalus Combination (*Ho Chu Ekki To* 補中益気湯)

- Ginseng and *Dang Gui* Ten Combination (*Juzen Taiho To* 十全大補湯)

- Ginseng Nutritive Combination (*Ninjin Yoei To* 人参養栄湯)

- Ginseng and Longan Combination (*Ki In To* 帰脾湯)

12. Lower Abdominal Fullness/Lower Abdominal Resistant Fullness 少腹満 / 少腹硬満 (*Sho Fuku Man/Sho Fuku Ko Man*)

Morphology

According to Dr. *Otsuka*:

The *Sho Fuku* means lower abdomen; the Man is fullness. In *Sho Fuku Ko Man*, the *Ko* signifies an objective hardness. Swollen abdomen/persistent swollen abdomen: in the *Sho Fuku Man*, the lower abdomen is said to be inflated; in the *Sho Fuku Ko Man*, it is inflated and shows resistance as well. This Abdominal Pattern 腹証 *Fukusho* appears often with *Oketsu* and sometimes with *Tan In*, 痰 飲 pathological fluids. For example, there is this old quote: "Cases of the resistant swollen abdomen and difficult urination occur without a blood dysfunction. But if the patient is behaving like a madman, then it is a blood pattern 血証 (*Ketsu Sho*), so that whether *Oketsu Sho* or *Tan In Sho* is present can be differentiated by whether the urination is scant and difficult, or normal."

Comment
The kind of resistance and obstruction felt by both patient and practitioner is similar to that in #2 Abdominal Fullness (*Fuku Man* 腹滿) (Figures 4.3 and 4.4). Here, however, the location is specifically in the lower abdomen.

Notes
This technique is done with Mid-level Pressure 中圧力 (*Chu Atsuryoku*), and the area of the lower abdomen will look distended and swollen even before palpating it. In either case, whether full (swollen) and hard (Figure 4.17) or full (swollen) and soft (Figure 4.18) to the touch, these findings belong to patterns of Fullness (*Jistu Sho* 実証).

Charting
These abdominal findings are charted as follows and care should be taken to distinguish between Figures 4.17 and 4.18 as their clinical interpretations are quite different (as we shall see):

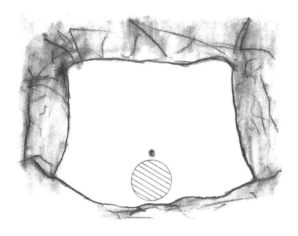

4.17

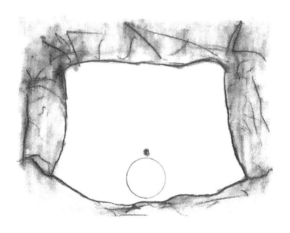

4.18

Clinical interpretation

These two findings are palpated as part of the same sequence (Figure 3.8) in the abdominal exam but are distinct from one another and have differing interpretations clinically. Nonetheless, both belong to Excess Patterns (*Jitsu Sho* 実証) either of Blood Stasis (*Oketsu* 瘀血) (Figure 4.17) or Toxic Water (*Sui Doku* 水毒) (Figure 4.18) respectively.

Both of these abdominal findings will only ever occur inside the:

- #2 Full Abdomen (*Fuku Man* 腹満) (Figures 4.3 and 4.4)

In the case of Figure 4.17, this abdomen will be found within the:

- #2a *Yang* Full Abdomen (*Yo Fuku Man* 陽腹満) (Figure 4.3)

whilst Figure 4.18 will tend to associate with the:

- #2b *Yin* Full Abdomen (*In Fuku Man* 陰腹満) (Figure 4.4)

Lower Abdominal Resistant Fullness (*Sho Fuku Ko Man* 少腹硬満) (Figure 4.17) is interpreted as a finding exclusively in Patterns of Excess (*Jitsu Sho* 実証) and specifically in those of Blood Stasis (*Oketsu* 瘀血). This finding is always associated with the symptom of constipation (due to Heat caused by *Oketsu*) and the other likely abdominal findings will include:

- #14 Lower Abdomen Spastic Knot (*Sho Fuku Kyu Ketsu* 少腹急結) (Figure 4.20)

- #10 Lower Abdominal Pulsations (*Sei Ka Ki* 臍下悸) (Figure 4.14)

This is an example of what might be called *Yangming* Stage (*Yomei Byo* 陽明病), in which the primary *Qi* Constraint, Heat and Excess symptoms will occur in the Lower *Jiao* (such as Abdominal Fullness, distention, pain, constipation and so on). Thus, formulas to Move and Regulate *Qi* (*Gyo Ri Ki* 行理氣), Harmonize *Qi* (*Wa Ki* 和気), Direct *Qi* Downward (*Fu Gyaku Ka Ki* 降逆下氣), Clear Heat (*Sei Netsu* 清熱) and Purge (*Tsu Ka* 通下) are needed such as Magnolia Bark (*Koboku* 厚朴), *Chi Shi* (*Ki Jitsu* 枳実), Rhubarb (*Daio* 大黄) and Mirabilitum (*Bo Sho* 芒硝) respectively in such example formulas as:

- Major Rhubarb Combination (*Dai Joki To* 大承気湯)

- Minor Rhubarb Combination (*Sho Joki To* 小承気湯)

or in milder cases:

- Apricot Seed and Linum Combination (*Ma Shi Nin Gan* 麻子仁丸), which includes Minor Rhubarb Combination

- Cimicifuga Combination (*Otsuji To* 乙字湯)

In other cases where this #12 Lower Abdominal Resistant Fullness (*Sho Fuku Ko Man* 少腹硬満) (Figure 4.17) is found along with either of the two findings:

- #5 Hypochondriac Painful Fullness (*Kyo Kyo Ku Man* 胸脅苦満) (Figure 4.7)

- #6 Hypochondriac Obstruction Resistance (*Kyo Ka Hi Ko* 脅下痞硬) (Figure 4.8)

then use other formulas for the #2a *Yang* Full Abdomen (*Yo Fuku Man* 陽腹満) such as:

- Major Bupleurum Combination (*Dai Saiko To* 大柴胡湯)

- Coptis and Rhubarb Combination (*San O Shashin To* 三黄瀉心湯)

- Capillaris Combination (*In Chin Ko To* 茵蔯蒿湯)

- Gentiana Combination (*Ryu Tan Sho Kan To* 龙胆泻肝汤)

Lower Abdominal Fullness (*Sho Fuku Man* 少腹満) (Figure 4.18) is also interpreted as a finding exclusively in Patterns of Excess (*Jitsu Sho* 実証), this time specifically in those of Toxic Water (*Sui Doku* 水毒). This finding is usually associated with Urinary Difficulty (*Rin Reki* 淋瀝) due to Heat in the Urinary Bladder (*Boko Netsu* 膀胱熱) and other likely abdominal findings would include:

- #14 Lower Abdomen Spastic Knot (*Sho Fuku Kyu Ketsu* 少腹急結) (Figure 4.20)

- #10 Epigastric Pulsations (*Shin Ka Ki* 心下悸) (Figure 4.14)

- #7 Epigastric Splash Sound (*Shin Ka Bu Shin Sui On* 心下部振水音) (Figure 4.9)

In such cases use example formulas to treat this Lower Abdominal Fullness (*Sho Fuku Man* 少腹滿) such as:

- Polyporus Combination (*Chorei To* 猪苓湯)

- Lotus Seed Combination (*Sei Shin Ren Shi In* 清心蓮子飲)

In other cases where this #12 Lower Abdominal Fullness (*Sho Fuku Man* 少腹滿) is found along with either of the two findings:

- #5 Hypochondriac Painful Fullness (*Kyo Kyo Ku Man* 胸脅苦滿) (Figure 4.7)

- #3 Epigastric Obstruction Resistance (*Shin Ka Hi Ko* 心下痞硬) (Figure 4.5)

then use other formulas for the #2b *Yin* Full Abdomen (*In Fuku Man* 陰腹滿) (Figure 4.4) such as:

- Hoelen 5 Combination (*Go Rei To* 五苓湯)

- Bupleurum and Hoelen Combination (*Sai Rei To* 柴苓湯)

- Siler and Platycodon Combination (*Bofutsu Sho To* 防風通聖散)

Refer to Figures 3.9a and 3.9b for the technique involved in palpating the two following possible findings.

13. Navel Spastic Knot Point 臍部急結 (*Sai Bu Kyu Ketsu*) Terasawa Oketsu (*Yu Xue*) 瘀血 Point
Morphology
According to Dr. *Otsuka*:

Sai 臍 means umbilicus and *Bu* 部 means a part of, so that this finding is located beside or around the navel. *Kyu Ketsu* 急結 indicates the same spastic knot described in Abdomen #14 below—Lower Abdominal Spastic Knot 少腹急結 (*Sho Fuku Kyu Ketsu*) which, whenever it is found, is typically associated with Blood Stasis 瘀血 (*Oketsu*).

Comment

There is tenderness around the umbilicus (*Saibu Atsu* 臍傍圧痛) upon pressure. This area is crowded with micro-circulatory vessels such as in the small intestine, mesentary (peritoneum) and caul (omentum). Thus, *Saibu Atsu* suggests the existence of a morbid state of blood occlusion due to a decrease in micro-circulation such as may occur in hemostasis or hyperemia. Even though the caul has a limited number of pain receptors, pain could derive from the small intestine or mesentary due to a morbid state of blood occlusion.

Notes

This technique is done with Mid-level Pressure 中圧力 (*Chu Atsuryoku*), as opposed to Abdomen #14 Lower Abdomen Spastic Knot 少腹急結 (*Sho Fuku Kyu Ketsu*) (Figure 4.20), which requires Deep Pressure 深圧力 (*Shin Atsuryoku*). The sensation felt on palpation is as if the fingers of the practitioner are suddenly prevented from penetrating deeper by a board-like obstruction. It is almost as if a flat, cylindrical object had been placed at the muscle level directly under the navel of the patient, preventing deeper pressure from being applied. There may or may not be pressure pain felt by the patient and it is the feeling of obstruction felt by the practitioner that confirms the finding, not any pain felt on pressure by the patient. This finding is considered one of Fullness 実 (*Jitsu*); however, it can be found in both Full 実 (*Jitsu*) and Empty 虚 (*Kyo*) Patterns 証 (*Sho*).

Charting

This abdominal finding (Figure 4.19) is charted as follows and care should be taken to reflect on the chart the exact location and intensity of the *Oketsu* findings. The marks can be made smaller or larger and drawn either to the left or right of the navel or below to reflect these differences:

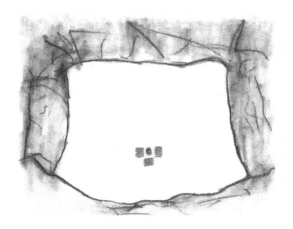

4.19

Clinical interpretation

This #13 Navel Spastic Knot (*Sai Bu Kyu Ketsu* 臍部急結) is a Blood Stasis (*Oketsu*) finding. However, unlike the #14 Lower Abdomen Spastic Knot (*Sho Fuku Kyu Ketsu* 少腹急結) (Figure 4.20), which confirms an Excess Blood Stasis finding, this one belongs to an Empty Pattern (*Kyo Sho* 虚証) of *Oketsu* (瘀血) in which the blood has become Dry (deficient) and no longer circulates freely.

Typically, this finding will occur within the #1b Tight and Powerless (*Fuku Bu Ko Ren Mu Ryoku* 腹部拘攣無力) Abdomen (Figure 4.2), which will likely also include the following additional findings:

- #9 Lower Abdominal Tight Spasm (*Sho Fuku Ko Kyu* 少腹拘急) (Figure 4.13)

- #10 Lower Abdominal Pulsations (*Sei Ka Ki* 臍下悸) (Figure 4.14)

In Weak Constitutions (*Kyo Taishitsu Sho* 虚体質証) such findings require *Yin* tonifying and Blood moistening and invigorating as well as gentle warming, circulating and softening with formulas containing Rehmannia (*Ji O* 地黄), *Dang Gui* (*Toki* 当帰), Cnidium

(*Sen Kyu* 川芎), Cinnamon (*Keishi* 桂枝) and Peony (*Shaku Yaku* 芍薬) in example formulas such as:

- Rehmannia Eight Combination (*Hachi Mi Jio Gan* 八味地黄丸腎気丸)

- Baked Licorice Combination (*Sha Kanzo To* 炙甘草湯)

- *Dang Gui* Four Combination (*Shi Motsu To* 四物湯)

- *Dang Gui* and Gelatin Combination (*Kyu Ki Kyogai To* 芎帰膠艾湯)

- *Dang Gui* and Jujube Combination (*Toki Shi Gyaku To* 当帰四逆湯)

- *Dang Gui*, Evodia and Ginger Combination (*Toki Shi Gyaku Ka Goshuyu Shokyo To* 当帰四逆加呉茱萸生姜湯)

If in such *Kyo* cases there is dry Blood Stasis and also some signs of heat *Nobose* (including insomnia and agitation) then formulas that also have a cooling and calming action may be needed according to the *Sho* such as:

- Coptis and Gelatin Combination (*Oren Akyo To* 黄連解毒湯)

- Ginseng and Zizyphus Combination (*Ten Noho Shin To* 天王补心湯)

- Scute Three Herb Combination (*San Motsu Ogon To* 三物黄芩湯)

- *Dang Gui* and Gardenia Combination (*Unsei In* 温清飲)

Sometimes within this #1b Tight and Powerless (*Fuku Bu Ko Ren Mu Ryoku* 腹部拘攣無力) abdomen (Figure 4.2) there will be deficiency in the Nutrient or *Ying Qi* (*Ei Ki* 栄気) causing the surface muscles on the abdomen to be dry, tight and cold leading to abdominal cramps and pain as well as loose stools. This can also give rise to the findings of this #13 Navel Spastic Knot (*Sai Bu Kyu Ketsu* 臍部急結) (Figure 4.19).

In this case, in addition to being #1b Tight and Powerless (*Fuku Bu Ko Ren Mu Ryoku* 腹部拘攣無力), this abdomen will also evidence:

- #8 Inside Spasm (*Ri Kyu* 裡急) (Figure 4.11) reflecting surface muscular tension due to deficient Dryness and sometimes Cold. There will be no splash sound as this is a Dry pattern but there will likely be gas accumulation in the upper left quadrant (part of the #7 finding, Figure 4.10)

Additionally, there will be:

- #10 Epigastric Pulsations (*Shin Ka Ki* 心下悸) (Figure 4.14) due to the tendency for Counterflow *Qi* (*Ki Nobose* 気のぼせ) caused by deficiency (inability of the *Qi* to root itself in the middle)

Such cases require gentle warming, circulating and softening with formulas containing Cinnamon (*Keishi* 桂枝) and Peony (*Shaku Yaku* 芍薬) in order to relax the vessels and improve blood flow in example formulas such as:

- Cinnamon Combination (*Keishi To* 桂枝湯)

- Cinnamon and Peony Combination (*Keishi Ka Shakuyaku To* 桂枝加芍薬湯)

However, in Moderate to Strong Constitutions (*Chu/Jitsu Taishitsu Sho* 中／実体質証), when they have evidence of this dry *Oketsu*, there will also be the need to "crack Blood" (*Ha Ketsu* 破血- break up Blood Stasis), which will call for herbs, in addition to those mentioned above, such as Persica Seed (*Tonin* 桃仁), Moutan Bark (*Bo Tan Pi* 牡丹皮) and even Safflower (*Koka* 紅花). An example formula in this case would be:

- Cinnamon and Persica Combination (*Sessho In* 折衝飲)

Refer to Figures 3.10a and 3.10b for the technique involved in palpating the two following possible findings.

14. Lower Abdomen Spastic Knot 少腹急結 (*Sho Fuku Kyu Ketsu*) *Otsuka Oketsu* (*Yu Xue*) 瘀血 Point

Morphology

According to Dr. *Otsuka*:

> As explained above in #9 Lower Abdomen Tight Spasm, 少腹拘急 (*Sho Fuku Ko Kyu*), *Sho Fuku* refers to the lower abdomen, and 急 *Kyu* means acute. Here 結 *Ketsu* refers to a knot, or a string. The Blood Stagnation point, 瘀血 *Oketsu*): this is the abdomen pattern 腹証 (*Fukusho*) for what is called *Oketsu* 瘀血 (blood stasis). This abdominal pattern most often occurs on the left side of the iliac fossa but may occur in the corresponding area on the right side, or around the navel. In response to rapid lateral pressure such as a strong stroke of the fingers across this area, there is sharp pain and a kind of resistance can be felt. The recommended way to examine for this is to have the patient lie with both legs extended. Quickly stroke the area proceeding obliquely from the navel to the left pelvic crest. If the *Oketsu* point is active there the patient will react by drawing up the knees, and will complain of sharp, acute pain there. This abdominal sign occurs more often in women than in men.

Comment

There is hyperalgesia due to referred pain and the strain of the abdominal wall. The types of pain include strong internal organ pain and referred pain related to the internal organ perceptive reflex. Anatomically speaking, the area in the left iliac fossa in a woman is known to approximate to a hypersensitive zone associated with the left ovary and uterine duct (fallopian tube); the area in the right iliac fossa is often associated with the ileocecal valve, appendix and ascending colon.

Notes

This technique is done with Deep Pressure 深圧力 (*Shin Atsuryoku*) and is the *only* part of the entire abdominal exam to require this level of pressure. As explained in Chapter 3, this level requires the practitioner to apply pressure that passes through the layers of adipose tissue and muscle down to the lower abdominal cavity itself. At that depth, a positive finding can only be charted when the following two pieces of evidence are established at the same time:

1. The practitioner can feel a hard, resistant knot (that may be as small as a pea or much larger)

and:

2. The moment this knot is palpated, the patient experiences a sudden, often sharp pain, which may cause their knees involuntarily to curl up towards their abdomen (as described above).

If the finding is established with the patient's legs extended, the exam should be repeated with the knees bent as this will relax any involuntary tension in the deep, smooth muscles of the lower abdomen which otherwise might be mistaken for *Oketsu*. If the finding is still present, it should then be charted.

Charting

This abdominal finding (Figure 4.14) is charted as follows and care should be taken to reflect on the chart both the location (either left or right side or both) and the relative strength of the *Oketsu* findings. The marks can be made smaller or larger to reflect these differences:

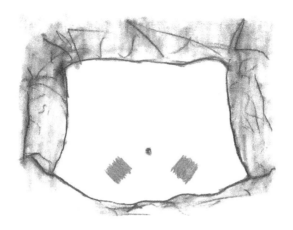

4.20

Clinical interpretation

This #14 Lower Abdomen Spastic Knot (*Sho Fuku Kyu Ketsu* 少腹急結) (Figure 4.20) is a Blood Stasis (*Oketsu*) finding like the #13 Navel Spastic Knot (*Sai Bu Kyu Ketsu* 臍部急結) (Figure 4.19). However, in that case the finding belonged to an Empty Pattern (*Kyo Sho* 虚証) of *Oketsu* (瘀血) in which the blood had become Dry (deficient) and could no longer circulate freely. In this case, the finding is a confirmation of an Excess Blood Stasis finding (*Jitsu Oketsu Sho* 実瘀血証), which typically involves Excess Heat Patterns (*Jitsu Netsu Sho* 実熱証) and sometimes Toxic Blood Patterns (*Ketsu Doku Sho* 血毒証).

This #14 Lower Abdomen Spastic Knot (*Sho Fuku Kyu Ketsu* 少腹急結) (Figure 4.20) is interpreted as a finding exclusively in Patterns of Excess (*Jitsu Sho* 実証) and specifically in those of Blood Stasis (*Oketsu* 瘀血) and it will occur inside an abdomen which is #2 Full (*Fuku Man* 腹満) and more specifically the #2a *Yang* Full Abdomen (*Yo Fuku Man* 陽腹満) (Figure 4.3).

When the following additional lower abdominal findings are also found:

- #10 Lower Abdominal Pulsations (*Sei Ka Ki* 臍下悸) (Figure 4.14)

- #12 Lower Abdominal Resistant Fullness (*Sho Fuku Ko Man* 少腹硬満) (Figure 4.17)

then formulas containing herbs that "crack Blood" (*Ha Ketsu* 破血—break up Blood Stasis) will need to be used such as Persica Seed (*Tonin* 桃仁), Moutan Bark (*Bo Tan Pi* 牡丹皮) and Safflower (*Koka* 紅花), and also ones that Purge Downward (*Tsu Ka* 通下) such as Rhubarb (*Daio* 大黄).

Example formulas according to their *Sho* (証) include:

- Major Rhubarb Combination (*Dai Joki To* 大承気湯)

- Minor Rhubarb Combination (*Sho Joki To* 小承気湯)

- Apricot Seed and Linum Formula (*Ma Shi Nin Gan* 麻子仁丸)

- Rhubarb and Mirabilitum Combination (*Cho I Joki To* 調胃承気湯)

- Rhubarb and Moutan Combination (*Daio Botan Pi To* 大黄牡丹皮湯)

- Persica and Rhubarb Combination (*Tokaku Joki To* 桃核承気湯)

- Cinnamon and Persica Combination (*Sessho In* 折衝飲)

However, in cases of #14 Lower Abdomen Spastic Knot (*Sho Fuku Kyu Ketsu* 少腹急結) (Figure 4.20) inside the same #2a *Yang* Full Abdomen (*Yo Fuku Man* 陽腹満) (Figure 4.3) when additional abdominal findings are not limited to the lower abdomen but also include any of the following:

- #3 Epigastric Obstruction Resistance (*Shin Ka Hi Ko* 心下痞硬) (Figure 4.5)

- #5 Hypochondriac Painful Fullness (*Kyo Kyo Ku Man* 胸脅苦満) (Figure 4.7)

- #8 Inside Spasm (*Ri Kyu* 裡急) (Figure 4.11)

then example formulas such as the following can be used according to their *Sho* (証):

- Major Bupleurum Combination (*Dai Saiko To* 大柴胡湯)

- Coptis and Rhubarb Combination (*San O Sshashin To* 三黄瀉心湯)

- Capillaris Combination (*In Chin Ko To* 茵蔯蒿湯)

Typically, as stated above, this #14 Lower Abdomen Spastic Knot (*Sho Fuku Kyu Ketsu* 少腹急結) (Figure 4.20) is found in abdomens which are *Yang* and Full (#2a *Yo Fuku Man* 陽腹滿). This abdominal finding suggests exclusively *Yang* interpretations involving a constitution of Strong *Yang Qi* (*Yo Ki Jitsu Sho* 陽気実証), Heat (*Netsu Sho* 熱症) and Dryness (*Kan Sho* 乾証)—all qualities of *Yang*. These are usually Blood Constitutional Types (*Ketsu Taishitsu Sho* 血体質証) and they suffer easily, as already stated, from Patterns of Blood Stasis (*Oketsu Sho* 瘀血証).

However, there are patterns of *Oketsu* in which there is also evidence of Toxic Water (*Sui Doku*), which can be confirmed by the abdominal finding:

- #7 Epigastric Splash Sound (*Shin Ka Bu Shin Sui On* 心下部振水音) (Figure 4.9)

In such cases the formula of choice in *Kampo* would be:

- Cinnamon and Hoelen Formula (*Keishi Bukuryo Gan* 桂枝茯苓丸)

SUMMARY OF FINDINGS

In the same way that we do not use individual herbs by themselves in treatment but rather prescribe combinations of ingredients in formulas, so in the clinical context, patients in the real world present with Abdominal Patterns (*Fukusho* 腹証) that include multiple findings, not just one.

Pulse Diagnosis (*Myaku Shin* 脈診) is the same in this respect whereby any given Pulse Pattern (*Myaku Sho* 脈証) will comprise several individual findings that co-exist in the same moment, likely reflecting a complex mix of Excess (*Jistu Sho* 実証) and Deficient (*Kyo Sho* 虚証) findings that may relate to chronic or more acute symptomology with either Root (*Hon* 本) or Branch (*Hyo* 表) etiologies in each case.

Thus, in clinical reality, the interpretation of findings from either the abdomen or the pulse, and for that matter the tongue also, will naturally require careful differentiation into their respective "Patterns" (*Sho* 証) in order to establish a hierarchy in the principle of treatment at any given time.

This is where a particular strength of the *Kampo* process lies. In focusing on identifying above all the Formula Patterns (*Yakusho* 薬証) in diagnosis, this process leads the practitioner naturally to prescribe the formula that most obviously matches the predominant *Sho* of the patient. As we have seen, this is referred to as "Matching Formula and Pattern" (*Ho Sho Iichi* 方証一致) and is a seminal feature of the *Kampo* dialectic essentially classifying the Disease Pattern (*Byo Sho* 病証) and the *Yakusho* as one and the same.

For example, if the abdomen #14 Lower Abdomen Spastic Knot (*Sho Fuku Kyu Ketsu* 少腹急結) (Figure 4.20) is palpated in the abdominal exam, this is interpreted as an indication for the use of Blood-cracking formulas. A specific formula will then be selected according to the Formula Pattern (*Yakusho* 薬証) that most closely matches that of the patient's presenting signs and symptoms. The Disease Pattern can be described as one of Blood Stasis (*Oketsu* 瘀血) but the diagnosis itself is identified by the name of the formula that is used to treat it.

In summarizing the 14 findings listed, it will be helpful therefore in attempting to streamline this process of matching abdomens to formulas, to group them into subcategories according to the differential diagnostic criteria most commonly used in *Kampo*. These are:

- Excess (*Jistu Sho* 実証) and Deficiency (*Kyo Sho* 虚証) findings

- *Qi*, Blood and Fluid (*Ki Ketsu Sui Sho* 気血水証) findings

- Herb or Formula "Family" findings

The following are several ways in which we might think about groups or families of findings that might help place them in a more clinical context and serve as a summary of the information provided in the preceding pages of this chapter.

1. Excess and Deficiency findings

Constitutional Pattern findings (*Tai Shitsu Sho* 体質証)

The Constitutional Strength of the patient can be assessed during the first part of the abdominal exam (using the technique in Figures 3.2a and 3.2b) and, as we have seen, will be categorized as either:

- #1 Weak Abdomen (*Fuku Ryoku Jyaku [Kyo]* 腹力弱 [虚]) (Figure 4.1)

- #2 Strong Abdomen (*Fuku Ryoku Jitsu* 腹力実) (Figure 4.2)

Each of these abdominal findings in turn can be further divided into *Kyo* 虚 and *Jitsu* 実 respectively. Thus, in summarizing overall constitutional Excess and Deficiency findings in the abdomen we can identify four distinct combinations of abdominal patterns as follows.

Empty (*Kyo* 虚証)
YIN WITHIN *YIN* (*IN CHU NO IN* 陰中の陰)

- #1a Lax and Powerless (*Fuku Bu Nan Jyaku Mu Ryoku* 腹部軟弱無力) (Figure 4.1)

This abdomen would likely include any or several of the following findings:

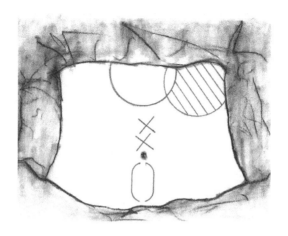

4.21

YANG WITHIN YIN (IN CHU NO YO 陰中の陽)

- #1b Tight and Powerless (*Fuku Bu Ko Ren Mu Ryoku* 腹部拘攣無力) (Figure 4.2)

This abdomen would likely include any or several of the following findings:

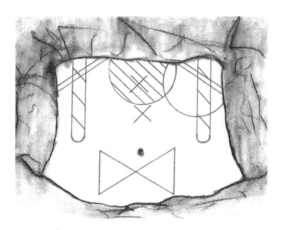

4.22

Full (*Jitsu*実証)

YANG WITHIN *YANG* (*YO CHU NO YO* 陽中の陽)

- #2a *Yang* Strong (*Yo Jitsu Sho* 陽実証) (Figure 4.3)

This abdomen would likely include any or several of the following findings:

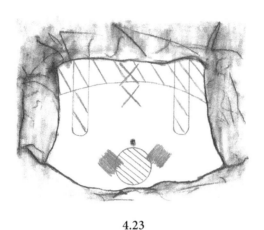

4.23

YIN WITHIN *YANG* (*YO CHU NO IN* 陽中の陰)

- #2b *Yin* Strong (*In Jitsu Sho* 陰実証) (Figure 4.4)

This abdomen would likely include any or several of the following findings:

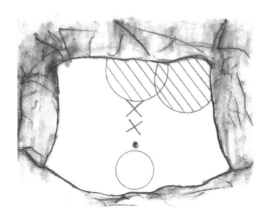

4.24

Disease Pattern findings (*Byo Sho* 病証)

These are assessed on the abdomen during the remainder of the exam (using the techniques in Figures 3.3–3.10).

They can be categorized as individual findings according to Excess (*Jitsu Sho* 実証) and Deficiency (*Kyo Sho* 虚証) in the following way.

EXCESS ABDOMINAL PATTERNS (*JITSU FUKUSHO* 実腹証)

- #3 Epigastric Obstruction Resistance (*Shin Ka Hi Ko* 心下痞硬) (Figure 4.5)

- #5 Hypochondriac Painful Fullness (*Kyo Kyo Ku Man* 胸脇苦満) (Figure 4.7)

- #12 Lower Abdomen Resistant Fullness (*Sho Fuku [Ko] Man* 小腹[硬]満) (Figure 4.17)

- #14 Lower Abdomen Spastic Knot (*Sho Fuku Kyu Ketsu* 小腹急結) (Figure 4.20)

DEFICIENCY ABOMINAL PATTERNS (*KYO FUKUSHO* 虚腹証)

- #4 Epigastric Obstruction (*Shin Ka Hi* 心下痞) (Figure 4.6)

- #9 Lower Abdominal Tight Spasm (*Sho Fuku Ko Kyu* 小腹拘急) (Figure 4.13)

- #11 Lower Abdomen Lacking Benevolence (*Sho Fuku Fu Jin* 小腹不仁) (Figure 4.15)

- #13 Navel Spastic Knot (*Saibu Kyu Ketsu* 臍部急結) (Figure 4.19)

EITHER EXCESS OR DEFICIENT ABDOMINAL PATTERNS

- #6 Hypochondriac Obstruction Resistance (*Kyo Ka Hi Ko* 脇下痞硬) (Figure 4.8)

- #7 Epigastric Splash Sound (*Shin Ka Bu Shin Sui On* 心下部振水音) (Figures 4.9 and 4.10)

- #8 Inside Spasm (*Ri Kyu* 裏急) (Figure 4.11)

- #10 Cardiac/Epigastric/Lower Abdominal Pulsations (*Shin Ki/Shin Ka Ki/Sai Ka Ki* 心悸 / 心下悸 / 臍下悸) (Figure 4.14)

2. Qi, Blood and Fluid findings

In *Kampo*, it is very common to interpret Disease Pattern findings (*Byo Sho* 病証) in the context of disharmonies of *Qi*, Blood and Fluids (*Ki Ketsu Sui Sho* 気血水証).

These patterns can be assessed using the abdominal exam and interpreted in the following manner providing yet another way of conceptualizing the *Fukushin* findings:

- #1a Lax and Powerless (*Fuku Bu Nan Jyaku Mu Ryoku* 腹部軟弱無力) (Figure 4.1)

  - *Yang Qi* Deficiency (*Yo Ki Kyo Sho* 陽気虚証)

  - Toxic Water (*Sui Doku Sho* 水毒証)

- #1b Tight and Powerless (*Fuku Bu Ko Ren Mu Ryoku* 腹部拘攣無力) (Figure 4.2)

  - *Ying Qi* Deficiency (*Ei Ki Kyo Sho* 営気虚証)

  - Blood Deficiency (Dryness) (*Kekkyo Sho* 血虚証)

- #2a *Yang* Strong (*Yo Jitsu Sho* 陽実証) (Figure 4.3)

  - *Yang Qi* Fullness (*Yo Ki Jitsu Sho* 陽気実証)

- Blood Stasis (*Oketsu Sho* 瘀血証)

- #2b *Yin* Strong (*In Jitsu Sho* 陽実証) (Figure 4.4)

  - *Yang Qi* Fullness (*Yo Ki Jitsu Sho* 陽気実証)

  - Toxic Water (*Sui Doku Sho* 水毒証)

- #3 Epigastric Obstruction Resistance (*Shin Ka Hi Ko* 心下痞硬) (Figure 4.5)

  - *Qi* Stasis (*Ki Tai Sho* 気滞証)

  - Possible Toxic Water (*Sui Doku Sho* 水毒証)

- #4 Epigastric Obstruction (*Shin Ka Hi* 心下痞) (Figure 4.6)

  - *Qi* Deficiency (*Ki Kyo Sho* 気虚証)

  - Toxic Water (*Sui Doku Sho* 水毒証)

- #5 Hypochondriac Painful Fullness (*Kyo Kyo Ku Man* 胸脇苦満) (Figure 4.7)

  - *Qi* Stasis (*Ki Tai Sho* 気滞証)—extreme

- #6 Hypochondriac Obstruction Resistance (*Kyo Ka Hi Ko* 脇下痞硬) (Figure 4.8)

  - *Qi* Stasis (*Ki Tai Sho* 気滞証)—moderate

- #7a Epigastric Splash Sound (*Shin Ka Bu Shin Sui On* 心下部振水音) (Figure 4.9)

  - Toxic Water (*Sui Doku Sho* 水毒証)

- #7b Epigastric Drumming Sound (*Shin Ka Bu "Don Don"* 心下部どんどん) (Figure 4.10)

  - *Qi* Stasis (*Ki Tai Sho* 気滞証)

- #8 Inside Spasm (*Ri Kyu* 裏急) (Figures 4.11 and 4.12)

  - *Qi* Stasis (*Ki Tai Sho* 気滞証)

- Nutritive *Qi* Deficiency (*Ei Ki Kyo Sho* 営気虚証)

- Blood Deficiency (Dryness) (*Kekkyo Sho* 血虚証)

- #9 Lower Abdominal Tight Spasm (*Sho Fuku Ko Kyu* 小腹拘急) (Figure 4.13)

  - *Yin* Deficiency (*In Kyo Sho* 陰虚証)

  - Blood Deficiency (Dryness) (*Kekkyo Sho* 血虚証)

- #10 Cardiac/Epigastric/Lower Abdominal Pulsations (*Shin Ki/Shin Ka Ki/Sai Ka Ki* 心悸／心下悸/臍下悸) (Figure 4.14)

  - *Qi* Counterflow (*Ki Nobose Sho* 気のぼせ証)—Cardiac Pulsations (*Shin Ki* 心悸)

  - Water Counterflow (*Sui Nobose Sho* 水のぼせ証)—Epigastric Pulsations (*Shin Ka Ki* 心下悸)

  - Blood Counterflow (*Ketsu Nobose Sho* 血のぼせ証)—Lower Abdominal Pulsations (*Sai Ka Ki* 臍下悸)

- #11 Lower Abdomen Lacking Benevolence (*Sho Fuku Fu Jin* 小腹不仁) (Figures 4.15 and 4.16)

  - *Yang Qi* Deficiency (*Yo Ki Kyo Sho* 陽気虚証)

- #12 Lower Abdomen Resistant Fullness (*Sho Fuku [Ko] Man* 小腹[硬]満) (Figures 4.17 and 4.18)

  - Blood Stasis (*Oketsu Sho* 瘀血証)—Lower abdominal Painful Fullness (*Sho Fuku Ko Man* 小腹硬満)

  - Toxic Water (*Sui Doku Sho* 水毒証)—Lower abdominal Fullness *Sho Fuku Man* 小腹満)

- #13 Navel Spastic Knot (*Saibu Kyu Ketsu* 臍部急結) (Figure 4.19)

  - [Deficiency] Blood Stasis ([*Kyo*] *Oketsu Sho* [虚]瘀血証)

- #14 Lower Abdomen Spastic Knot (*Sho Fuku Kyu Ketsu* 小腹急結) (Figure 4.20)

  - [Excess] Blood Stasis (*[Jitsu] Oketsu Sho* [実]瘀血証)

3. "Herb family" findings

Yet another way to relate to the abdominal findings presented in this book is to associate each one with a particular herb or herbs which such a finding may point to. This method may be referred to as "Abdominal findings related to herb families." These associations apply to each abdominal finding as follows:

- #1a Lax and Powerless (*Fuku Bu Nan Jyaku Mu Ryoku* 腹部軟弱無力) (Figure 4.1)

  - Ginseng (*Nin Jin* 人参): Aconite (*Bushi* 附子) families

- #1b Tight and Powerless (*Fuku Bu Ko Ren Mu Ryoku* 腹部拘攣無力) (Figure 4.2)

  - Cinnamon (*Keishi* 桂枝); Peony (*Shaku Yaku* 芍薬); Maltose (*Koi* 膠飴); Rehmannia (*Jio* 地黄) families

- #2a *Yang* Strong (*Yo Jitsu Sho* 陽実証) (Figure 4.3)

  - Bupleurum (*Saiko* 柴胡); Pinellia (*Hange* 半夏); Coptis (*Oren* 黄連); Rhubarb (*Daio* 大黄) families

- #2b *Yin* Strong (*In Jitsu Sho* 陽実証) (Figure 4.4)

  - Bupleurum (*Saiko* 柴胡); Pinellia (*Hange* 半夏); Hoelen (*Bukuryo* 茯苓); Atractylodes (*Jutsu* 朮); Alisma (*Taku Sha* 沢瀉); Polyporus (*Chorei* 猪苓) families

- #3 Epigastric Obstruction Resistance (*Shin Ka Hi Ko* 心下痞硬) (Figure 4.5)

  - Pinellia (*Hange* 半夏) family

- #4 Epigastric Obstruction (*Shin Ka Hi* 心下痞) (Figure 4.6)

- Ginseng (*Ninjin* 人参) family

- #5 Hypochondriac Painful Fullness (*Kyo Kyo Ku Man* 胸脇苦満) (Figure 4.7)

  - Bupleurum (*Saiko* 柴胡) family—acute/Full

- #6 Hypochondriac Obstruction Resistance (*Kyo Ka Hi Ko* 脇下痞硬) (Figure 4.8)

  - Bupleurum (*Saiko* 柴胡) family—chronic/Full or Empty

- #7a Epigastric Splash Sound (*Shin Ka Bu Shin Sui On* 心下部振水音) (Figure 4.10)

  - Hoelen (*Bukuryo* 茯苓); Atractylodes (*Jutsu* 朮); Alisma (*Taku Sha* 沢瀉); Polyporus (*Chorei* 猪苓) families

- #7b Epigastric Drumming Sound (*Shin Ka Bu "Don Don"* 心下部どんどん) (Figure 4.10)

  - Bupleurum (*Saiko* 柴胡); Cinnamon (*Keishi* 桂枝); Peony (*Shaku Yaku* 芍薬); *Chi Shi* (*Ki Jitsu* 枳実) families

- #8 Inside Spasm (*Ri Kyu* 裏急) (Figures 4.11 and 4.12)

  - Bupleurum (*Saiko* 柴胡); Cinnamon (*Keishi* 桂枝); Peony (*Shaku Yaku* 芍薬); Maltose (*Koi* 膠飴) families

- #9 Lower Abdominal Tight Spasm (*Sho Fuku Ko Kyu* 小腹拘急) (Figure 4.13)

  - Rehmannia (*Jio* 地黄) family

- #10 Cardiac/Epigastric/Lower Abdominal Pulsations (*Shin Ki/Shin Ka Ki/Sai Ka Ki* 心悸 / 心下悸 / 臍下悸) (Figure 4.14)

  - Dragon Bone (*Ryu Kotsu* 竜骨); Oyster Shell (*Borei* 牡蠣); Cinnamon (*Keishi* 桂枝) families—Cardiac pulsations (*Shin Ki* 心悸)

- Hoelen (*Bukuryo* 茯苓); Atractylodes (*Jutsu* 朮) families—Epigastric pulsations (*Shin Ka Ki* 心下悸)

- Persica Seed (*To Nin* 桃仁); Moutan Bark (*Bo Tan Pi* 牡丹皮); Safflower (*Ko Ka* 紅花) families—Lower Abdominal Pulsations (*Sai Ka Ki* 臍下悸)—Excess

- Rehmannia (*Jio* 地黄); Cnidium (*Sen Kyu* 川芎); *Dang Gui* (*Toki* 当帰) families—Lower Abdominal Pulsations (*Sai Ka Ki* 臍下悸)— Deficiency

- #11 Lower Abdomen Lacking Benevolence (*Sho Fuku Fu Jin* 小腹不仁) (Figures 4.15 and 4.16)

  - Aconite (*Bushi* 附子); Rehmannia (*Jio* 地黄) families

- #12 Lower Abdomen Resistant Fullness (*Sho Fuku [Ko] Man* 小腹[硬]満) (Figures 4.17 and 4.18)

  - Rhubarb (*Daio* 大黄); Persica Seed (*To Nin* 桃仁); Moutan Bark (*Bo Tan Pi* 牡丹皮); Safflower (*Ko Ka* 紅花) families—Lower Abdominal Painful Fullness (*Sho Fuku Ko Man* 小腹硬満)

  - Hoelen (*Bukuryo* 茯苓); Atractylodes (*Jutsu* 朮); Alisma (*Taku Sha* 沢瀉); Polyporus (*Chorei* 猪苓) families—Lower Abdominal Fullness (*Sho Fuku Ko Man* 小腹満)

- #13 Navel Spastic Knot (*Saibu Kyu Ketsu* 臍部急結) (Figure 4.19)

  - Rehmannia (*Jio* 地黄); Cnidium (*Sen Kyu* 川芎); *Dang Gui* (*Toki* 当帰) families

- #14 Lower Abdomen Spastic Knot (*Sho Fuku Kyu Ketsu* 小腹急結) (Figure 4.20)

  - Rhubarb (*Daio* 大黄); Persica Seed (*To Nin* 桃仁); Moutan Bark (*Bo Tan Pi* 牡丹皮); Safflower (*Ko Ka* 紅花) families

5

CONCLUSION

"Medical art is understanding. Understanding arrives through learning. There are no old or new formulas, only efficacious ones."

Kamei Nanmei亀井南冥 (1743–1814), a Japanese Confucian
scholar physician from the late *Edo* period, quoted in the author's
preface of *30 Years of Kampo: Selected Case Studies of an Herbal
Doctor*, Otsuka, K., publ. Oriental Healing Arts Institute, 1984)

WHY I WROTE THIS BOOK

In taking on this project I was faced from the outset with an undeniable paradox: how to write a book (that one reads) focusing on a skill (that one practices). In Chapter 3 I rather disingenuously referred to the fact that the discipline of *Fukushin* cannot truly be learned from a book and requires years of committed practice, preferably alongside a mentor. I stand by that assertion, but nevertheless would argue the case for a book such as this for several reasons.

The first is that our field has a general paucity of such material (especially in English), the kind that focuses on a practical manual discipline and examines it from a cultural, historical, anthropological and medical perspective that includes its direct and specific application in clinical practice. As such, assuming this book does in fact fulfill those claims, I hope it will add to the small library of existing texts dedicated to the subject of the abdomen in traditional medicine.

Secondly, it is my sincere hope to provoke some interest amongst professionals in all disciplines in the growing field (in the West) of what I have tended to refer to as Traditional Japanese Medicine (TJM) and in particular *Kampo*. I appreciate that many readers will be more likely to have a background in Traditional Chinese Medicine (TCM), which in turn would suggest a familiarity with *Pinyin*, the system of romanization of Chinese characters based on their pronunciation. It will not have escaped their attention that this book predominantly uses *Romaji* (the romanization of the Japanese language), and this is a deliberate choice of mine when using medical or historical terms and proper names including those of the formulas. I have done so in the belief that during its 1500 years of sustained cultivation and development, from its initial transmission from and continued interaction with the Chinese mainland, *Kampo* has established its own unique position within the umbrella of East Asian Traditional Medicine. I am borrowing this term from Margaret Lock, Professor of Anthropology at McGill University in Montreal, to denote the plurality of traditional medical practices common to East Asia (*East Asian Medicine in Urban Japan*, 1980, publ. University of California Press). As such, it deserves to be studied and practiced on its own terms, following its own unique linguistic, philosophical and practical landscape, of which *Fukushin* is one (particularly unique) part.

Finally, in developing a passion for *Fukushin* and being someone who originally came into this medicine from a very practical, tactile discipline (*Shiatsu*), I have always had the highest regard for the role of touch in clinical practice. One of my most fervent hopes is that this book may in some small way further the interest in how a practical art such as this can become indispensable in the clinical setting and can act as a transformative experience for patient and practitioner alike. In an era when apparently many of us are all too ready to surrender our hard-earned tactile diagnostic abilities to data-driven technology, to trade our hands-on skills for numbers and images, I hope that this kind of material might spark an interest amongst readers to maintain and improve their own palpation skills.

THE IMPORTANCE OF *SHO* (証)

The concept of *Sho*, as I have attempted to demonstrate in this text, is the cornerstone of the *Kampo* edifice, providing the foundation upon which the entire clinical paradigm is set. The orientation of the structure and process of patient diagnosis and treatment will be determined precisely by one's understanding of this term. In making this claim, I would like in these concluding remarks to examine carefully what exactly we mean by *Sho*, how we define it and in what ways we prejudice and prioritize aspects of its meaning in a clinical setting.

Allow me, in doing so, to summarize some of the things already stated on this topic earlier in this text.

There are multiple translations for the term *Sho* including "Conformation" (Hsu H.Y., 1980), "Pattern" (Kaptchuk T., 2000), "Presentation" (Mitchell *et al.*, 1999) and the ubiquitous "Syndrome" (as used throughout contemporary TCM literature).

In the Japanese *Kampo* tradition, as we have seen, clinical evidence or "proof" is collectively termed the *Sho*, or more properly the *Shokogun* 症候群, a cluster (*Gun*) of symptoms (*Sho*) and prodromes (*Ko*). The Japanese *Kanji* (ideograph) for *Sho* literally suggests a "departure from the norm," deriving from the Daoist concept of illness as representing a deviation from the right(eous), upright or correct path, and is distinguished in Japanese from the term *Byo* 病 (illness). In *Kampo*, the patient *Sho* refers both to the constellation of presenting clinical signs and symptoms including the constitutional strength of the individual (see Chapter 1, "The purpose of the abdominal exam" section for a discussion of Constitutional Patterns (*Taishitsu Sho* 体質証) and Disease Patterns (*Byo Sho* 病証).

As I have suggested, a *Kampo* practitioner's skill lies in their ability to identify a Formula Pattern (*Yakusho* 薬証) in the form of an existing historical prescription that most closely corresponds to the patient *Sho* (the conformation of signs and symptoms including their constitutional tendencies). This process revolves around matching clinically established knowledge (the formula) with the lesser-known variable (the patient) and is wholly dependent on the subjective scrutiny of the clinical gaze. *Sho* thus translates ultimately as a method of treatment rather than referring to either a disease name or a pathological syndrome.

EVIDENCE IS MORE POWERFUL THAN LOGIC?

My deliberate use of this phrase refers to the familiar Japanese proverb, "*Ron Yori Shoko,*" which is one of the 48 proverbs in the *Iroha Karuta*, a Japanese card game dating from the *Tokugawa* Shogunate (1603–1868), which is still used as a way of learning the Japanese phonetic alphabet. There are many literal translations of this proverb, for example, "Proof rather than argument" (Buchanan D., 1987), "A single fact is worth a shipload of arguments" (*Bulletin of the Language Institute of Gakushuin University*, 1998). The closest English vernacular parallel would probably be, "The proof of the pudding is in the eating."

I have generally tended to translate *Sho* as "Pattern" (see the "Glossary of Selected Terms") but in many ways the term "Evidence" is both more accurate and explicit. Whether classifying constitution or disease, whether identifying differential diagnosis or defining treatment strategies, all can be expressed, as we have seen, in terms of their respective *Sho*, which is none other than the empirical "Evidence" put forward to justify any one or all of them.

The abdominal "Evidence" presented in these pages provides one particular lens through which we can better approach an understanding of health and disease. In my humble opinion it happens to be a relatively simple, extremely direct, hands-on way in which to gather clinical evidence in a manner that strikes immediately to the core of one's sensibilities, rather like great music or wine, piercing through intellectual filters, beyond language and reasoning, and registering a rich tapestry of tactile impressions that in turn will ultimately and necessarily submit themselves to scrutiny and interpretation.

I actually began writing this book as a means of motivating myself to consider the various ways in which I myself tend to privilege clinical evidence in my own practice, particularly in regard to tactile evidence and especially in terms of abdominal palpation and findings. My aim was to identify the origin and nature of at least some of my clinical bias and examine its influence on my clinical judgment. I soon realized the enormity of this task as I began grappling with the powerful cultural, linguistic, historical, philosophical and socio-political implications of what constitutes evidence in any discipline, especially one that derives from a culture and is expressed in a language other than one's own.

This, in turn, led me to consider the qualities unique to the two primary paradigms that seem pertinent to this issue: empirical evidence, deriving directly from the senses, and deductive evidence, which is based on logical analysis and reasoning. It is clear to me at this point that my own clinical judgment operates with a healthy measure of bias towards the former, though I am quick to acknowledge that it is this very recognition that happily prevents me from dismissing the value of the latter.

So it is that I often find myself shuffling between privileging evidence I have experienced first-hand in the presence of a patient, versus that which has been transmitted through teachers, texts, related disciplines and other received wisdom emanating from the general discourse of East Asian Medicine. The paradoxical respect I have for both these modes of finding meaning in my work also propels me to treat, teach and occasionally attempt to write.

Choosing to focus on a specific clinical topic through which to frame this enquiry was a deliberate one. As I have attempted to argue in this book, palpation of the abdomen has, since the earliest beginnings of this medicine in *Han* dynasty China, served a significant role in the entire diagnostic and treatment processes of all the major disciplines that make up our medicine. Its continued evolution and survival into the present day in its many forms and iterations is testimony to its clinical effectiveness and enduring appeal to practitioners who value the importance of empirical sensory evidence alongside analytical reasoning in their clinical decision-making.

In the process of writing this text, I have come to a deeper appreciation of my own clinical bias as well as respectfully noting those of others from different traditions. I suspect I have raised many issues that deserve fuller attention elsewhere, but if I have managed to address even some of these interrelated but highly complex issues in a way that seems at least marginally useful to the practicing clinician, I will be happy. The only criticism I will make in this regard is that I cannot agree with any form of conscious and deliberate privileging of what might be characterized as an attempt to distinguish between more or less "valid" evidence. Such entitled claims are newcomers to the history of medical discourse and have yet to demonstrate outcomes that justify such a hierarchical position with regard to ascribing relative validity to differing expressions of evidence.

DEFINITIONS OF EVIDENCE

Evidence is defined generally as information upon which to base a conclusion. Empirical evidence refers in particular to that which can be verified without recourse to theoretical or deductive constructs (*Webster's New World Dictionary*, 2003). The *Kampo* use of the term *Sho* reflects a philosophy, deeply woven into the fabric of Japanese culture, that experience (things that can be seen, smelled, tasted, touched) is able to somehow offer richer intrinsic value to human existence than abstract ideas. This notion of what types of human experience (evidence) are to receive privileged attention permeates Japanese life until today.

One example in the popular culture, which accounts for its enduring significance in the practice of medicine, is of course the symbolic significance of the *Hara* (abdomen) as discussed in detail in Chapter 1. As I have suggested, the locus of feelings within the abdomen is literally evidenced by the use of this term within the framework of the language itself, the implication being that to get to the truth of the matter in any human endeavor, one should trust one's gut instinct rather than one's reasoned explanation.

This example of cultural bias in Japan toward empirical over abstract evidence extends very naturally and explicitly into the realm of medicine. Many of the distinguishing features of *Kampo*, as I have attempted to suggest, reflect this empirical bias and have tended to subjugate the role of abstract theoretical methods of constructing evidence in the clinical setting.

The belief that clinical evidence is most accurately derived from concrete sensory experience runs deep in East Asian Medicine as a whole and is clearly favored in many of the formative classical texts. For example, throughout the text of the *Sho Kan Ron* and *Kin Ki Yo Raku* (see the "Glossary of Selected Terms"), *Zhang Zhong Jing* offers little by way of treatment rationale, preferring instead to suggest succinct descriptions of the empirical evidence in the form of practitioner and patient signs and symptoms and proceeding directly to the appropriate herbal formula that "masters" the situation.

This trend is also found in the indigenous Japanese religion *Shinto* 神道, which influenced the very earliest shamanistic practices pre-dating the arrival of the first medical teachings and texts from mainland China into Japan in the 6th century CE. Even in Japanese *Zen* 禅 we find a reluctance to demonstrate anything other than passing interest in the more abstract Buddhist *Dharma* (teachings), such as reincarnation for example, preferring instead to concentrate practice on the search for attaining Illumination (*Kensho Godo* 見性悟道), in the here-and-now, as an experience that lies within the nature of literally every "sentient being."

When it comes to identifying bias in defining clinical evidence in Japanese medical discourse, as I have attempted to suggest, it could perhaps best be characterized by a statement from one of its more prominent and controversial figures (first introduced in Chapter 2), *Yoshimasu Todo* 吉益東洞. He was influential in reviving an interest amongst *Edo* period *Kampo* practitioners in the Chinese *Han* dynasty classics, epitomized in his exhortation directed at colleagues to "return to the classics." (This slogan was notably adopted by *Yanagiya Sorei* 柳谷素霊 [see Chapter 2] almost 200 years later in his founding of the *Keiraku Chiryo* 経絡治療 movement in early 20th century Japanese Acupuncture circles).

Yoshimasu emphasized empirical focus on the clinical signs and symptoms as representing concrete evidence for the use of a specific matching formula without the need for detailed rationales of etiology and pathogenesis. This method of "Matching Pattern and Treatment (Formula)" (*Ho Sho I Chi* 方証一致) profoundly impacted the *Kampo* community of his day and remains at the core of how we practice now. He relied heavily in this process on empirical evidence derived principally from *Fukushin*, about which he wrote extensively as we have seen (Chapter 2). One of his more famous remarks, said to be his personal motto, will serve here as a summary of this attempt to define the term "evidence" in general, and how it is specifically interpreted in the context of *Kampo*: "Do not speak of what is invisible" (Yasui, 2007).

EVIDENCE IN THE CLINICAL SETTING

This book then is about evidence—in this case, practical evidence in the form of findings obtained from the abdominal exam, the stuff more generally we as clinicians seek to grasp, define, collect, analyze and interpret. It manifests as signs and symptoms, often in the most incoherent of narratives, fueled by snippets of raw, shapeless experience that nonetheless imprint themselves (more randomly than we might admit) on our discriminating sensibilities. It is processed by privileged personal and collective filters into algorithms with sufficient coherence to differentiate a treatment rationale. All this is under the formidable orchestration of what Michel Foucault has famously (and critically) called "the clinical gaze" (Foucault M., 1963).

One way we define clinical evidence is the detailed identification, cataloging and analysis of signs and symptoms. This is precisely the definition of the *Kampo* use of the term *Sho*. In the case of *Fukushin*, as the focus of this book has hopefully demonstrated, each abdominal *Sho* can be defined according to its specific cluster of findings which in turn will correspond sometimes precisely (or at least in part) to matching Formula Evidence (*Yakusho*). This process might unfold equally in either a "context of discovery" or a "context of justification" depending on our biases. For me, any claim for empirical evidence must ultimately survive the litmus test of clinical outcome in order truly to qualify as useful both to the practitioner and the patient. As *Kamei Nanmei* (1743–1814), a Japanese Confucian scholar physician from the late *Edo* period, remarked (quoted above at the beginning of this chapter), "Medical art is understanding. Understanding arrives through learning. There are no old or new formulas, only efficacious ones."

In my definition of clinical evidence as outcome-based, however, I am anxious to distance myself from the term "evidence-based medicine" in its contemporary definition as "the integration of best research evidence with clinical expertise and patient values" (Sackett D., 2000). Not because this description is unappealing (it actually seems to capture a sense of the complex nature and plurality of factors that constitute clinical evidence), but because of the qualitative hierarchy it employs in apparently privileging some findings over others. My problem with this definition of evidence is that it favors "hypothesis-testing systematic research" as yielding knowledge that is more generalizable and therefore in some way more clinically relevant than the anecdotal experiences of "hypothesis-generating clinical experience" (Hoffman I., 2009). Whilst apparently offering a balanced, inclusive definition of clinical evidence, one that would seem to embrace the relative validity of multiple perspectives, it seems to me to point instead to a world of prescriptive authority in healthcare rather than one that generates new and exciting possibilities. I cannot but be reminded of *Animal Farm*'s Napoleon, who Boxer claims "is always right," when he eventually comes up with the commandment to (literally) trump all others, "All animals are created equal, but some are more equal than others" (Orwell G., 1945).

It is my discomfort with this epistemological approach, in which the categorization of clinical evidence into a systematic body of knowledge inevitably leads to standardized diagnoses and interventions, that has always steered me towards the more practical, hands-on methods of obtaining such clinical evidence. For me, *Fukushin* is precisely interesting because of its ability to provide direct sensory input that "opens up" rather than "nails down," that poses rather than answers questions. Indeed, in the diagnostic process, I firmly believe in the power of doubt (and I use the constructive Buddhist definition of the word here as in the three essential conditions for *Zen* practice: Great Faith, Great Doubt, Great Determination) to provide more enriching and nuanced interpretations of clinical evidence than conviction. A line from *In Praise of Shadows* seems relevant here: "We do not dislike everything that shines, but we prefer a pensive shadow to a thin transparence" (Tanizaki J., 1933).

EVIDENCE AND CONTEXT

In this Conclusion, I have tried to emphasize the problematic issue of offering up any iteration of clinical evidence, from whatever tradition, in which one's aim is merely to categorize, explain and justify. I acknowledge the potential danger in this enterprise, seeming as it might to destabilize the carefully crafted relationship between our rational and sensory abilities in clinical work. In my case, far from undermining clinical confidence, this effort has so far contributed in tangible and exciting ways to the quality and satisfaction of my professional life. It is my profound hope that a re-examination of our conceptual and practical relationship to the "evidence" we claim for our work and the factors that determine it, will be of concern, interest and use to colleagues in the field.

As some have pointed out more convincingly than I, there has always existed in the history of recorded medicine a productive tension between medical practice and knowledge when it comes to the validation of clinical evidence (Farquhar J., 1992). Lock, quotes Dubos (the great American microbiologist and experimental pathologist) as identifying these viewpoints as "ontological" versus "physiological," either one being emphasized depending on the prevailing ideas of the time (Lock M., 1980). Some examples might include the rational (Dogmatic) and Empirical schools of Greece and Rome, the Classical (*Koho-Ha*) and Later Generation School (*Gosei-Ha*) Schools of *Kampo* in *Edo* period Japan, or perhaps in the modern era the emergence of "Functional" versus "Biomedical" paradigms.

History, it would seem, has amply exposed the hollowness of successive attempts at privileging any particular expression of clinical evidence at any given point in time. Yet perhaps the most glaring modern example of an attempt to do just that can be found in the very *Hara* of our own profession in the hegemonic narrative of TCM which others have noted has appealed so seductively to the "unambiguous, standardized, packaged approach" inherent in the modern mindset (Fruehauf H., 1999).

Lest I appear overly judgmental, I should acknowledge that I am also of course privileging evidence myself according to my own historical and current biases. As will be apparent to readers, and as I have acknowledged elsewhere, my perspective has been strongly influenced by the philosophy and methodology of the *Koho-Ha* (Classical School) of *Kampo*, which I have attempted to suggest in this book has a highly pragmatic approach to the practice of medicine emphasizing as it does reliance on readily observable and palpable phenomena through skills such as *Fukushin*.

Thus, I am calling attention here to a conscious bias amongst *Kampo* practitioners like myself in favor of clinical findings that can be evidenced through direct contact with the patient over interpretations of a more abstract nature. In particular, my focus on this type of sensory evidence experienced in the moment of the clinical encounter relies heavily on the use of abdominal palpation (*Fukushin*).

EVIDENCE AND SCIENCE

This discussion now assumes a perspective that many contemporary social scientists, historians and philosophers have adopted in challenging the theory of modernization in general and that of scientific knowledge in particular (Leslie, C. and Young, A. 1992). This perspective, post-modern if you will, takes issue with the very notion of "objective" evidence in the physical world, preferring instead the struggle for meaning where universally valid answers do not exist (Weisskopf V., 1972).

Within the social sciences in particular and nowhere more so than in the field of psychoanalysis, the struggle to acknowledge the relative nature of what may be called "evidence," clinical or otherwise, is readily apparent even from the time of Freud. From *Becoming Freud* (Phillips, A. 2016), a recent publication about the early life of the founder of the psychoanalytic movement:

> Freud would let people speak, but be speaking on their behalf when he thought he knew what they were talking about. Science was the kind of knowledge that allowed scientists to speak on other people's behalf, to know better. The doctor knows more about the patient's body than the patient does but there are many ways in which the patient knows and experiences his body in ways the doctor can't. It was this essential perplexity that crystallized in Freud…and that would be the heart of the matter for psychoanalysis.

A propos, in an essay entitled "Attention and Interpretation" appearing in *Clinical Seminars and Other Works* (Bion, W. 2019), examining the nature and expression of the encounter between the psychoanlytic method and science itself, Wilfred Bion concludes:

> What is required is not a base for psycho-analysis and its theories but a science that is not restricted by its genesis in knowledge and sensuous background. It must be a science of at-one-ment. It must have a mathematics of at-one-ment, not identification. There can be no geometry of "similar," "identical" or "equal"; only of analogy.

Indeed, Relativist thinking in modern scientific discourse is quite recent, though already prevalent, inevitably challenging the view of progress in "normal" science (Kuhn T., 1962). Of particular relevance here is the effect such a radical paradigm shift has had on cultural studies of traditional Asian medical systems, the first groundbreaking example of which is found in the Introduction to *Asian Medical Systems* (Leslie C., 1976). Other medical anthropologists have since contributed in important ways to this epistemological debate (Kleinman A., 1980; Lock M., 1980; Ohnuki-Tierney E., 1984), as well as sinologists (Porkert M., 1974; Unschild P., 1988) and historians, amongst whom the work of Joseph Needham is too prolific and influential to begin to quote here. More recently, clinical scholars in our own field have entered the debate (Scheid V., 2002 and 2007; Bensky D., 1990; Fruehauf H., 2010) broadening the scope of the discourse to include concrete clinical issues.

Referring to exactly those issues, in particular the perception and application of evidence in *Kampo* medicine as applied to the practice of *Fukushin*, I want to make a further observation— namely, that this paradigm shift is not limited to the social sciences nor to how their contribution has helped reframe consideration and legitimization of some medical traditions from other parts of the world. It has been taking place within the prevailing medical establishment for some time already here in the West and is fast gathering momentum. In the field of psychology, even in Freud's lifetime, there were those who questioned the validity of one of his models of clinical evidence (dream analysis), proposing instead a less abstract relational methodology of practice focusing on sensory participant observation (Sullivan H., 1953).

Indeed, Hans Strupp, a German psychologist and analyst who fled Nazi Germany to study psychology at George Washington University (whose Department of Psychiatry had been founded by Sullivan) claimed: "Given the uniqueness of every therapeutic dyad and the multitude of relevant interacting variables influencing the course of treatment, the 'empirical validation' of any therapy is utterly illusory." This quote appeared in a brilliant article by Irwin Hoffman, "Double-thinking our way to 'scientific' legitimacy: the desiccation of human experience," in which he argues an even more interesting and controversial point: "Is it desirable, clinically, for a practitioner to have a mind-set in which he or she even aspires to 'know' what 'standard intervention' to apply in working with a particular patient at a particular moment?" (Hoffman I., 2009).

He goes on to perfectly capture the essence of the paradigm shift referred to here as suggestive of a move away from mere analysis and justification toward a more constructive, relational engagement between the patient and practitioner. He points out that this inevitably requires more, not less, subjective reflection and criticism between and by both parties toward an inclusive, not exclusive therapeutic end.

I will conclude this examination of some of the recent attention to genuinely alternative ways of thinking that exist in orthodox medical circles, even in the most hallowed halls and classrooms of renowned medical institutions here in the US, with a reference that really surprised me in several ways. In a relatively recent article in the *New England Journal of Medicine*, a well-published and not uncontroversial husband and wife team, both M.D.s at Beth Israel Deaconess Medical Center in Boston (Harvard Medical School's teaching hospital), raised some striking concerns about the current state of modern medical practice in the US (Hartzband P. and Groopman J., 2011). I will not attempt here to do justice to this provocative and courageous article, but in essence, these esteemed authors, champions themselves of the prevailing medical establishment, dared to question both the ethical and clinical validity of modern medicine from the linguistic, economic and socio-political perspective. The alarm has been raised, the post, post-modern era in medicine is upon us!

PARTING WORDS

I have tried in my concluding remarks to reach out in a number of directions, perhaps too many for one single chapter. My main intention was to point to the inherent biases of the clinical filters we all use to confirm what we refer to as evidence in all its forms. I have tried to suggest that the only real evidence of which we can authentically speak with any conviction is that of the patient's progress. My method of attempting to achieve this has been to subvert the tendency to categorize and explain clinical outcomes within some kind of uber-rational paradigm. Instead I have put forward the practice of *Fukushin* as a practical method of gathering sensory clinical evidence that can be formulated as an open-ended expression of multiple possible interpretations on multiple dimensions of human experience as it relates to health and disease.

In this enterprise, I have to thank my many teachers, colleagues and students for constantly offering unique and unexpected challenges to the accepted wisdom that the richer one's clinical experience, the more positive will be the clinical outcome. Not necessarily. "But habit is a great deadener," says Vladimir in *Waiting for Godot* (Beckett S., 1952), and "experience" can surely sometimes pass for a whole lot of unchallenged and repeated mistakes, especially in spaces where powerful transference is at work. I am also deeply indebted to Dr. Orna Guralnik for the amazing gift of demonstrating to me the concrete benefits of serious interdisciplinary study in lending meaning to the life of the practicing clinician. I have been inspired by her seamless and skillful application of conspicuously abstract theories drawn from the contemporary post-modern discourse (in particular those deriving from structuralist and cultural theory), in her work as an analyst and clinical psychologist and in her considerable body of published work, amongst which perhaps her most recent is quite related to this chapter (Guralnik O., 2011). This has encouraged me to re-examine my own relationship to clinical evidence from the perspective of language, culture and society and, I believe, to begin to open up a space for myself to experiment, reflect and begin to truly learn.

On that note, and in the spirit of self-reflection, I will be curious to hear my college-aged daughter's response to these concluding remarks. I can already imagine her having quite a stern reaction to what she (and other generation y/z'ers) might claim as the epitome of "cultural appropriation," in this case committed by her father, a white male, in respect to his characterization of and pronouncements about aspects of a culture other than his own. I'm not sure I am equipped with an adequate defense in that particular case.

Meanwhile, my current interpretation of the earlier subheading in this conclusion, "Evidence is more powerful than logic?" (deliberately posed as a question), no longer reflects a belief that practical experience is somehow intrinsically more legitimate than abstract thinking, rather that they exist on the same continuum, constantly complementing, opposing and interacting with one another. With this in mind, I refer the reader back to a quote, once again from Dr. *Otsuka*, I offered at the beginning of Chapter 3: "Skill comes before study, and lack of skill is just like a fading flower for it looks pitiful."

In apparent contradiction to what I may seem to have been arguing throughout these conclusory remarks, I will allow myself to attempt an interpretation of this quote, as I believe it may carry some unwarranted and misleading emphasis in translation. I prefer to think that Dr. *Otsuka*, his own life-example an epitome of inclusive respect for medical diversity and tradition, is not commenting here on the hierarchical importance of skill (we might say sensory experience) over study (we might say abstract logic), rather that when the realm of ideas is firmly couched within the immediacy of one's authentic, lived experience, as opposed to shaping and directing it, the richness, color and fragrance of the resulting bloom will effortlessly overshadow its impermanence.

It is significant to me that *Otsuka* clearly held both a deep respect for the purist ways of his teacher, *Kyushin Yumoto* 湯本求真 (1876–1941), as well as a willingness to break with tradition and attempt more diversity in his own clinical process. This commitment to plurality in medical practice can be perceived in his positive response to a challenging question put to him by one of his later teachers, *Kenji Kakuya*, quoted in his preface to *30 Years of Kampo* (Otsuka K., 1984): "You say that you belong to the school of old formulas, a school that tolerates no dissent from other schools. Don't you think this is a weakness of the school of the old formulas?"

So, in concluding this discussion on evidence and indeed the wider presentation in this book of *Fukushin* as one of the key protagonists in the process of gathering such evidence, I would humbly suggest that to practice *Kampo* without palpating the abdomen is to me like watching a nature program on a screen. Of course, you can get a sense of being there, even perhaps claim you can almost "feel" its qualities and power, yet how much richer and deeper the experience of actually stepping outside your door! Touching another is a direct and very real human encounter that does not eclipse an intellectual response but stands alongside it as a rich sensory complement to the overall human experience. I hope this book will in some way contribute to the depth and richness of that experience for you.

Selected Bibliography

Agnes, M. (2003) *Websters New World Dictionary*. New York, NY: Pocket Books.

Angurarohita P. (1989). Buddhist influence on the neo-Confucianist concept of the sage. *Sino-Platonic Papers* 10 June, 20.

Aryoshi S. (1966). *The Doctor's Wife*. New York: Kodansha International (1978).

Basho M. (1693). The Rustic Gate. In W. De Bary, D. Keene and R. Tsunoda (eds.) *Sources of Japanese Tradition*, Vol. 2. New York: Columbia University Press (2005).

Beckett S. (1952). *Waiting for Godot*. New York: Grove Press.

Bensky, D. and Barolet, R. (1990) *Chinese Herbal Medicine: Formulas and Strategies* (English and Chinese Edition). Seattle, WA: Eastland Press.

Bion W. (2019). *Clinical Seminars and Other Works*. London: Routledge.

Buchanan D. (1987). *Japanese Proverbs and Sayings*. Norman: University of Oklahoma Press.

Bulletin of the Language Institute of Gakushuin University (1998) No.22, 40–62.

Daidoji K. (2013). The adaptation of the treatise on cold damage in eighteenth century Japan. *Asian Medicine* 8, 2, 361–393.

Dann, J. (2005) Koshi-Balancing – a method of structural alignment and therapy. *North American Journal of Oriental Medicine*, 12, 34, 17.

Dawes N. (2002). Kampo medicine: ancient art, modern science #1. *NAJOM* 9, 25, 22.

Dawes, N. (2012). Evidence is more powerful then logic. *The Lantern, 9 1*,10.

Dogen, E. (1766) "The Treasury of the True Dharma Eye" (*Shōbōgenzō* 正法眼蔵), compiled between 1231-1253, first published in Japanese in 1766.

Durckheim K. (1956). *Hara—The Vital Center of Man* (English translation from German). Rochester: Inner Traditions (2004).

Farquhar J. (1992). Time and Text: Approaching Chinese Medical Practice through Analysis of a Published Case. In C. Leslie and A. Young (eds.) *Paths to Asian Medical Knowledge*. Berkeley: University of California Press, p.62.

Foucault M. (1963). *Naissance de la Clinique*. Paris: Presses Universitaires de France.

Fruehauf H. (1999). Chinese medicine in crisis: science, politics and the making of TCM. *The Journal of Chinese Medicine* 61, 6–14.

Guralnik O. (2011). Raven: Travels in Reality. In M. Dimen (ed.) *With Culture in Mind: Psycholanalytical Stories*. New York: Routledge.

Hartzband P. and Groopman J. (2011). The new language of medicine. *New England Journal of Medicine* 365, 1372–1373.

Hoffman I. (2009). Double-thinking our way to "scientific" legitimacy: the desiccation of human experience. *Journal of the American Psychiatric Association* 57, 1043.

Hsu H.-Y. (1980). *Commonly Used Chinese Herbal Formulas with Illustrations*. Long Beach: Oriental Healing Arts Institute.

Hsu H.-Y. (1990). *Commonly Used Chinese Herbal Formulas with Illustrations—Companion Handbook*. Long Beach: Oriental Healing Arts Institute.

Hsu H.-Y and Preacher W. (1981). *Shang Han Lun—The Great Classic of Chinese Medicine* (English translation from Japanese by K. Otsuka). Long Beach: Oriental Healing Arts Institute.

Hsu H.-Y. and Wang S.-Y. (1983). *Prescriptions from the Golden Chamber* (English translation from Chinese). Long Beach: Oriental Healing Arts Institute.

Hsu H.-Y. and Wang S.-Y. (1985). *The Theory of Feverish Diseases and Its Clinical Applications*. Long Beach: Oriental Healing Arts Institute.

Huang H. (2009). *Ten Key Formula Families in Chinese Medicine*. Seattle: Eastland Press.

Huang H. (2009). *Zhang Zhong Jing's Clinical Application of 50 Medicinals*. Beijing: People's Medical Publishing House.

Huang H. (2011). *Huang Huang's Guide to Clinical Application of Classical Formulas*. Beijing: People's Medical Publishing House.

Inaba K. B. (1800). *Extraordinary Views of Abdominal Patterns: Fukusho—Kiran*. Transl. J. Kageyama Portland: The Chinese Medicine Database (2018).

Kaibara E. (1991). *Lessons for Nourishing Life, 1713*. Reprint annotated by K. Ishikawa. Tokyo: Iwanami.

Kaptchuk T. (2000). *The Web That Has No Weaver*. New York: Contemporary Books.

Karchmer E. (2013). Ancient formulas to strengthen the nation: healing the modern Chinese body with the treatise on cold damage. *Asian Medicine* 8, 2, 394–422.

Keijuro W. (1910). A bibliographic sketch of Master Todo Yoshimasu #20. *NAJOM* 10, 29, 26.

Kleinman A. (1980). *Patients and Healers in the Context of Culture*. Los Angeles: University of California Press.

Kuhn T. (1962). *The Structure of Scientific Revolutions*. Chicago: University of Chicago Press.

Kuriyama S. (1997). On Stiff-shoulders. In K. Yamada and S. Kuriyama (eds.) *Illness and Medicine in History*. Kyoto: Shibunkaku, pp.37–62.

Kyushin, (1908) Sino-Japanese Medicine Akashi shuppan, Tokyo, 2018.

Leslie C. (1976). *Asian Medical Systems*. Berkeley: University of California Press.

Leslie C. and Young A. (eds) (1992). *Paths to Asian Medical Knowledge*. Berkeley: University of California Press.

Liao Y. (1997). The Characteristics of Early Abdominal Diagnosis Texts. In K. Yamada and S. Kuriyama (eds.) *Illness and Medicine in History*. Kyoto: Shibunkaku, pp.343–369.

Lock M. (1980). *East Asian Medicine in Urban Japan*. Berkeley: University of California Press.

Lu, Y., 陆 渊雷, 1931. Shanghan lun jinshuo 伤寒论今释 ("A Modern Interpretation of the Treatise on Cold Damage") Boo Yanju, 鲍 艳举, Baojin Hua, 花宝金, Wei Hou, 炜 侯., editors. Beijing: Academy Press.

Manase D. (1986). The Illustrations and Explanations of a Hundred Patterns of Abdomen. In *The Compilation of Japanese Abdominal Diagnosis Texts 6*. Osaka: Orient Shuppan.

Matsumoto K. and Birch S. (1988). *Hara Diagnosis: Reflections on the Sea*. Taos: Paradigm Publications.

Mitchell C., Ye F. and Wiseman N. (1999). *Shang Han Lun: On Cold Damage, Translation and Commentaries*. Taos: Paradigm Publications.

Ogyū S. (2006). *Ogyū Sorai's Philosophical Masterworks: The Bendō and Benmei*. Translation of annotated eighteenth-century edition with an introduction by John A. Tucker, transl. Hawaii: University of Hawaii Center for Korean Studies.

Ohnuki-Tierney E. (1984). *Illness and Culture in Contemporary Japan*. Cambridge: Cambridge University Press.

Orwell G. (1945). *Animal Farm*. London: Secker and Warburg.

Ōtsuka, K. (1934) 大塚 敬節. Ruisho *Kanbetsu Kani Yoketsu* (*Leizheng jianbie hanyi yaojue*) 類證鑒別漢醫要訣 (The Key to Classifying and Discriminating Presentations in Kampo Medicine) In: *Shenfang Tang*, 唐 慎坊., translators. *Suzhou Guoyi Zazhi* 蘇州國醫雜誌 (*Suzhou* Journal of National Medicine) 2, 4.

Otsuka K. (1956). *Kampo: A Clinical Guide to Theory and Practice*. Transl. G. De Soriano and N. Dawes. Oxford: Churchill Livingstone (2010). London: Singing Dragon (2017).

Otsuka K. (1979). Commentary on Yoshimazu Todo #20. *NAJOM* 10, 29, 26.

Otsuka K. (1981). Annotation on Yoshimasu Tōdō. In *Compilation of Japanese Philosophy 63: Modern Science Philosophy Vol. 2*. Tokyo: Iwanami.

Otsuka K. (1984). *30 Years of Kampo: Selected Case Studies of an Herbal Doctor*. Long Beach: Oriental Healing Arts Institute.

Otsuka Y. (1976). Chinese Traditional Medicine in Japan. In C. Leslie (ed.) *Asian Medical Systems*. Berkeley: University of California Press, pp.322–340.

Pert C. (1997). *Molecules of Emotion: Why You Feel the Way You Feel*. New York: Simon and Schuster.

Phillips A. (2016). *Becoming Freud: The Making of a Psychoanalyst* (Jewish Lives). New Haven: Yale University Press.

Porkert M. (1974). *Theoretical Foundations of Chinese Medicine* (East Asian Science). Cambridge: MIT Press.

Sackett D. (2000). Evidence-Based Medicine: How to Practice and Teach. In *Evidence Based Medicine*, 2nd edn. Edinburgh: Churchill Livingstone.

Scheid V. (2002). *Chinese Medicine in Contemporary China: Plurality and Synthesis*. Durham: Duke University Press.

Scheid V. (2004). Restructuring the field of Chinese medicine: a study of the Menghe and Ding scholarly currents, 1600–2000 (Part 1). *East Asian Science, Technology and Medicine* 22, 10–68.

Scheid V. (2007). *Currents of Tradition in Chinese Medicine 1626–2006*. Seattle: Eastland Press.

Scheid V. (2013). Patterns, syndromes, types: who should we be and what should we do? *European Journal of Oriental Medicine* 7, 3, 10–21.

Scheid V. (2013). Transmitting Chinese medicine: changing perceptions of body, pathology and treatment in late Imperial China. *Asian Medicine* 8, 2, 299–360.

Scheid V. (2013). The treatise on cold damage as a window on emergent formations of medical practice in East Asia. *Asian Medicine* 8, 2, 295–298.

Scheid V. (2014). Convergent lines of descent: symptoms, patterns, constellations, and the emergent interface of systems biology and Chinese medicine. *East Asian Science, Technology and Society* 8, 1, 107–139.

Scheid V., Bensky D., Ellis A. and Barolet R. (2009). *Chinese Herbal Medicine, Formulas and Strategies*, 2nd edn. Seattle: Eastland Press.

Sella, Y. (2018). *From Dualism to Oneness in Psychoanalyisis*. Oxford: Routledge.

Sullivan H. (1953). *Interpersonal Theory of Psychiatry*. New York: Norton.

Suzuki S. (1998). *Zen Mind, Beginner's Mind*. New York: Weatherhill.

Tanizaki J. (1933). *In Praise of Shadows*. Sedgwick: Leete's Island Books (1977).

Terasawa K. (2012). *A Study of Yoshimasu Tōdo: The Idea of Creating Japanese Kanpo*. Tokyo: Iwanami.

Unschuld P. (1988). *Medicine in China: A History of Ideas*. Berkeley: University of California Press.

Wada T. (1821). "Idle Talk Under Palm Trees." Facsimiled in 2001. 4th edn (Vol. 15). Pittsburgh: KKIS.

Watanabe K. (2013). *Clinical Pearls for Kampo Medicine*. Tokyo: Nankodo.

Weisskopf V. (1972). *Physics in the 20th Century: Selected Essays by Victor Frederick Weisskopf*. Cambridge: MIT Press.

Westen D. (2002). The language of psychoanalytic discourse. *Psychoanalytic Dialogues* 12, 857–898.

Willberg P. (2003). *Head, Heart and Hara: The Soul Centres of West and East*. UK: New Gnosis Publications.

Wiseman N. (2014). *A Practical Dictionary of Chinese Medicine*. Boulder: Paradigm Publications.

Yakubo S., Ito M., Ueda Y., Okamoto H., *et al.* (2014). Pattern classification in Kampo medicine. *Evidence-Based Complementary and Alternative Medicine*, https://dx.doi.org/10.1155%2F2014%2F535146

Yamada T. (2009). All about abdominal palpation: the traditional diagnosis method. *Kampo Medicine* 60, 6.

Yasui H. (2007). History of Kampo medicine. *KAIM* 1 (Special edition), 3–9.

Yasui, H. (2007) Medical History in Japan – Todo Yoshimasu and his Medicine. *KAIM* 2, 32.

Yoshimasu T. *Abdominal Diagnosis of Master Tōdō's School: Theory and Illustrations*. Facsimile available at Kyoto University Digital Library, http://m.kulib.kyotou.ac.jp/webopac/ufirdi.do?ufi_target=catdbl&ufi_locale=ja&pkey=RB00000283

Romaji/Pinyin/English Formula Cross-Reference

Romaji Japanese name	Kanji Characters	Pinyin Chinese name	*Commonly Used Chinese Herbal Formulas with Illustrations* (Hong-Yen Hsu 1980)	*Chinese Herbal Medicine, Formulas and Strategies* (Scheid *et al.* 2009)
Anchu San	安中散	*An Zhong San*	Cardamom and Fennel Combination pp.366	Calm the middle powder p.268
Bakumondo To	麦門冬湯	*Maimendong tang*	Ophiopogon Combination p.537	Ophiopogonis Decoction pp.670–673
Bofutsu Sho San	防风通圣丸	*Fang Feng Tong Sheng San*	Siler and Platycodon Combination p.119	Saposhnikovia Powder that Sagely unblocks pp.290–292
Boi Ogi To	防已黄耆湯	*Fang Ji Huang Qi Tang*	Stephania and Astragalus Combination p.477	Stephania and Astragalus Decoction pp.735–737
Bukuryo In	茯苓飲	*Fu Ling Yin*	Hoelen Combination p.485	Omitted. Rx from the *Kin Ki Yo Ryaku* 金匱要略
Bukuryo Takusha To	茯苓泽瀉湯	*Fu Ling Ze Xie Tang*	Alisma and Hoelen Combination p.483	Omitted. Rx from the *Kin Ki Yo Ryaku* 金匱要略

Romaji Japanese name	Kanji Characters	Pinyin Chinese name	Commonly Used Chinese Herbal Formulas with Illustrations (Hong-Yen Hsu 1980)	Chinese Herbal Medicine, Formulas and Strategies (Scheid et al. 2009)
Bun Sho To	分消湯	Fen Xiao tang	Hoelen andf Alisma Combination p.205	Separate and Reduce Decoction p.689
Bushi Richu To	附子理中湯	Fu Zi Li Zhong Tang	Aconite, Ginseng and Ginger Combination p.287	Aconite Accessory Root Pill to Regulate the Middle p.261
Bushi To	附子湯	Fu Zi Tang	Aconite Combination p.288	Aconite Accessory Root Decoction pp.747–749
Byaku Ko To	白虎湯	Bai hu Tang	Gypsum Combination p.185	White Tiger Decoction pp.150–154
Chi Baku Hachimi Gan	知柏八味丸	Zi Bo Ba Wei Wan (Zhi Bai Di Huang Wan)	Anemarrhena, Phellodendron and Rehmannia Formula p.230	Anemarrhena, Phellodendron and Rehmannia Pill p.369
Chikuyo Sekko To	竹葉石膏湯	Zhu Ye Shi Gao Tang	Bamboo Leaves and Gypsum Combination p.220	Lophatherum and Gypsum Decoction pp.155–157
Choijoki To	调胃承气汤	Tiao Wei Cheng Qi Tang	Rhubarb and Mirabilitum Combination p.154	Regulate the Stomach and Order the Qi Decoction p.67
Chorei To	猪苓湯	Zhu Ling Tang	Polyporus Combination p.472	Polyporus Decoction pp.729–731
Choto San	釣藤散	Gou Teng San	Gambir Formula p.386	Uncaria Powder p.813
Chu Ken Chu To	中建中湯	Zhong Jian Zhong Tang	Omitted. Dr. Otsuka's Middle Build the Middle Formula	Omitted. Made by combining Dai Kenchu To with Sho Kenchu To
Dai Jyoki To	大承気湯	Da Cheng Qi Tang	Major Rhubarb Combination p.145	Major Order the Qi Decoction pp.63–66

Dai Kenchu To	大建中湯	Da Jian Zhong tang	Major Zanthoxylum Combination p.315	Major Construct the Middle Decoction pp.268–270
Daio Botanpi To	大黄牡丹皮湯	Da Huang Mu Dan (Pi) tang	Rhubarb and Moutan Combination p.626	Rhubarb and Moutan Decoction pp.880–882
Dai Saiko* To	大柴胡湯	Da Chai Hu Tang	Major Bupleurum Combination p.128	Major Bupleurum Decoction pp.286–289
En-nen Hange To	延年半夏湯	Yan Nian Ban Xia Tang	Evodia and Pinellia Combination p.411	Pinellia Decoction to Extend Life p.264
Eppi Ka Jutsu To	越婢加朮湯	Yue Bi Jia Zhu Tang	Atractylodes Combination p.523	Maidservant from Yue's Decoction plus Atractylodes p.185
Go*rei San	五苓散	Wu Ling San	Hoelen Five Combination p.516	Five Ingredient Powder with Poria pp.724–728
Go Sha Jin Ki gan	牛車腎気丸	Niu Che Shen Qi Wan	Achyranthes and Plantago Formula p.247	Omitted. From the Ji Sheng Fang by Yan Yonghe (Jin-Yuan period)
Go*shuyu To	呉茱萸湯	Wu Zhu Yu Tang	Evodia Combination p.325	Evodia Decoction pp.261–264
Hachimi Gan (Hachimi Jio Gan, Jinki Gan)	八味丸（八味地黄丸、腎気丸）	Ba Wei Di Huang Wan (aka Ba Wei Wan or Jin Gui Shen Qi Wan)	Rehmannia Eight Combination p.250	Eight-Ingredient Pill with Rehmannia p.369
Hange Byakujutsu Tenma To	半夏白朮天麻湯	Ban Xia Bai Zhu Tian Ma Tang	Pinellia and Gastrodia Combination p.561	Pinellia, White Atractylodes Macrocephala and Gastrodia Decoction pp.811–812
Hange Koboku To	半夏厚朴湯	Ban Xia Hou Pu Tang	Pinellia and Magnolia Combination p.395	Pinellia and Magnolia Bark Decoction pp.516–519

Romaji Japanese name	Kanji Characters	Pinyin Chinese name	*Commonly Used Chinese Herbal Formulas with Illustrations* (Hong-Yen Hsu 1980)	*Chinese Herbal Medicine, Formulas and Strategies* (Scheid *et al.* 2009)
Hange Shashin To	半夏瀉心湯	*Ban Xia Xie Xin Tang*	Pinellia Combination p.105	Pinellia Decoction to Drain the Epigastrium pp.127–130
*Ho*chu Ekki To*	補中益気湯	*Bu Zhong Yi Qi tang*	Ginseng and Astragalus Combination p.255	Tonify the Middle and Augment the *Qi* Decoction p.317–322
Ho In to	補陰湯	*Bu Yin Tang*	*Tang-Kuei* and Rehmannia Combination p.259	Omitted. From the *Wan Bing Hui Chun* compiled by *Gong Tingxian* in the *Ming* dynasty
Hon Ton To	奔豚湯	*Ben tun Tang*	Pueraria and Ginger Combination	Omitted. Rx from the *Kin Ki Yo Ryaku* 金匱要略 (chapter on *Ben Tun*)
Inchin Gorei San	茵蔯五苓散	*Yin Chen Wu Ling San*	Capillaris and Hoelen Combination p.521	Virgate Wormwood and Five Ingredient Powder with Poria p.729
Inchinko To	茵蔯蒿湯	*Yin Chen Hao Tang*	Capillaris Combination p.519	Virgate Wormwood Decoction pp.710–712
I Rei To	胃苓湯	*Ping Wei San*	Magnolia and Hoelen Combination p.512	Calm the Stomach Powder pp.687–688
Isho Ho	痿証方	*Wei Zheng Fang*	Eucommia and Achyranthes Combination p.274	Omitted. Japanese Rx by *Hukui Futei* appearing in *Kampo Shinryo Iten* compiled by *Domei Yakazu et al.*

Ji In Ko Ka To	滋陰降火湯	*Zi Yin Jiang Huo Tang*	Phellodendron Combination p.199	Decoction to Enrich *Yin* and Direct Fire Downward pp.388–389
Ju Mi Bai Doku to	十味敗毒湯	*Shi Wei Bai Du Tang*	Bupleurum and Schizonepeta Combination p.624	Ten Ingredient Powder to Overcome Toxicity pp.872–873. Experimental Formula by *Hanaoka Seshu* (1760–1835)
*Ju*zen Taiho* To*	十全大補湯	*Shi Quan Da Bu Tang*	Ginseng and Tang-Kuei Ten Combination p.262	All Inclusive Great Tonifying Decoction pp.348–350
Kami Kihi To	加味帰脾湯	*Jia Wei Gui Pi Tang*	Ginseng, Longan and Bupleurum Combination p.416	Omitted. Augmented Restore the Spleen Decoction
Kami Shoyo San	加味逍遥散	*Jia Wei Xiao Yao San*	Bupleurum and Peony Combination p.87	Augmented Rambling Powder p.124
Kanbaku Taiso To	甘麦大棗湯	*Gan Mai Da Zao Tang*	Licorice and Jujube Combination p.347	Licorice, Wheat and Jujube Decoction pp.471–474
Kanzo Bushi To	甘草附子湯	*Gan Cao Fu Zi Tang*	Licorice and Aconite Combination p.298	Licorice and Aconite Accessory Root Decoction p.749
Kanzo Shashin To	甘草瀉心湯	*Gan Cao Xie Xin Tang*	Pinellia and Licorice Combination p.103	Licorice Decoction to Drain the Epigastrium p.130
Keishi Bukuryo Gan	桂枝茯苓丸	*Gui Zhi Fu Ling Wan*	Cinnamon and Hoelen Combination p.423	Cinnamon Twig and Poria Pill pp.583–586
Keishi Ka Bushi To	桂枝加附子湯	*Gui Zhi Jia Fu Zi Tang*	Cinnamon and Aconite Combination p.302	Cinnamon Twig plus Aconite Accessory Root Decoction p.19

Romaji Japanese name	Kanji Characters	Pinyin Chinese name	*Commonly Used Chinese Herbal Formulas with Illustrations* (Hong-Yen Hsu 1980)	*Chinese Herbal Medicine, Formulas and Strategies* (Scheid *et al.* 2009)
Keishi Ka Ryukotsu Borei To	桂枝加竜骨牡蠣湯	*Gui Zhi Jia Long Gu Mu Li Tang*	Cinnamon and Dragon Bone Combination p.351	Cinnamon Twig Decoction plus Dragon Bone and Oyster Shell pp.439–441
Keishi Ka Shakuyaku To	桂枝加芍薬湯	*Gui Zhi Jia Shao Yao Tang*	Cinnamon and Peony Combination p.60	Cinnamon Twig Decoction plus Peony p.18
Keishi To	桂枝湯	*Gui Zhi Tang*	Cinnamon Combination p.63	Cinnamon Twig Decoction pp.13–18
Ki Pi to	帰脾湯	*Gui Pi Tang*	Ginseng and Longan Combination p.425	Restore the Spleen Decoction pp.353–355
Ko Sha Rikkunshito	香砂六君子湯	*Xiang Sha Liu Jun Zi Tang*	Cardamom and Saussurea Combination	Six Gentlemen Decoction with Aucklandia and Amomum p.312
Kyu Ki Kyogai To	芎帰膠艾湯	*Xiong Gui Jiao Ai Tang*	*Dang Gui and Gelatin Combination p.576*	Omitted. Rx from the *Kin Ki Yo Ryaku* 金匱要略
Mao Bushi Kanzo To	麻黄細辛甘草湯	*Mahuang Fu Zi Gan Cao tang*	Mahuang Aconite and Licorice Combination p.74	Ephedra, Aconite Accessory Root and Licorice Decoction p.52
Mao Bushi Sai Shin To	麻黄細辛附子湯	*Mahuang Xixin Fu Zi Tang*	Mahuang and Asarum Combination p.72	Ephedra, Aarum and Aconite Accessory Root Decoction pp.50–52
Ma Shi Nin Gan	麻子仁丸	*Ma Zi Ren Wan*	Apricot Seed and Linum Formula p.535	Hemp Seed Pill pp.81–83
Ninjin To (Richu To)	人参湯(理中湯)	*Ren Shen Tang (Li Zhong Tang)*	Ginseng and Ginger Combination p.295	Regulate the Middle Pill pp.257–260

Ninjin Yoei To	人参養榮湯	*Ren Shen Yang Rong Wan*	Ginseng Nutritive Combination p.239	Ginseng Decoction to Nourish Luxuriance pp.350–352
Ogi Kenchu To	黄耆建中湯	*Huang Qi Jian Zhong Tang*	Astragalus Combination p.293	Astragalus Decoction to Construct the Middle p.267
Oren Akyo To	黄連阿膠湯	*Huang Lian E Jiao Tang*	Coptis and Gelatin Combination p.97	Coptis and Ass-Hide Gelatin Decoction pp.469–470
Oren Gedoku To	黄連解毒湯	*Huang Lian Jie Du Tang*	Coptis and Scute Combination p.175	Coptis Decoction to Resolve Toxicity pp.167–169
Oren To	黄連湯	*Huang Lian Tang*	Coptis Combination p.98	Coptis Decoction pp.131–133
Otsuji To	乙字湯	*Yi Zi Tang*	Cimicifuga Combination p.613	Decoction "B" p.607. Japanese Rx from the *Asada No Shoho* by *Asada Sohaku*
Rikkunshi To	六君子湯	*Liu Jun Zi Tang*	Major-Six Herb Combination p.242	Six Gentlemen Decoction pp.311–312
Rokumijiogan	六味地黄丸	*Liu Wei Di Huang Wan*	Rehmannia Six Combination p.245	Six Ingredient Pill with Rehmannia pp.365–368
Ryo Kei Jutsu Kan To	苓桂朮甘湯	*Ling Gui Zhu Gan Tang*	Atractylodes and Hoelen Combination p.493	Poria, Cinnamon Twig, Atractylodes and Licorice Decoction pp.738–741
Ryo Kei Kanso To	苓桂甘棗湯	*Ling Gui gan Cao tang*	Hoelen, Licorice and Jujube Combination p.495	Omitted. Rx from the *Kin Ki Yo Ryaku* 金匱要略 (chapter on *Ben Tun*)
Ryutan Shokan To	龙胆泻肝汤	*Long Dan Xie Gan Tang*	Gentiana Combination p.181	Gentiana Decoction to Drain the Liver p.201

Romaji Japanese name	Kanji Characters	Pinyin Chinese name	Commonly Used Chinese Herbal Formulas with Illustrations (Hong-Yen Hsu 1980)	Chinese Herbal Medicine, Formulas and Strategies (Scheid et al. 2009)
Sai Boku To	柴朴柴	Chai Pu Tang	Bupleurum and Magnolia Combination	Omitted. Combination of Sho Saiko To and Hange Ko Boku To
Sai Kan To	柴陥柴	Chai Xian Tang	Bupleurum and Scute Combination p.543	Omitted. From the Shen Shi Zun Sheng Shu compiled by Shen Qian-Lu
Saiko* Ka Ryukotsu Borei To	柴胡加竜 骨牡蠣湯	Chai Hu Jia Long Gu Mu Li Tang	Bupleurum and Dragon Bone Combination p.340	Bupleurum plus Dragon Bone and Oyster Shell Decoction pp.113–116
Saiko* Keishi Kankyo To	柴胡桂枝 乾姜湯	Chai Hu Gui (Zhi) (Gan) Jiang Tang	Bupleurum, Cinnamon and Ginger Combination p.85	Bupleurum, Cinnamon Twig and Ginger Decoction pp.140–142
Saiko* Keishi To	柴胡桂枝 湯	Chai Hu Gui Zhi Tang	Bupleurum and Cinnamon Combination p.117	Bupleurum and Cinnamon Twig Decoction pp.109–110
Saiko Seikan To	柴胡清肝 湯	Chai Hu Qing Gan Tang	Bupleurum and Rehmannia Combination p.160	Bupleurum Decoction to Clear the Liver pp.202–203
Saiko Sokan San	柴胡疎肝 散	Chai Hu Shu Gan San	Bupleurum and Cyperus Formula	Bupleurum Powder to Dredge the Liver pp.512–513
Sairei To	柴苓湯	Chai Ling Tang	Bupleurum and Hoelen Combination p.464	Omitted. Combination of Sho Saiko To and Go Rei San.
Sanmotsu Ogon To	三物黄芩 湯	San Wu Huang Qin Tang	Scute Three Herb Combination p.192	Omitted. Rx from the Kin Ki Yo Ryaku 金匱 要略

San O Shashin To	三黄瀉心湯	San Huang Xie Xin Tang	Coptis and Rhubarb Combination p.190	Omitted. Rx from the *Kin Ki Yo Ryaku* 金匱要略
Sei Shin Ren Shi In	清心蓮子飲	Qing Xin Lian Zi Yin	Lotus Seed Combination p.164	Clear the Heart Drink with Lotus Seed pp.197–199
Sen Puku Ko Tai Shoseki To	旋覆代赭石湯	Xuan Fu Dai Zhe Shi Tang	Inula and Hematite Combination p.384	Inula and Hematite Decoction pp.542–544
Sessho In	蛰虫飲	Zhe Chong Yin	Cinnamon and Persica Combination p.573	Drink to Turn back the Penetrating (Vessel) p.586. Japanese Rx from the *San Ron* by *Kagawa Genyetsu*
Shakanzo To	炙甘草湯	Zhi Gan Cao Tang	Baked Licorice Combination p.529	Prepared Licorice Decoction pp.356–359
Shi Gyaku Ka Ninjin To	四逆加人參湯	Si Ni Jia Ren Shen Tang	Ginger, Licorice and Aconite Combination with Ginseng p.311	Frigid Extremities Decoction plus Ginseng p.277
Shigyaku San	四逆散	Si Ni San	Bupleurum and Chi Shi p.112	Frigid Extremities Powder pp.116–120
Shigyaku To	四逆湯	Si Ni Tang	Aconite, Ginger and Licorice Combination p.313	Frigid Extremities Decoction pp.274–277
Shikunshi To	四君子湯	Si Jun Zi Tang	Four Major Herb Combination p.264	Four Gentlemen Decoction pp.309–311
Shimotsu To	四物湯	Si Wu Tang	*Dang Gui* Four Combination p.432	Four Substance Decoction pp.333–336
Shinbu To	真武湯	Zhen Wu Tang	Vitality Combination p.278	True Warrior Decoction pp.744–747

Romaji Japanese name	Kanji Characters	Pinyin Chinese name	Commonly Used Chinese Herbal Formulas with Illustrations (Hong-Yen Hsu 1980)	Chinese Herbal Medicine, Formulas and Strategies (Scheid et al. 2009)
Shiun Ko	紫雲膏	Zi Yun Gao	Lithospermum Ointment	Omitted. "Purple Cloud Ointment" Modified by Hanaoka Seichu from Wai Ke Zheng Zong compiled by Chen Shi-Gong. Original name: Run Ji Gao.
Sho Joki To	小承気湯	Xiao Cheng Qi Tang	Minor Rhubarb Combination p.141	Minor Order the Qi Decoction pp.66–67
Sho Kenchu To	小建中湯	Xiao Jian Zhong Tang	Minor Cinnamon and Peony Combination p.291	Minor Construct the Middle Decoction pp.264–267
Sho Kyo Shahsin To	生姜瀉心湯	Sheng Jiang Xie Xin Tang	Pinellia and Ginger Combination p.110	Fresh Ginger Decoction to Drain the Epigastrium p.130
Sho Saiko* To	小柴胡湯	Xiao Chai Hu Tang	Minor Bupleurum Combination p.91	Minor Bupleuerum Decoction pp.104–109
So Kan To	疎肝湯	Shu Gan tang	Bupleurum and Evodia Combination p.432	Dredge the Liver Decoction pp.513–514
Ten Noho Shin To	天王补心湯	Tian Wang Bu Xin Dan	Ginseng and Zizyphus Combination p.270	Emperor of Heaven's Special Pill to Tonify the Heart pp.459–461
Tokaku Joki To	桃核承気湯	Tao He Cheng Qi Tang	Persica and Rhubarb Combination p.435	Peach Pit Decoction to Order the Qi pp.559–562

Toki Kenchu To	当帰建中湯	Dang Gui Jian Zhong Tang	Tang-Kuei, Cinnamon and Peony Combination p.317	Omitted. Rx from the Kin Ki Yo Ryaku 金匱要略
Toki Shakuyaku San	当帰芍薬湯	Dang Gui Shao Yao San	Tang-Kuei and Peony Formula p.585	Tang-Kuei and Peony Powder pp.587–590
Toki Shigyaku Ka Goshuyu Shokyo To	当帰四逆加呉茱萸生姜湯	Dang Gui Si Ni Jia Wu Zhu Yu Sheng Jiang Tang	Tang-Kuei, Evodia and Ginger Combination p.319	Tang-Kuei Decoction for Frigid Extremities plus Evodia and Fresh Ginger p.255
Toki Shigyaku To	当帰四逆湯	Dang Gui Si Ni Tang	Tang-Kuei and Jujube Combination p.321	Tang-Kuei Decoction for Frigid Extremities pp.252–255
Tsu Sen San	通仙散	Tong Xian San	No equivalent	Created as an anesthetic by the surgeon Hanaoka Seishu 華岡青洲 (1760–1846), based on an original formula by Hua To 華佗 called Ma Fei San 麻沸散.
Unkei To	温経湯	Wen Jing Tang	Dang Gui and Evodia Combination p.588	Flow-warming Decoction pp.577–580
Unsei In	温清飲	Wen Qing Yin	Dang Gui and Gardenia Combination p.439	Warming and Clearing Derink p.337
Untan To	温胆汤	Wen Dan Tang	Bamboo and Hoelen Combination p.114	Warm Gall Bladder Decoction pp.786–789
Yokukan San	抑肝散	Yi gan San	Bupleurum Formula p.343	Restrain the Liver Powder p.124
Yokukan San Ka Chin Pi Hange	抑肝散加陳皮半夏	Yi gan San Jia Ban Xia Chen Pi	Bupleurum, Citrus and Pinellia Formula p.346	Omitted. From Ren Zhai Zhi Zhi compiled by Yang Shi-Yi

Glossary of Selected Terms

Romaji	Kanji	Pinyin	English	Definition in this text
Akabane Kobei	赤羽幸兵衛	*Qi Yu Xing Bing Wei*	*Kobe Akabane*	Japanese doctor in the 20th century famous for his *Akabane* Test, a diagnostic protocol measuring pain threshold's temperature sensitivity at the "Entry–Exit" points of each meridian using a heat source (usually a lighted incense stick). Also known for his use of *Hinaishin* (皮内鍼) or Intradermal (embedded) needles in his Acupuncture practice
Ampuku	按腹	*An Fu*	Abdominal Palpation	A form of traditional Japanese abdominal massage first mentioned in *Ampuku Zukai* (1827) by *Ota Shinsai*
Anma	按摩	*An Mo*	*Anma* Massage	The traditional massage system of East Asia; part of a wider system of preventive healthcare referred to as *Do In An Kyo*
Anmashi	按摩師	*An Mo Shi*	*Anma* therapist	A person trained and qualified as a practitioner of *Anma* Massage

Romaji	Kanji	Pinyin	English	Definition in this text
Asada Shohaku	浅田宗伯	*Qian Tian Zong Bai*	Dr. *Shohaku Asada*	1815–1894. Another of the *Kampo* doctors of the *Secchu-Ha,* his life spanned the final stages of the Edo period and into the *Meiji* by which time the traditional practice of *Kampo* was under threat from the rise of Western medicine. He was amongst the very few traditionally trained *Kampo* specialists to survive this transition in which previously held traditional licenses of those who had no Western training were revoked. He was a prolific author and also wrote several important prescriptions such as *Nyo Shin San* 女神散 (see Chapter 2, "The Eclectic School" section)
Asuka Jidai	飛鳥時代	*Fei Niao Shi Dai*	*Asuka* period	539–710 CE. A period of continued assimilation of Chinese Medical knowledge into Japan
Atsuryoku Shindo	圧力深度	*Ya Li Shen Du*	Depth of pressure	Referring to the depth of pressure used in the *Fukushin* exam
Azuchi Momoyama Jidai	安土桃山時代	*An Tu Tao Shan Dai*	*Azuchi-Momoyama* period	1573–1600. This period of political unification followed the *Muromachi* and in turn led up to the establishment of the *Tokugawa Bafuku* or *Edo Jidai*
Basho	芭蕉	*Ba Jiao*	*Basho*	The pen name of the famous *Edo* period poet whose real name was *Matsuo Chuemon Munefusa* 松尾忠右衛門宗房
Bi Myaku	微脈	*Wei Mai*	Faint Pulse	Also called the Minute Pulse. It indicates the waning of the essential Vital energy (*Sei Ki*)
Bo shin	望診	*Wang Zhen*	Observational Diagnosis	The visual exam as part of the 4 Pillars of diagnosis based on observation by the naked eye

Budo	武道	*Wu Dao*	martial arts	Literally meaning "Martial Way" or *Bujutsu* 武術 meaning "martial technique," collectively used to refer to the martial arts in Japan
Bun Shin	聞診	*Wen Zhen*	Listening Diagnosis	The auditory exam; diagnosis by means of the auditory and olfactory senses
Byo	病	*Bing*	Disease	Distortion of normal functional activities of the body
Byo Ki	病気	*Bing Qi*	Illness	Distorted *Ki*; illness, the *Byo* above plus *Ki*
Byo Sho	病証	*Bing Zheng*	Disease Pattern	A cluster of signs and symptoms that correspond to and identify a named disease or pattern of disharmony
Chin Myaku	沈脈	*Chen Mai*	Deep pulse	Sometimes called sunken. Indicates the disease has penetrated deeper into the body. Can be Excess (*Jitsu*) or Deficiency (*Kyo*)
Chi No Michi Sho	血の道証	*Xue Dao Zheng*	*Chi No Michi*	Literally "way of the blood." This is an autonomic nervous and hormonal disorder, and not a primary blood disorder. It equates partially to peri-menopausal syndrome and its symptoms
Cho Netsu	潮熱	*Chao Re*	Tidal fever	Fever without chills that may take hold of the person suddenly like a wave; typically a sign of the *Yo Mei Byo*
Chu Atsu	中圧	*Zhong Ya*	Mid-level Pressure	The type of pressure used in the *Fukushin* exam that is applied at the level of the fascia and muscle layers
Chu Fuh	中風	*Zhong Feng*	Acute febrile disease of moderate severity	One of the evil wind conditions of the *Sho Kan Ron* of moderate severity, between strong severity and weak severity. Not to be confused with internal wind or apoplexy

Romaji	Kanji	Pinyin	English	Definition in this text
Chu Shin	中心	*Zhong Xin*	Core	Center and heart of one's being; described as a base for understanding *Kampo* in *Otsuka's Kampo Igaku* (see the section "Notes on How to Study Kampo")
Dejima	出島	*Chu Dao*	Exit Island	The Dutch trading post in *Nagasaki* bay through which the *Tokugawa* Shogunate retained contact with the Western world during the isolationist *Edo* period (1603–1868)
Do In An Kyo	導引按蹻	*Daoyin Anmo*	*Doin Ankyo*	The traditional system of breathing, movement, massage and meditation exercises of East Asia derived from Yoga. Influenced development of *Taiji Quan* and *Tuina* in China and later *Shiatsu* and other bodywork and movement forms in Japan
Do Ki	動悸	*Dong Ji*	Pulsations	Also called *Shin Ki*, these are subjectively or objectively detected pulsations felt on the abdomen
Edo Ji Dai	江戸時代	*Jiang Hu Shi Dai*	*Edo* period	Historical era which began in 1603; the capital of Japan was Tokyo (*Edo*); also known as the *Tokugawa* period, 德川時代, *Tokugawa jidai*, 1603–1868. Medical historians hypothesize that Abdominal Diagnosis (*Fuku Shin*) came to prominence during *Edo* due to socio-economic changes and changes in the way medicine was taught and practiced
Ei Ki	営気	*Ying Qi*	Nutritive *Qi*	Sometimes called "construction *Ki*," it originates from the raw nutrients obtained from food that go to make up the blood

Ei Yo	栄養	*Rong Yang*	Nourishment	A subjective definition of good health, such as that of being well nourished. This helps to determine *Kyo* and *Jitsu*
Fu Jin	不仁	*Bu Ren*	Numbness	A tingling feeling, numbness or palsy, described as feeling as though the area does not belong to you; a *Kyo* state
Fujiwara Sadaie	藤原定家	*Teng Yuan Ding Jia*	*Sadaie Fujiwara*	Also known as *Teika*, an imperial court poet (1162–1241), known for his personal diary the "Record of the Clear Moon" (*Meigetsu* 明月記) in which he makes multiple references to the abdomen in regard to assessment and treatment of medical problems. See Chapter 2, "The abdomen in Acupuncture" section
Fuku (Bu)	腹部	*Fu (Bu)*	The Abdomen (Area)	Literally "abdominal sac"; abdominal area or part of the body
Fuku Bu Bo Man	腹部膨満	*Fu Bu Peng Man*	Distended Abdomen	An abdomen that is bloated or distended
Fuku Bu Ko Ren Mu Ryoku	腹部拘攣 無力	*Fubu Ju Luan Wu Li*	Tight and Powerless	Abdomen #1b, Figure 4.2. This is the *Yang* within *Yin* abdomen, thin, tight and weak
Fuku Bu Mu Ryoku	腹部無力	*Fu Bu Wu Li*	Powerless Abdomen	An abdominal wall without proper tone, although there may be strength in the depths
Fuku Bu Nan Jyaku Mu Ryoku	腹部軟弱 無力	*Fu Bu Ruan Ruo Wu Li*	Lax and Powerless Abdomen	#1a Lax and Powerless Abdomen (Figure 4.1), like that described above, without strength in the depths
Fuku Choku Kin No Ren Kyu	腹直筋の 攣急	*Fu Zhi Jin Luan Ji*	Ropy Abdomen	Rectus abdominis spasm; a cramp in the musculature of the abdominal wall which usually denotes *Kyo*. A manifestation of the *Ri Kyu* abdomen (#8, Figure 4.11)
Fuku Chu Rai Mei	腹中雷鳴	*Fu Zhong Lei Ming*	Abdominal Thunder	Borborygmus, a loud noise in the hollow organs of the abdomen, usually denoting stagnant gas or *Ki*

Romaji	Kanji	Pinyin	English	Definition in this text
Fuku Man	腹満	*Fu Man*	Full Abdomen	An abdomen which appears replete and firm; this fullness can be either *Yang* (#2a Figure 4.3) or *Yin* (#2b Figure 4.4); it can also be either *Jitsu or Kyo*
Fuku Ryoku Jitsu	腹力実	*Fubu Li Shi*	Strong Abdomen	Constitutional reference to the abdomen strength
Fuku Ryoku Kyo	腹力虚	*Fubu Li Kyo*	Weak Abdomen	Constitutional reference to the abdomen strength
Fukushima Kodo	福島弘道	*Fu Dao Hong Dao*	*Kodo Fukushima*	1911–1992. Blind Acupuncturist and founder of the *Toyohari* system
Fuku Shin	腹診	*Fu Zhen*	Abdominal Diagnosis	A specialized *Kampo* tactile diagnosis
Fukusho	腹証	*Fu Zheng*	Abdominal Pattern	A tactile diagnostic pattern, differentiated according to the cumulative findings of the Abdominal Exam (*Fuku Shin*)
Fukusho Ki Ran	腹証奇覧	*Fu Zeng Qi Lan*	*Extraordinary Views of Abdominal Patterns*	Written by *Inaba Katsubunrei* (circa 1800) at the behest of his students, this text remains one of the richest extant sources of material related to the practice of abdominal diagnosis and the prescription of matching classical formulas. It has shaped much of the current practice of *Fukushin* in the modern *Koho-Ha* tradition and provided a rich source of reference for the author of this book
Fu (Myaku)	浮	*Fu (Mai)*	Floating (Pulse)	A pulse or structure that has lost its "anchor" due to pathology, and appears to float like wood on water
Fu Ri	不利	*Bu Li*	Urinary Block	Urinary impairment (does not flow)
Fu Shitsu	風湿	*Feng Shi*	Wind and damp	The evil forces of wind and damp together are used to describe rheumatism

Gai	外	Wai	Outside or back of body	External (to the body); factors from outside the body; dorsal. Care is taken when using the pairings *Gai/Nai* versus *Hyoh/Ri*
Gai Gyaku (Jo Ki)	咳逆(上気)	Ke Ni (Shang Qi)	Counterflow cough	Coughing attack caused by upward movement of *Ki*
Gai In	外因	Wai Yin	External causes	Disease causes which are external such as the 6 external pathogenic factors, trauma
Gai Jya (Ja)	外邪	Wai Xie	External Evil	External pathogenic factor, in the language of the *Sho Kan Ron* (flu, abdominal typhus, bloody flux, cholera, smallpox, common cold, viruses, dampness, heat, cold, allergic substance, environmental pollution)
Gai Sho	外証	Wai Zheng	Superficial symptoms	Symptoms in the superficial layer; the surface of the body
Gai Sho/Gai Kan	外感/外傷	Wai Shang	Pathogen damage entering from outside the body at the superficial level	*Gai*, as distinct from *Nai*, refers to the source of an acute illness manifested on the body surface, whereas *Nai* refers to the organs. In contrast *Hyo* is the site of an injury by an external pathogen, and *Ri* an internal pathogen. External injury, surface wound, traumatic injury, wound are *Gai Shoh*; *Gai Kan* is an illness that begins with a fever pattern such as the *Shang Han*

Romaji	Kanji	Pinyin	English	Definition in this text
Gan Jin	鑒真	Jian Zhen	Jian Zhen	Chinese Buddhist monk (688–763 CE) arrived in Japan in 752 along with many medical texts and students. Responsible for the dissemination of many Chinese Medicine teachings in *Nara* period Japan. There had been others brining Chinese medical teachings before him, notably the monk *Zhicong* (智聰)in 562 (see Chapter 2, "Early development (6th–13th centuries CE)" section)
Gen Bu To	玄武湯	Xuan Wu Tang	Gen Bu To	Following the death of Emperor *Gen* (483–515 CE) of the Northern *Wei* dynasty, this formula was renamed *Shin Bu To* (Vitality Combination)
Gen Ki	元気; 原気	Yuan Qi	Original or Source *Ki*	*Ki primum* or original, primordial *Ki*; the most fundamental Vital energy of the body; the combination of the innate and acquired *Ki*
Gen Myaku	弦脈	Xuan Mai	Wiry Pulse	Sometimes called the Bowstring pulse. In the *Sho Kan Ron* this pulse can indicate pain but often reflects deficiency of digestive function and sometimes accumulation of pathological fluids (*Tan In*)
Ge Sho	下焦	Xia Jiao	Lower burner	The lower part of the body; the umbilicus and lower abdomen
Go	合	He	(Combined) With	Character used when combining two formulas; Combined formula
Goju Kata	五十肩	Wu Shi	Fifty-Year Shoulder	Frozen shoulder

Gosei-Ha	後世派	*Hou shi pai*	The *Gosei* (Later Generation) school	Founded by *Sanki Tashiro* (1465–1537) influenced by the Chinese *Jin-Yuan* dynasty (1115–1368) physicians *Li Dong Yuan* (1180–1251) and *Zhu Dan Xi* (1281–1358); promoting, respectively, the importance of Spleen and Stomach digestive functions and nourishing *Yin*
Goto Konzan	後藤艮山	*Hou Teng Gen Shan*	Dr. *Gonzan Goto*	*Edo* period Japanese *Kampo* physician (1659–1733). Founder of the *Kohoh-Ha* (Classical School). He is known for the theory that blockage of the flow of *Ki* is the cause of all illness. Had many prominent students, amongst them: *Kagawa Shuan* 香川修庵 (1683–1755), *Yoshimasu Todo* 吉益東洞 (1702–1773) and *Yamawaki Toyo* 山脇東洋 (1705–1762)
Goyozei-Tenno	後陽成天皇	*Hou yangcheng tianhuang*	Emperor *Go-Yozei*	1571–1617; reigned 1586–1611
Gyaku	逆	*Ni*	Counterflow	A reversal of the normal flow; flowing backwards (usually upwards), also called a regurgitation
Gyaku Ki	逆気	*Ni Qi*	Counterflow *Ki*	Pathogenic state of *Ki* in which there is counterlflow
Gyaku Rei	逆冷	*Ni Leng*	Counterflow Cold	See also *Ketsu Rei* (厥冷) where the limbs are icy cold
Gyo Ki	行気	*Xing Qi*	Activate *Qi*	Treatment method to activate or move the *Qi*
Hakkan	発汗	*Fa Han*	Sweating	May be a sign of generalized *Ki* deficiency or in the *Tai Yo Byo* the need for formulas containing Cinnamon (*Keishi*)
Hakko Ben Sho	八綱弁証	*Ba Gang Bian Zheng*	8 Parameters	Also known as the 8 principles used in differential diagnosis. They are: *Yin/Yang*; Exterior/Interior; Excess/Deficiency; Hot/Cold

Romaji	Kanji	Pinyin	English	Definition in this text
Han	煩	Fan	Troublesome Distress	Vexation, disquiet, restless sensations of discomfort and dryness; it combines with other sensations (see below); this term appears in the Sho Kan Ron in the In stages and can be accompanied by cold
Hanaoka Seishu	華岡青洲	Hua Gang Qing Zhou	Dr. Seishu Hanaoka	1760–1846. Another Secchu-Ha doctor famous for his surgery (partial mastectomy) performed under herbal anesthetic in 1804—the first ever recorded in modern medical history. He had several students, also surgeons, amongst them Honma Soken 本間棗軒 (1804–1872) and Nakagawa Shutei 中川壺山, who also used herbal anasthetics in their surgeries
Han Gai Han Ri Sho	半外半裏証	Ban Wai Ban Li Zheng	Half-outside, half-inside Sho	Symptoms of an outside pathogen plus symptoms of internal Sho
Han Netsu	煩熱	Fan Rre	Troublesome Heat	Han: feeling of discomfort, irritation or vexation arising spontaneously on a body surface, such as the soles of the feet, or the palms of the hands
Han So	煩躁	Fan Zao	Troublesome plus restless movement	Described in the Sho Kan Ron as two kinds of discomfort occurring together: Han, troublesome pain, plus So, painful spontaneous fidgeting/restlessness of the hands and feet
Hara	腹	Fubu	Abdomen/Belly	Refers physically to the abdomen but also metaphysically to the Heart, Mind or Spirit
Haramaki	腹巻	Fu Juan	Belly band	Originally worn as a piece of armor, in modern times a wrap used for health purposes (to keep the belly warm) and as a fashion item

Hara Nanyo	原南陽	Yuan Nan Yang	Dr. Nanyo Hara	1752–1820. A physician from the *Secchu-Ha* famous for his creation of the topical "Purple Cloud" ointment *Otsujito* 乙字湯 which appeared in his book *Experimental Prescriptions of Hara Nanyo* (*Hara Nanyo Keikenho* 原南陽経験方)
Hara Shin	腹診	Fu Zhen	Abdominal Diagnosis	Distinguished from *Fukushin* (same characters) as being a more "energetic" assessment of the abdomen
Hari	針	Zhen	Acupuncture	The insertion of fine needles at specific points throughout the body for the purposes of regulating the flow of *Ki* to bring it into balance for better health. Used along with Moxibustion (*Kyu*)
Heian Jidai	平安時代	Ping An Shi Dai	The *Heian* period	794–1185CE. Japan ceased exchange with China in the middle of this era and went into the first of two major isolation periods, this one finishing with the advent of the *Kamakura* period
Hie	冷え	Leng	Icy Feeling (noun)	This differs from *Kan* (cold). This patient is icy to the touch, but subjectively feels only a vague cold sensation. It differs from the chills which accompany fevers
Hie Sho	冷え症	Leng Zheng	Icy Constitution	From Japanese Folk Medicine; a constitutional type distinguished by a tendency to feel a vague chill, separate from environmental coldness and lacking a robust nature
Hi Jyaku	菲弱	Fei Ruo	Delicate and Weak	The Veneer Abdomen: a tactile diagnostic term for a condition requiring tonics (*Hozai*)
Hi Man Tai Shitsu	肥満体質	Fei Man Ti Zhi	Fat and Full	A constitutional type, typically denoting *Jitsu* Fullness

Romaji	Kanji	Pinyin	English	Definition in this text
Hi So	肥瘦	*Fei Shou*	Thick or Thin	Diagnostic assessment of constitutional body type, for use with the three substances (*Ki Ketsu Sui*)
Ho Ho	補法	*Bu Fa*	Tonification Method	A method of treatment used to tonify or reinforce
Hon	本	*Ben*	Root	The root cause of a disease as opposed to its Branch manifestation (*Hyo*)
Hon Ji Ho	本治法	*Zhi Ben Fa*	Root Treatment	Treatment aimed at correcting the underlying causes of disease manifestation
Hon Ton Byo	奔豚病	*Ben Tun Bing*	Running Piglet disease	Panic attack, involving palpitations progressing upwards from the hypogastrium to the cardiac area and also palpable near the lower part of the navel; mentioned in the "Prescriptions from the Golden Cabinet" (*Kin Ki Yo Ryaku*)
Hon Ton Sho	奔豚証	*Ben Tun Zheng*	Running Piglet *Sho*	The symptom complex (pattern) described above
Honzo Komoku	本草綱目	*Ben Cao Gang Mu*	*Compendium of Materia Medica*	Written by the famous *Ming* dynasty (1368–1644) herbalist *Li Shi Zhen* 李時珍 (1518–1593). Referencing 1892 medicinal substances (1094 herbs, 276 minerals and 444 animal products and other substances) used in 11,096 different formulas and recipes
Ho Sho I Chi	方証一致	*Sui Zheng Zhi Liao*	Matching Pattern and Formula	The method of matching the *Sho* of the patient with the *Sho* of the Formula. *Yoshimasu Todo's* system of naming the treatment and the diagnosis as one and the same, i.e. the formula name itself
Ho Sho So Tai	方証	*Sui Zheng*	Pattern Based Treatment	The same meaning as *Ho Sho I Chi* (see above)

Hotei	布袋	Budai	Hotei	A *Zen* monk from the 10th century, whose image became popular in *Edo* period folklore in Japan and was associated with a jovial attitude and a sense of contentment as illustrated by his large belly and smiling face. In Chinese he is often known as the laughing Buddha, 笑佛 *Xiao Fo*. Some traditions in Buddhism even identify him with *Maitreya*, Sanskrit for "loving Kindness," the name given to the future Buddha, who is prophesied to manifest in the world at a time when the teachings of the historical (*Shakyamuni*) Buddha are no longer adhered to in the world. The only historical figure amongst the 7 Gods of Fortune (*Shichifukujin*)
Ho Zai	補劑	Bu Ji	Tonic	Refers to groups of herbal formulas that have a tonic effect
Hsu Hong-Yen	許鴻源	Xu Hong Yuan	Dr. *Hong-Yen Hsu*	Taiwanese Pharmacy Doctor, trained in Japan and a colleague of Dr. *Otsuka Keisetsu*. Went on to found Sun Ten Pharmaceutical Company and was an international scholar, publishing 24 books on *Kampo*, and held many prestigious posts in Asia including president of the Taiwan Pharmaceutical Association for 30 years
Hyo	標	Biao	Branch	The symptomatic manifestation of a disease as opposed to its Root cause (*Hon*)
Hyo	表	Biao	Exterior surface	Ectodermal, external, superficial surface layer of the body

Romaji	Kanji	Pinyin	English	Definition in this text
Hyoh Sho	表証	Biao Zheng	Exterior Pattern	A pattern of symptoms of the body's exterior layer calling for the appropriate action or treatment pattern
Hyo Ji Ho	標治法	Zhi Biao Fa	Branch Treatment	Treatment aimed at correcting the superficial symptoms of disease manifestation
Hyomen Atsu	表面圧	Biao Mian	Superficial pressure	The type of pressure in the *Fukushin* exam that only penetrates the superficial layers of the dermis
Hyo Ri	表裏	Biao Li	Exterior/ Interior	A diagnostic paradigm; an illness engages either from the body's exterior defenses or from the interior. Alternatively, the depth of illness: *Hyo* is shallow and *Ri* is deep
Iaido	居合道	Ju He Dao	The Way of the Sword	A Japanese martial art that literally means "the way of mental presence and immediate reaction" referring to the state of mind and body required to be prepared for any attack at any time
Ibukuro	胃袋	Wei Dai	Stomach organ	The anatomical stomach organ. Can also refer to "tripe" in butchery
I Cho Kyo Jaku/Jyaku	胃腸虚弱	Wei Chang Xu Ruo	Gastrointestinal tract *Kyo* and weak	Weak and empty stomach and intestinal function leading to poor absorption. This is a reference to constitution (*Taishitsu*)
In	陰	Yin	Yin	The cool, still, primary energy in opposition to *Yo* (*Yang*). Symbolized by the shady side of the mountain. The final three stages in the six divisions diagnosis pattern

Inaba Katsubunrei	稲葉克文禮	Dao Ye Ke Wen Li	Dr. Katsubunrei Inaba	Edo period Kampo practitioner who focused in particular on the use of Fukushin in practice. Author of the seminal Edo text on Fukushin: Extraordinary Views of Abdominal Patterns (Fukusho Kiran). Later, one of Inaba's students Wakuda Yoshitora (和久田叔虎) wrote an addendum to his teacher's text: Fukusho Ki Ran Yoku (腹証奇覽翼)
I Nai Tei Sui	胃内停水	Wei Nei Ting Shui	Pathogenic water	An abnormal fluid and gas retention in the stomach as confirmed by Fuku Shin. See abdomen #7 (Figure 4.9)
Inaka	田舎	Tian She	Countryside	Part of the "inner Japan" Ura Nihon, as discussed in Chapter 1, "Form and function" section
In Chu No In	陰中の陰	Yin Zhong Zhi Yin	Yin within Yin	The Yin aspect of a Yin phenomenon, e.g. abdomen #1a Lax and Powerless in Figure 4.1
In Chu No Yo	陰中の陽	Yin Zhong Zhi Yang	Yang within Yin	The Yang aspect of a phenomenon that is classified as Yin, e.g. abdomen #1b Tight and Powerless in Figure 4.2
In Fuku Man	陰腹満	Yin Fu Man	Yin Full Abdomen	This is abdomen #2b in Figure 4.4. It is the Yo Chu No In abdomen
Ingyo Tenno	允恭天皇	Yun Gomg Tian Huang	Emperor Ingyo	During his reign (412–453 CE) the very first record of the arrival of medical information from China into Japan came via the physician Kim Moo (金武)
In Sho	陰証	Yin Zheng	Yin Pattern	Signs and symptoms of an In Sho, or Yin disease pattern

Romaji	Kanji	Pinyin	English	Definition in this text
In Yo Setsu	陰陽説	*Yin Yang Shuo*	*Yin/Yang Theory*	One of the basic theories of Chinese Medicine. Inseparable and contradictory opposites symbolized by the sunny side and shady side of the mountain whose images (bright and dark) are contained within the characters
Iokai	医王会	*Yi Huang Hui*	Medicine King Institute	*Iokai Shiatsu* Center established in 1968 by its founder *Masunaga Shizuto*. Continues to promote treatment, training and research into *Masunaga's* Meridian style of *Shiatsu* in Tokyo, which is typically known as *Zen Shiatsu*
Iryakusho	医略抄	*Yi Lue Chao*	"Selected Therapies"	Text by *Tamba Masatada* (1081)
Ishimpo	醫心方	*Yi Xin Fang*	*The Essentials of Medicine*	Compiled in 984 CE by *Tamba Yasuyori*. Thirty volumes from excerpts from Chinese medical classics of the *Han*, *Sui*, *Tang* and *Song* dynasties. Comprised an encyclopedia of Chinese medical knowledge that had reached Japan by that time. Japan's oldest extant medical classic dating from the *Heian* period (794–1185 CE)
Ishizaka Sotetsu	石坂宗哲	*Shi Ban Zong Zhe*	Dr. *Sotetsu Ishizaka*	1770–1841. *Secchu-Ha* doctor known for his integration of modern anatomy into Acupuncture practice and for his exchanges with Philipp Franz von Siebold (1796–1866), a German physician and botanist who lived on Exit Island (*Dejima*) in the 1820s
Ji Jyun	滋潤	*Zi Run*	Luxuriating and moistening	An attribute of certain crude drugs used in *Kampo* which moisten and nourish. A cure for Dryness, a supplement for ageing

Jin Kan	腎間	Shen Jian	Moving Qi between the Kidneys	Abdominal area around the umbilicus and above the level of the kidneys, where an aortic pulse can be detected
Jin Ki Gan	腎気丸	Shen Qi Wan	Kidney Ki pills	Modern Chinese name for the formula: Rehmannia Eight Combination (Hachi Mi Gan)
Jitsu	実	Shi	Jitsu	Fullness or Excess; a robust constitutional type; in contrast to Kyo
Jitsu Sho (Jissho)	実証	Shi Zheng	Jitsu Sho	Fullness pattern; in illness this may be a transient hyperfunctioning stage or it may also describe a constitutional type who is strong
Joriki	定力	Ding Li	Mind Power	The kind of single-minded concentration that can be developed through Zen practice
Jya/Ja	邪	Xie	Pathogen	Pathogen, evil, stress, chaos, wrongdoing
Jya ki	邪気	Xie qi	Pathogenic Ki	Pathogenic factors (physical or metaphysical) which distort the natural healthy energy of the body (Shoki 正気) and can cause disease
Jyaku/Jaku	弱	Ruo	Weak	Pulse; body type
Ka	加	Jia	Plus	In writing the name of a formula, the character Ka indicates an additional ingredient is added, e.g. KF32–35

Romaji	Kanji	Pinyin	English	Definition in this text
Kagawa Shuan	香川修庵	*Xiang Chuan Xiu An*	Dr. *Shuan Kagawa*	1683–1755. One of *Goto Konzan's* main students along with *Yoshimasu Todo* and *Yamawaki Toyo* in the *Koho-Ha* faction. Unlike his teachers who had valued the classics *Ko Tei Nai Kyo* and *Ko Tei Hachijuichi Nan Gyo*, he dismissed them and held the *Sho Kan Ron* as the only worthy authority in Herbal Medicine. He also went by the name *Ippondo* and wrote two significant *Koho* texts "Ippondo's Notes on Medicine" (*Ippondo Gyoigen*) and "Ippondo's Notes on Drugs" (*Ippondo Yakusen*)
Kaitai Shinsho	解体新書	*Jie Ti Shin Shu*	"New Text on Anatomy"	The seminal anatomy textbook by *Sugita Genpaku* along with *Maeno Ryotaku*, published in 1774. It was based on a translation of the Dutch version (1734) of the original German anatomical text (1722) written by Johann Adam Kulmus (1689–1745). A pivotal medical text of the period and one which hastened the move towards Western medical thinking founded on basic anatomy.

Kajiwara Shozen	梶原性全	*Wei Yuan Xing Quan*	*Shozen Kajiwara*	A monk with a deep knowledge of medicine who lived in *Kamakura* (1266–1337) during the later *Kamakura* period (*Kamakura Jidai*, 1185–1333). He wrote two highly influential medical texts: the *Tonisho* (1302–1304) and the *Manampo* (1313). His was a prime example of the new generation of monk scholars who contributed to the transmission of medical knowledge away from the court aristocracy to student monks and thus to the general population
Ka (Ke) Ho	家方	*Jia Fang*	Family formula	Secret formula traditionally not shared with outsiders
Kaku Ran	霍乱	*Huo Luan*	Sudden Turmoil	Urgent diarrhea and stomach pain as in food poisoning or other infectious diseases affecting the gut. Also the term used for cholera
Kaku Taiei	鶴泰栄	*He Tai Rong*	*Taiei Kaku*	The teacher of *Inaba Katsubunrei*
Kampo Igaku	漢方医学	*Han Fang Yi Xue*	*Kampo* Medicine	A modern *Kampo* classic written in 1956 by *Otsuka Keisetsu*, this text has been translated into English as: *Kampo: A Clinical Guide to Theory and Practice* by Gretchen De Soriano and Nigel Dawes, 1st publ. Churchill Livingstone, 2010; 2nd edn. publ. Singing Dragon, 2017
Kampo (Kan Po)	漢方	*Han Fang*	Sino–Japanese Medicine	Japanese traditional medicine, rooted in clinical use of classic texts and teachings from China's *Han* dynasty (206 BCE–220 CE) and enriched by cultural and medical experience from Japan
Kampo To Min Kan Yaku Hyakka	漢方と民間薬百科	*Han Fang Min Jian Yao Bai Ke*	*An Encyclopedia of Kampo and Folk Medicine*	By *Otsuka Keisetsu*, publ. *Shu Fu no Tomo Sha*, 1966

Romaji	Kanji	Pinyin	English	Definition in this text
Kampo Yaku	漢方薬	*Han Fang Yao*	*Kampo* Herbal Medicine	As distinct from *Kampo* on its own, whose original meaning referred to any and all of the disciplines within "Chinese Medicine"
Kan	寒	*Han*	Cold	Objective plus subjective feelings of coldness; the pathogen from the *Sho Kan Ron*
Kan	勘	*Kan*	Intuition	A diagnostic tool based not upon objective findings but on other skills of the physician such as insight, intuition, a "sixth sense"
Kan Cho	漢朝	*Han Chao*	*Han* dynasty	Ancient China's second imperial dynasty (206 BCE–220 CE). Many significant medical classics were written during this period, notably: "Treatise on Cold Damage" (*Sho Kan Ron*); *The Yellow Emperor's Classic of Internal* Medicine (*Ko Tei Nai Kyo*) and the "Classic of Difficulties" (*Nan Gyo*). These texts later became the foundation of *Kampo* in Japan
Ka Shitsu Gyo Ki	化湿行気	*Hua Shi Xing Qi*	Resolve dampness to activate *Qi*	A therapeutic method to treat *Qi* stagnation by resolving dampness
Kata	型	*Xing*	Form	The term used especially in the martial arts to refer to a particular choreographed sequence or pattern of movements through which the art takes form and is practiced. It includes the timing, sequence, posture, attitude and intentional aspects that define the practical expression of particular disciplines in the martial, fine and healing arts in East Asia

Kata Kori	肩こり	N/a	Stiff Shoulders	A native Japanese description for stiff neck and upper back; refer to the writings of *Kuriyama Shigehisa*, "The Historical Origins of Katakori" (1997), *Japan Review* 9, 127–149
Katsu Ki (Kakki)	活気	Huo Qi	Vital energy	The *Ki* of life
Kei Ho	経方	Jing Fang	Classical Formulas	Formulas from the *Han* dynasty. In contrast to Contemporary Formulas (*Shi Fang* 时方) and Modern Formulas (*Jin Fang* 今方)
Keiraku Chiryo	経絡治療	Jing Luo Zhi Liao	Meridian Therapy	Style of Acupuncture founded by *Yanagiya Sorei* in the early part of the 20th century
Keiraku Shin	経絡診	Jing Luo Zhen	Meridian Diagnosis	A method of energetic assessment and diagnosis using meridian palpation
Kei Ren	痙攣	Jing Luan	Spasm	A twitch, cramp or spasmodic attack or seizure; the origins may be *Kyo* or *Jitsu*
Keitai Tenno	継体天皇	Ji Ti Tian Huang	Emperor *Keitai*	Reign: 507–531 CE
Kenka Goshi	喧嘩腰	Xuan Hua Yao	Fighting waist	Someone who in their posture demonstrates that they are seriously ready for a fight
Kensho Godo	見性悟道	Jian Xing Wu Dao	Insight/ Illumination	An initial awakening or insight into the nature or essence of things in Buddhist practice
Ketsu	厥	Jue	Pivotal	The pivotal one of the three *In* disease stages; a syncope (transient loss of consciousness with inability to maintain postural tone that is followed by spontaneous recovery)
Ketsu	血	Xue	Blood	Blood as a substance from among the three substances (*Ki Ketsu Sui*), or as a circulatory function

Romaji	Kanji	Pinyin	English	Definition in this text
Ketsu Byo	血病	*Xue Bing*	Blood-related Illness	An illness due to properties of the blood or ingredients of the blood; hormones, lipids, from the *Sho Kan Ron* (theory of three substances)
Ketsu Gyaku	厥逆	*Jue Ni*	Counterflow in the *Yin* Stage	Cold extremities, as a morbid condition occurring in the final stages of the six divisions
Ketsu In (Kecchin)	厥陰	*Jue Yin*	Absolute *Yin*	"Certain *yin*"; the final *In/Yin* Stage, also referred to as "terminal" or "absolute"
Ketsu In (Kecchin) Byo	厥陰病	*Jue Yin Bing*	Absolute *Yin* illness	An illness conforming to the "Certain *Yin*" Stage; the final stage of the six divisions
Ketsu Kan (Kekkan)	厥寒	*Jue Han*	*Ketsu* Cold	Feeling cold subjectively (and objectively) in the body or limbs; contrast with *Ketsu Rei*
Ketsu Kyo (Kekkyo)	血虚	*Xue xu*	Blood Deficiency	A defect of the individual blood cells, their constituents, or the whole of the liquid blood
Ketsu Netsu	血熱	*Xue Re*	Blood Heat	Heat in the blood, as the cause or as the result of illness
Ketsu Rei	厥冷	*Jue Leng*	Frigid Extremities	*Ketsu rei* describes the *In* Stage when limbs are cold to the touch but the patient has no sensations of cold; it is considered more severe than *Ketsu Kan*
Ketsu Sho (Kessho)	血証	*Xue Zheng*	Blood Pattern	Symptom complex originating with blood pathology
Ketsu Shoku (Kesshoku)	血色	*Xue Se*	Complexion	Literally "blood color," as an indicator of health
Ki	気	*Qi*	*Ki*	Vital energy, the basic function for existence. *Ki* is one of the primary three substances
Ki	悸	*Ji*	Subjective Palpitations	These are complaints by the patient which may not be felt by the physician; compare with *Do Ki* (動悸)

Ki Byo	気病	*Qi Bing*	*Ki* Disease	An illness whose root cause is blockage in the flow or function of *Ki*. *Ki* slumped, interned, stopped, delayed, or stagnated; a primary dysfunction of *Ki*
Ki Gyaku	気逆	*Qi Ni*	Counterflow *Ki*	An upward surge of *Ki* due to illness. These characters are also translated as Counterflow *Ki*, Rebellious *Ki*, Regurgitation of *Ki*. This is often part of a disease process recognizable in the *Sho Kan Ron*. Contrast this movement to *Nobose*, which is a dysfunction of a primary substance
Ki Kai	気海	*Qi Hai*	Sea of *Ki*	The character for *Ki* 気 translates most typically as "Vital energy" while *Kai* 海 translates as "Sea." Located in the area of the Acupuncture point Re.6, on the abdominal midline, three finger widths below the navel
Ki Ketsu Sui	気血水	*Qi Xue Shui*	*Ki*, Blood and Fluids	The three substances; the diagnostic 'hinge' of the *Kin Ki Yoh Ryaku*
Kin	緊	*Jin*	Tense/tight	May refer to pulse or to musculature
Kin Cho	緊張	*Jin Zhang*	Tense and stretched	A measure of muscle strength or tension; it may be Strong (*Jitsu*) or Weak (*Kyo*)
Kinhin	経行	*Jing Xing*	Walking Meditation	In *Zen* practice this form of Walking Meditation usually follows each period of sitting (*zazen*) or can be practiced on its own
Kin Ki Yo Ryaku	金匱要略	*Jin Gui Yao Lue*	"Prescriptions from the Golden Cabinet"	A text devoted to the treatment of chronic disease; comprises the second section of the *Shan Han Za Bing Lun* 傷寒雜病論 by *Zhang Zong Jing* in the 3rd century CE
Kinmei Tenno	欽明天皇	*Ming Ming Tian Huang*	Emperor *Kinmei*	Reign: 539–571 CE

Romaji	Kanji	Pinyin	English	Definition in this text
Ki Rin	氣淋	*Qi lin*	Strained urination	Strangury, the symptom of painful, frequent urination of small volume; spastic dysuria, when due to a *Ki* disorder
Ki Ryoku	氣力	*Qi Li*	Strength of *Ki*	Diagnostic measure used for assessing the three substances. The *Ki Ryoku* can be replete or waning; contrast to *Tai Ryoku*, body strength
Kissa Yojoki	喫茶養生記	*Chi Cha Yang Sheng Ji*	"Treatise on Tea Drinking for Good Health"	The first known Japanese text devoted to the art of tea written in 1193 by *Myoan Eisai*
Ki Tai	氣滞	*Qi Zhi*	*Ki* slumped	*Ki* slumped; a primary dysfunction of *Ki*
Kitao Shunpo	北尾春圃	*Bei Wei Chun Pu*	Dr. *Shunpo Kitao*	1658–1741. Developed a method of abdominal diagnosis based on assessing the strength or otherwise of the "Movement between the Kidneys" (腎間動氣)—a *Gosei-Ha* approach to *Fukushin*
Kitasato Kenkyujo	北里研究所	*Bai Li Yan Jiu Suo*	Kitasato Institute	Established in 1914 as the first private medical research facility in Japan, including for *Kampo* research
Ki Utsu	氣鬱	*Qi Yu*	*Ki* depression	*Ki* depressed; the blues, depression
Ki Utsu Tai (Uttai)	氣鬱滞	*Qi Yu Zhi*	*Ki* interned	*Ki* stagnation plus *Ki* depression
Ki Zai	氣剤	*Qi Ji*	*Ki* regulator	A prescription aimed at restoring the flow of *Ki*, or crude drugs for modulating psychoactivity
Kobayashi Shoji	小林詔司	*Xiao Lin Zhao Si*	*Shoji Kobayashi*	Contemporary Acupuncturist known for his *Shakuju* style
Kofun Jidai	古墳時代	*Gu Fen Shi Dai*	The *Kofun* period	250–538 CE. The earliest arrival of Chinese medical teachings into Japan occurred during this time

Koho-Ha	古方派	Gu Fang Pai	Classical School	A 17th-century school of *Kampo*, started by *Goto Gonzan*, advocating a return to the practical medicine of the *Sho Kan Ron*, opposing the *Gosei-Ha* faction; *Otsuka* was a proponent of the modern *Kohoh-Ha*
Ko Kan	口乾	Kou Gan	Dry Mouth	Dry mouth due to scant secretions, common in the elderly. Distinguish from actual thirst *Ko Katsu*—see below
Ko Kan I Gaku	皇漢医学	Huang Han Yi Xue	*Handbook of Chinese Medicine*	An early modern *Kampo* guidebook written by *Yumoto Kyushin* 湯本求真 (1876–1941), the principal teacher of *Otsuka Keisetsu*
Ko Katsu	口渇	Kou Ke	Thirst	An active desire to drink water, different from Dry Mouth
Kokoro	心	Shin	Heart	Referring to the metaphysical sense of the heart in terms of spirit, compassion and sensitivity
Ko Kyu	拘急	Ju Ji	Strained Resistance	Muscular tension and strain at the surface of the body
Ko Myaku	洪脈	Hong Mai	Surging pulse	Often the pulse of the *Yo Mei Byo*
Komyo Kogo	光明皇后	Guang Ming Huang Hou	Empress *Komyo*	701–760 CE. Dedicated the treasures in the Treasure House (*Shosoin*) in *Nara* to her husband upon his death
Ko Ren	拘攣	Ju Luan	Myotonia	Muscle tension that is slow to relax
Koshi	腰	Yao	Lower Back and Hips	The "outward structural source of support and motive power in the human body" (see Chapter 1, "Form and function")

Romaji	Kanji	Pinyin	English	Definition in this text
Koshi Balancing	No equivalent	No equivalent	No equivalent	A method of structural alignment and therapy founded by Jeffrey Dann, PhD, L.Ac., a medical anthropologist and licensed Acupuncturist since 1984. He has lectured in the Beijing University of Chinese Medicine on Japanese Acupuncture and structural Acupuncture. He is an adjunct faculty in the post-doctoral Japanese Acupuncture program at Tristate College of Acupuncture (New York) and the American College of Traditional Chinese Medicine (San Francisco). He studied bodywork and the martial arts of the *Mito Tobukan* where he achieved a 4th dan in *Kendo*, *nidan* in *Iaido* and *shodan* in *Naginatado*. His Aloha Wellness clinic is in Boulder, Colorado
Koshinuke	腰抜け	*Yao Ba*	Spineless	Cowardly or lacking determination and resolve as in a "weak" person (*Yowa goshi*) as opposed to a "fearless" person (*Kenka Goshi*)
Kosho-Ha	考証派	*Jiao Shi Pai*	School of Textual Analysis	Existed alongside the *Secchu-Ha* in the later *Edo* and early *Meiji* and dedicated itself to the commentary on and compilation and dissemination of scholarly works on *Kampo*
Ko Tei Hachijuichi Nan Gyo	黄帝八十一難經	*Huang Di Baishiyi Nan Jing*	"The Yellow Emperor's Classic of 81 Difficult Questions"	The full name of the "Classic of Difficulties" (*Nan Gyo*), one of the great *Han* dynasty classical texts alongside the *Ko Tei Nai Kyo* and the *Sho Kan Ron*

Ko Tei Nai Kyo	黄帝内経	Huang Di Nei Jing	The Yellow Emperor's Classic of Internal Medicine	A Chinese medical text that has formed the fundamental doctrinal source material for Kampo for over two millennia; generally dated from 2nd century BCE and comprising two texts: the "Basic Questions," 素問 So Mon (Japanese), Su Wen (Chinese); and the "Spiritual Pivot," 靈框 Ling Shu (Chinese). Note the unusual reading of the characters
Ko Ten No Ki	後天之気	Hou Tian Zhi Qi	Acquired Energy	Sometimes referred to as "Post-Heaven Essence," derived from the combined environmental resources of food (all nutritional substances transformed as part of the digestive process governed by the Spleen/Stomach) and air (primarily oxygen absorbed by the Lungs)
Ko Waku Byo	狐惑病	Hu Huo Bing	Fox Demon Possession	From the Kin Ki Yoh Ryaku, a type of psychopathy with confusion, uneasiness and restlessness. Alternatively, aphthous ulcers of the mouth and genital regions or sudden, unexplained abdominal cramps as in the formula Kanzo Shashin To
Kyo	去	Qu	Minus	A term used in writing formulas to denote a variation of a classical formula where one ingredient is removed
Kyo	虚	Xu	Empty	A constitution or condition requiring tonics; lacking tone; asthenia, deficiency
Kyo Fuku Man	虚腹満	Xu Fu Man	Kyo Full Abdomen	This is a Fuku Man but in a Deficient Pattern where the fullness is a result of weak digestion with resulting gas and fluid accumulation. Not to be confused with abdomen #2b, Figure 4.4, Yin Full Abdomen (In Fuku Man) which is a truly strong abdomen though often soft to the touch

Romaji	Kanji	Pinyin	English	Definition in this text
Kyo Han	虚煩	Xu Fan	Kyo Troublesome Restlessness	Restlessness or vexation accompanying chronic or consumptive illness; alternatively, mental exhaustion
Kyo Jyaku (Jaku)	虚弱	Xu Ruo	Kyo and Weak	A pulse or body type both Kyo and weak (occurring together); asthenia, hypofunctioning, debility
Kyo Jyaku Tai Shitsu	虚弱体質	Xu Ruo Ti Zhi	Kyo, weak body type	Deficient body constitutional type, requiring tonics
Kyo Ka Hi Ko	脇下痞硬	Xie Xia Pi Ying	Hypochondriac Obstruction Resistance	Abdomen #6, Figure 4.8. This is where the hypochondriac area on one or both sides of the patient feels tight to the touch (with or without discomfort)
Kyo Kan	虚寒	Xu Han	Kyo and Cold	Kyo and cold (occurring together) asthenia: cold
Kyo Kyo Ku Man	胸脇苦満	Xiong Xie Ku Man	Hypochondriac Painful Fullness	Abdomen #5, Figure 4.7. As opposed to Kyo Ka Hi Ko (above) there is an extreme form of tenderness, discomfort or distress either spontaneously or when pressure is applied in the hypochondriac area. This finding is always bilateral and may include the chest area also
Kyo Ro	虚労	Xu Lao	Kyo Troubles	Chronic consumptive disease; asthenia of the viscera; weakness and fatigue from overwork
Kyo Sho	虚証	Xu Zheng	Kyo Shoh	Hypofunctioning, asthenia, deficiency, emptiness, needing tonics; a Kyo symptom pattern
Kyu	灸	Jiu	Moxibustion	The dried leaves of Mugwort (Artemesia vulgaris) burned on or near the skin at specific points. An integral part of meridian-based treatment along with Acupuncture (Hari)

Li Zhu Igaku	李朱醫學	Li Zhu Yi Xue	Li Zhu Medicine	The medicine of *Li Dong Yuan* (1180–1251) and *Zhu Danxi* (1281–1358)
Manaka Yoshio	間中善雄	Jian Zhong Shan Xiong	Dr. *Yoshio Manaka*	1911–1989. Medical doctor and influential figure in 20th century Japanese Acupuncture circles with his innovative legacy including the Ion-Pumping cords, 8 Extraordinary Channels abdominal diagnosis and many other techniques and protocols, some of which are included in the text *Chasing the Dragon's Tail*, Birch S. and Itaya K., publ. Paradigm Publications, 1995
Manampo	万安方	Wan An Fang	Treatise on Infinite Peace	The second major work written in 62 volumes (started in 1313) by the monk physician *Kajiwara Shozen*, this time in Chinese characters as a textbook for student monks. Mostly based on materials from the *Seizai Soroku* 聖済総録 only recently printed in *Yuan* dynasty China in 1300. In contrast to his other populist text the *Tonisho*, this one was intended for scholarly study of the medicine by student monks
Manase Dosan	曲直瀬道三	Qu Zhi Lai Dao San	Dr. *Dosan Manase*	1507–1594. Student of *Sanki Tashiro* and considered one of the early pioneers of the *Gosei-Ha* (Later Generation) school, along with his successor *Manase Gensaku* 曲直瀬玄朔 (1549–1631)
Manase Gensaku	曲直瀬玄朔	Qu Zhi Lai Xuan Shuo	Dr. *Gensaku Manase*	1549–1631. Successor to *Manase Dosan* (see above)
Masunaga Shizuto	増永静人	Zeng Yong Jing Ren	Shizuto Masunaga	1925–1981. Originator of the *Zen Shiatsu* style and founder of *Iokai Shiatsu* Institute in Tokyo. Teacher, practitioner and author. One of his many students, *Suzuki Takeo*, was the author's *Shiatsu* teacher

Romaji	Kanji	Pinyin	English	Definition in this text
Matsumoto Kiiko	松本岐子	*Song Ben Qi Zi*	*Kiiko Matsumoto*	Contemporary Japanese Acupuncturist, teacher and author based in the US now teaching her own system internationally (KM style); influenced by the "family style" of one of her teachers, *Nagano Kiyoshi* 永野晴
Meiji Ishin	明治維新	*Ming Zhi Wei Xin*	*Meiji* Restoration	Followed directly the *Edo* period beginning in 1868–1912 and forming the first half of the Empire of Japan, which came to an end after the Second World War with the establishment of the Japanese constitution in 1947. *Meiji* marked the opening up of Japan to the Western world with all the many and profound social, cultural, political and economic changes that accompanied it. This period was succeeded by the *Taisho* period (1912–1926)
Men (Mei) Gen	瞑眩	*Ming Xuan*	Treatment reaction	A temporary adverse-like reaction to a formula during the course of treatment; commonly described in Folk Medicine rather than in *Kampo*. Sometimes referred to as "Healing Crisis"
Minamoto no Sanetomo	源実朝	*Yuan Shi Chao*	*Sanetomo Minamoto*	Born in 1192 he became the third Shogun of the *Kamakura* period (1185–1333), though his reign was short as he was assassinated at the *Hachiman* shrine in *Kamakura* in 1219. Famously, *Myoan Essai* dedicated his book "Treatise on Tea Drinking for Good Health" (*Kissa Yojoki*) to him in 1193
Min Kan Yaku	民間薬	*Min Jian Yao*	Folk Medicine	The domestic medicine of Japan, apart from *Kampo*

Misono Isai	御薗意斎	Yu Yuan Yi Zhai	Isai Misono	Acupuncturist in the second half of the 16th century. Son of *Misono Mubunsai*, and author of the *Shindo Hiketsu Shu* (later published by his student in 1685)
Misono Mubunsai	御薗夢分斎	Yu Yuan Meng Fen Zhai	Mubunsai Misono	Acupuncturist and court physician in the *Muromachi* period and founder of the *Mubun* style of Acupuncture (*Mubunryu*). Well-known for his chart of the abdomen (see Figure 2.3). Father to and teacher of *Misono Isai*
Mon Shin	問診	Wen Zhen	The Questioning Exam	The verbal aspect of *Kampo* diagnosis; the skilled questioning of the patient
Mubunryu	夢分流	Meng Fen Liu	Mubun style	The pre-*Edo* period style of Acupuncture developed by *Misono Mubunsai* involving the use of a Big Needle (*Da Shin* 大針) and Small Mallet (*Kozuchi* 小槌). See Chapter 2, "The abdomen in Acupuncture" section
Mu Kan	無汗	Wu Han	Absence of Sweating	A sign of strong *Yo Ki* and the need for sudorifics
Muromachi Jidai	室町時代	Shi Ting Shi Dai	Muromachi period	A period of Japanese medieval history (1336–1573) also known as the *Ashikaga* Shogunate (*Ashikaga bakufu* 足利幕府) or the *Muromachi* Shogunate (*Muromachi bakufu* 室町幕府)
Myaku Shin	脈診	Mai Zhen	Pulse Diagnosis	One part of the tactile diagnosis, well developed in *Kampo* practice. Originally involving the palpation of the pulses in nine different regions of the body, but more usually in contemporary practice focused on those felt along the radial artery of both wrists

Romaji	Kanji	Pinyin	English	Definition in this text
Myoan Eisai	明菴栄西	Ming An Rong Xi	Eisai Myoan	Studied Zen (Chan) Buddhism in China on Tiantai mountain in Zhejiang province. Returned to Japan in 1193 to write the "Treatise on Tea Drinking for Good Health" (Kissa Yojoki) dedicated to Minamoto no Sanetomo 源実朝 (1192–1219), the third Shogun of the Kamakura Shogunate
Nagata Tokuhon	永田徳本	Yong Tian De Ben	Dr. Tokuhon Nagata	1513–1630. Another student of Tashiro Sanki in the Gosei-Ha tradition, also a Buddhist and Confucian scholar. Along with Tashiro and Manase Dosan they were known collectively as the "three venerable physicians" (Sansei 三聖) of the Gosei-Ha
Nagoya Geni	名古屋玄医	Ming Gu Wu Xuan Yi	Dr. Geni Nagoya	1628–1696. The first prominent advocate of what was to become the Classical School of Kampo (Koho-Ha) though it is generally agreed that the actual founder of that faction was Goto Konzan
Nai In	内因	Nei Yin	Interior Etiology	Disease causes which are internal such as the 7 emotions
Nai Sho	内傷	Nei Shang	Internal Damage	Pathogenic factors causing damage to the viscera, or chronic illness arising from internal imbalance or disorder
Nai (Uchi)	内	Nei	Inside or Interior	Nai/Gai refer to inside/outside, as Hyo/Ri refer to interior/exterior; body locations for locating and treating the active pathogen within the six divisions. See Hyo, Ri and Gai in this glossary

Nakagami Kinkei	中神琴渓	*Zhong Shen Qin Xi*	Dr. *Kinkei Nakagami*	1744–1833. A student of *Yoshimasu Todo* who famously converted to the *Secchu-Ha* from the *Koho* tradition of his teacher. He criticised the literal or dogmatic use of *Sho Kan Ron* prescriptions, arguing instead in favor of what he called the "unfettered remedy" approach, meaning a more liberal clinical interpretation of each formula that does not adhere to fixed rules or interpretations
Namikoshi Tokujiro	浪越徳 治郎	*Lang Yue De Zhe Lang*	*Tokujiro Namikoshi*	1905–2000. Well-known *Shiatsu* practitioner, teacher and author who founded the Japan *Shiatsu* College in 1940, which helped establish what has become known as the *Namikoshi* style
Nan Gyo	難経	*Nan Jing*	"Classic of Difficulties"	An ancient *Han* dynasty text said to be the original source of Acupuncture, along with the *Ko Tei Nai Kyo*, believed to date from 2nd to 1st century BCE. Full name: *Ko Tei Hachijuichi Nan Gyo*
Nan Jyaku Mu Ryoku	軟弱無力	*Ruan Ruo Wu Li*	Lax and Powerless	Soft, weak and no strength (abdomen); refer to *Fuku Bu Nan Jyaku Mu Ryoku*
Netsu	熱	*Re*	Outbreak of fever	A subjective or objective feeling of heat; a rise in body temperature or feeling hot. In the *Sho Kan Ron*, it refers to actual fever
Netsuri	熱利	*Re Li*	Hot diarrhea	The diarrhea that can occur in a (toxic) heat pattern
Nin Myaku	任脈	*Ren Mai*	Conception Vessel	The Acupuncture meridian along the anterior midline channel called the Conception Vessel or *Renmai*. One of the 8 Extraordinary Channels (*Qi Jing Ba Mai* 奇經八經) used in Acupuncture, and martial and meditative arts

Romaji	Kanji	Pinyin	English	Definition in this text
Nizuma Ke	新妻家	*Xin Qi Jia*	*Nizuma* family	A Kyoto lineage known for their prescriptions
Nobose	のぼせ	*Japanese term*	Headrush	*Nobose* is a folk term for the rising of *Ki*, and results from *Qi* Slumping (*Ki Tai*). *Nobose* can occur within any of the three substances of *Ki*, water and blood and can be either Excess (*Kyo*) or Deficient (*Jitsu*) in nature. It can be felt as a rush of blood to the head, a rush of warmth or a light-headed feeling (seeing stars), and can include symptoms of dizziness, tinnitus, headache, anxiety and so on. Contrast *Nobose* to Counterflow *Qi* (*Ki Gyaku*) where the treatments are different
Nyo Hei	尿閉	*Niao Bi*	Blocked Urination	Lack of flow of urine due to an accident or trauma
O Fu	悪風	*Wu Feng*	Evil Wind	This is aversion, fear or hate of wind, moving air, draughts; a pathogenic factor from the *Sho Kan Ron*
Ogino Gengai	荻野元凱	*Di Ye Yuan Kai*	Dr. *Gengai Ogino*	1737–1806. Early *Secchu-Ha* doctor who was famous as a pioneer in the practice of bloodletting
O Kan	悪寒	*Wu Han*	Evil Cold	This is aversion, fear or hate of cold, cold sensation or chills; a pathogenic factor from the *Sho Kan Ron*
Oketsu	瘀血	*Yu Xue*	Blood Stasis	Blood stagnation itself or set of symptoms caused by blood stagnation. There can be *Jitsu* or *Kyo* patterns
Oketsu Sho	瘀血証	*Yu Xue Zheng*	Blood stagnation pattern	A set of signs and symptoms denoting a pathology in the quality and/or movement of the blood

Omote	表	Biao	Visible	Meaning "surface," "exterior" or "front" implying that which is seen or obvious. What can be perceived from the outside or surface of a particular phenomenon, the obvious superficial aspect
O Naka	お腹	Wu Fu	Belly	The "honorable middle" referring to one's stomach, belly or "tummy"
On Po	温補	Wen Bu	Warm and Replenish	A form of tonification therapy, as a general term for formulas that tonify
Oogimachi-Tenno	正親町天皇	Zheng Qin Ting Tian Huang	Emperor Oogimachi	1517–1593; reigned 1557–1586
O Rai Kan Netsu	往来寒熱	Wang Lai Han Re	Alternating Chills and Fever	A fever pattern associated with the Shaoyang Stage (Sho Yo Byo)
Ota Shinsai	太田晋斎	Tai Tian Jin Zhai	Shinsai Ota	First known reference to Ampuku in his book Ampuku Zukai 按腹図解 (publ. 1827)
Otsuka Keisetsu	大塚敬節	Da Zhong Jing Jie	Dr. Keisetsu Otsuka	A renowned Classical School (Koho-Ha) physician whose life spanned the late Meiji, Taisho and Showa periods from 1900–1980. Author of numerous influential texts on Kampo including Kampo Igaku. For a brief biography refer to the English translation of this text by Gretchen De Soriano and Nigel Dawes: Kampo: A Clinical Guide to Theory and Practice (see "Selected Bibliography")
Otsuka Yasuo	大塚恭男	Da Zhong Gong Nan	Dr. Yasuo Otsuka	1930–2009. Japanese medical historian; physician and son of Otsuka Keisetsu. He joined the Research Institute of Oriental Medicine at the Kitasato Institute in 1972 and served as its president from 1986 to 1996

Romaji	Kanji	Pinyin	English	Definition in this text
Poka Poka	ポカポカ	*Japanese term*	Uncomfortable Warmth	Japanese onomatopoeic phrase from *Folk Medicine*; a discomfort relieved by slapping the fingers to the palms of the hands; this relieves *Han Netsu*
Rangaku	蘭学	*Lan Xue*	Dutch Studies	Referring essentially to "Western Medicine" defined by the arrival of medical texts and teachings through the Dutch trading post of *Dejima* (出島) in the bay of *Nagasaki* during the *Edo* period. Hence this "new" medicine was commonly referred to at the time in Japan as *Rampo* (蘭方) or "Dutch Medicine." It had initially been called "Medicine of the Red-haired People" (*Komo Igaku* 薦菰医学) and prior to that at the time of the initial Portuguese arrival into Japan in the early 16th century it had been known as "Barbarian Medicine" (*Nanban Igaku* 南蛮医学)
Rei Kan	冷感	*Leng Gan*	Frigid Extremities	Chilly extremities
Ren Kyu	攣急	*Luan Ji*	Acute spasm	Muscle stiffness or spasm
Ri	裏	*Li*	Internal, interior	Endodermal. A pathogen coming from outside the body elicits a defence mechanism internally at this level; also means the site of chronic disease
Rikishi	力士	*Li Shi*	Men of power	Referring to *Sumo* wrestlers
Ri Kyu	裏急	*Li Ji*	Inside Spasm	Abdomen #8, Figures 4.11 and 4.12. Literally "internal emergency"; a spasm; as an abdominal diagnostic sign it usually designates *Kyo* and can take two forms: involuntary tension in the rectus abdominis muscle (Figure 4.11) or so-called "jumping fishes" (Figure 4.12). Alternatively, it refers to painful excretion of stool with diarrhea

Ri Kyu Ko Ju	裏急後重	Li Ji Hou Zhong	Internal spasm, heavy afterward	An acute spasm of pain followed by a bearing-down sensation, as in colitis; tenesmus
Rin	淋	Lin	Straining to Urinate	Also described as spastic dysuria, strangury, painful urge to urinate
Ri No Kan	裏の寒	Li Han	Internal Cold	Cold symptoms in the interior
Rin Reki	淋瀝	Lin Li	Sparse Urine	Slow or painful discharge of urine due to spasm; strangury; *Shiburi*
Ri Shitsu	痢疾	Li Ji	Diarrhea	Could be symptomatic of any number of infectious diseases such as cholera, dysentery or chronic diseases such as colitis, Crohn's, IBS. Can also refer just to dysentery
Ri Sho	裏証	Li Zheng	Internal Pattern	Symptoms in the interior, the viscera; endodermal symptoms
Roku Byo I Sho	六病位証	Liu Bing Zheng	Six Stage Theory	Also known as the six divisions described in the *Sho Kan Ron* as six distinct stages of disease manifestation and their respective treatment
Ruijyuho	類聚方	Lei Ju Fang	*A Variety of Assembled Formulas*	The text of *Todo Yoshimasu's* study of the formulations of the *Sho Kan Ron* from 1764. In it he proposed new and hitherto undocumented interpretations of each of the Formula Patterns from *Zhang Zhong Jing's* classic, emphasizing the signs and symptoms that comprise the *Sho* rather than any intellectual interpretation according to the theory of the six divisions (*Roku Byo Sho*)
Ruijyuho Ko Gi	類聚方 広義	Lei Ju Fang Jiang Yi	*An Overview of the Ruijyuho*	This text is *Yodo Odai's* (1856) annotations on the text *Ruijyuho* by *Todo Yoshimasu* (1751). [AQ] The term *Ko Gi* denotes an overview (see above)

Romaji	Kanji	Pinyin	English	Definition in this text
Ruijyuho Shu Ran	類聚方 集覧	*Lei Ju Fang Ji Lan*	*An Inspection of the Rui Jyu Ho*	The term *Ko Gi* denotes an overview of, or commentary on, in this case the original *Ruijyuho* 類聚方 (see above)
Ryo Ji Sa Dan	療治茶談	*Liao Zhi Cha Tan*	*Discussion on Medical Treatment over Tea*	A medical manual by *Tsuda Gensen* (1737–1809), written in 1770
Ryu Tai	溜滞	*Liu Zhi*	Accumulation and slumped *Ki*	*Ryu* denotes accumulation, while *Tai* is a slump (stagnation) in the flow. *Ki* is accumulating and slumped (stuck)
Sado	茶道	*Cha Dao*	The Way of Tea	The art of the Japanese Tea Ceremony
Sai Bu De Do Ki	臍部で 動悸	*Qi Bu Dong Ji*	Navel Pulsation	A clearly detected pulsation of the umbilicus
Sai Bu Kyu Ketsu	臍部急結	*Qi Bu Ji Jie*	Navel Spastic Knot Point	Abdomen #13, Figure 4.19. These are pulsations felt either side of the navel or just below it and usually relate to the finding of *Oketsu* with accompanying *Ketsu Nobose* symptoms
Saika Tanden	臍下丹田	*Qi Xia Dantian*	Cinnabar or Elixir Field	The center of Vital energy below the navel related to the "movement of *Ki* between the Kidneys" (see the definition of *Fukushin* in Chapter 1). Another name for the lower *Dantian* in Chinese is the "Golden Stove" or *Jin Lu* 金炉 identifying the process of purification and refining of energy taking place there as a kind of alchemic cauldron
Saku Myaku	数脈	*Shuo Mai*	Rapid Pulse	Usually a sign of heat. With a floating (*Fu*) pulse it means outside fever (*Hyo Netsu Sho*) and with a deep (*Chin*) pulse it means inside fever (*Ri Netsu Sho*); with a thin (*Sai*) and Weak (*Kyo*) pulse it means waning of the *Yin* (*In*)

Samu Ke	寒気	Han Qi	Cold shivers	A chill, or alternatively a cold climate, from the *Kin Ki Yo Ryaku* and the *Sho Kan Ron*. Take care to differentiate types of cold and chills when selecting treatment. Shivering with cold when attributed to *Okan* or *Ofuh* calls for distinctive treatment
San In San Yo	三陰三陽	San Yin San Yang	The three *Yins* and three *Yangs*	The diagnostic paradigm of the *Sho Kan Ron*, also known as the six divisions (*Roku Byo Sho*)
Satsu Ho Ben Chi	弁証論治	Bian Zheng Lun Zhi	Pattern Recognition and Treatment Determination	Differential diagnosis and treatment according to patterns of disharmony
Secchu-Ha	折衷派	Zhe Zhong Pai	Eclectic School	The *Kampo* school of "Compromise" beginning at the end of the *Edo* period and continuing into the *Meiji* period (1868–1912). It attempted to form a bridge between the teachings of the oppositional *Gosei-Ha* and *Koho-Ha* Schools that preceded it
Sei	精	Jing	Essence	The essence of life; the substance related to reproduction and metabolism, semen; alternatively, spirit
Sei Ka Fu Jin	臍下不仁	Qi Xia Bu Ren	Lower Abdominal Numbness	Numbness in the lower abdomen, which can progress to the lower body. This appears frequently in treatment patterns related to the formula *Hachi Mi Gan*
Sei Ka Ki	臍下悸	Qi Xia Ji	Pulsations around the navel	Abdomen #10, Figure 4.14. These are felt distinctly during the tactile diagnosis, directly beside or below the navel, and are usually found in patterns of *Oketsu* with *Ketsu Nobose* symptoms

Romaji	Kanji	Pinyin	English	Definition in this text
Sei Ki	生気	*Sheng Qi*	Life *Ki*, essential *Ki*	The fundamental Vital energy (*Ki*) of life; precaution is taken in selecting a formula not to disrupt its functioning
Sei Shin	精神	*Jing Shen*	Spirit or Mood	Mental state, state of the soul
Seitai Ho	整体法	*Zheng Ti Fa*	*Seitai* Therapy	Initially founded by *Takahashi Michio* in the 1920s, the term, which means literally "properly ordered body," was coined by *Noguchi Haruchika* (1911–1976) to describe a series of techniques he developed designed to free up the activity of the life force (*Ki*) by re-adjusting the physiology of the body. This could be done on another person as a form of treatment as in *Seitai Ho* 整体法 or on oneself as forms of self-adjustment such as *Seitai Taiso* 整体体操 or *Katsugen Undo* 活元運, a method based on spontaneous, free-form movement designed to reveal and nurture the underlying natural rhythms of the body/mind
Seiza	正座	*Zheng Zuo*	Right Sitting	The correct or "proper" manner of sitting in Japan used in formal circumstances
Sen Sei	先生	*Xian Sheng*	Teacher	A term of respect for a teacher; "those who were born before"
Sen Tsu	疝痛	*Shan Tong*	Mountain of Pain	Colic pain; severe pain confined to one spot. Can include hernia
Setsu	切	*Qie*	Touch (deep)	Literally "to cut (through)." The type of deep, penetrating pressure used in the *Fukushin* exam. Contrasts with *Shoku* that is used as the initial "contact" pressure at the beginning of the exam

Setsu Shin	切診	Qie Zhen	The Tactile Exam	The hand of the physician examining the body of the patient; one of the 4 Pillars of Diagnosis (*Shi Shin*) that includes abdominal palpation, pulse-taking and meridian palpation
Sha Ho	瀉法	Xie Fa	Reducing Method	A method of treatment used to reduce or drain
Shakuju Chiryo	積聚治療	Ji Zhu Zhi Liao	*Shakuju* Therapy	A modern Acupuncture style and system developed by *Kobayashi Shoji*
Shiatsu Ho	指圧法	Zhi Ya Fa	*Shiatsu* Therapy	Finger Pressure Massage. Derived from the traditional massage and breathing exercise system of Japan, *Do In Ankyo* 导引按摩, focusing on the application of static pressure applied to the meridians and points to regulate energetic flow as well as gentle stretches and manipulations that restore harmony to the system
Shichifukujin	七福神	Qi Fu Shen	7 Gods of Fortune	Believed to bring good luck in Japanese mythology. Amongst the 7, all were mythical gods except for *Hotei*
Shin	心	Xin	Heart	The organ of the heart, or the functions of the heart in the *Sho Kan Ron*, the area of the body where this organ is located
Shin Atsuryoku	深圧力	Shen Ya Li	Deep Pressure	The type of pressure used in the *Fukushin* exam that penetrates beyond the skin, fascia and muscle layers into the abdominal cavity
Shindo Hiketsu Shu	鍼道秘訣集	Zhen Dao Mi Jue Di	Compilation of Secrets of Acupuncture	Important *Edo* period Acupuncture text published (1685) as a compilation of the works of *Misono Isai* 御薗意斎 (1557–1616) by one of his students
Shin Ka Bu	心下部	Xin Xia Bu	Epigastrium	Literally "the area beneath the Heart"; the solar plexus; the epigastric area

Romaji	Kanji	Pinyin	English	Definition in this text
Shin Ka Bu Shin Sui On	心下部振水音	*Xin Xia Bu Zhen Shui Yin*	Epigastric Splash Sound	Abdomen #7, Figure 4.9. The sound made when tapping the area of the abdomen described as "beneath the heart," on the left side, denoting the pathogenic accumulation of fluid (*Suidoku*)
Shin Ka Gyaku Man	心下逆満	*Xin Xia Ni Man*	Counterflow fullness in the epigastrium	*Kampo* terms: *Shin Ka*—the area beneath the heart; *gyaku*—counterflow movement; *man*—a feeling of fullness. This sensation applies to formulas such as *Hange Shashin To* or *Go Shuyu To*
Shin Ka Hi	心下痞	*Xin Xia Pi*	Epigastric Obstruction	Abdomen #4, Figure 4.6. The patient has a feeling of subjective obstruction in the epigastrium (*Shin Ka Bu*), which cannot be confirmed objectively through touch by the physician. Also known as *Shin Ka No Tsukae*, a constricted feeling in the epigastrium
Shin Ka Hi Ken	心下痞堅	*Xin Xia Pi Jian*	Epigastric Hardness	Similar to *Shin Ka Hi Ko* (below)
Shin Ka Hi Ko	心下痞硬	*Xin Xia Pi Ying*	Epigastric Obstruction Resistance	Abdomen #3, Figure 4.5. The patient has a feeling of subjective obstruction and pain in the epigastrium (*Shin Ka Bu*) which is confirmed objectively through touch by the physician
Shin Ka Ki	心下悸	*Xin Xia Ji*	Epigastric Pulsations	Abdomen #10, Figure 4.14. These are pulsations seen or felt in the epigastric area (*Shin Ka Bu*) which may be termed either *Kyo* or *Jitsu* and are usually found in Toxic Water Patterns (*Suidoku Sho*) with *Sui Nobose*

Shin Ka Man	心下満	*Xin xia man*	Epigastric Fullness	Fullness felt in the *Shin Ka Bu*, epigastric area, which may be deemed either *Kyo* or *Jitsu* but is generally subjective patient sensation
Shinkantaza	只管打坐	*Zhi Guan Da Zuo*	Silent Illumination	Literally "merely sitting in meditation," suggesting a reflective state of mind rather than a focused one such as in *Zazen*, with no particular point of attention (mantra, breath or otherwise)
Shin Kei	神経	*Shen Jing*	A nerve	Term used for diseases of the nervous system as well as psycho-emotional conditions. This *Shin* describes the *Kampo* term for the soul/mind/spirit, which is housed in the "heart." The *Kei* is the same character as in *Kei Raku*, the term for Acupuncture meridians or pathways
Shin Kei Shitsu	神経質	*Shen Jin Zhi*	Neurotic Sensitivity	Neurosis or nervous sensitivity; constitutional reference to a personality type who is easily affected by all manner of stimulation to the nervous system
Shin Kei Sho	神経症	*Shen Jing Zheng*	Nervous Disorder	A neurotic or nervous condition or Pattern (*Sho*)
Shin Kei Sho Jyo	神経症状	*Shen Jing Zheng Zhuang*	Neurotic Symptoms	A collection or series of neurotic symptoms that belong to a nervous disorder (*Shin Kei Sho*)
Shin Ki	心悸	*Xin Ji*	Cardiac Pulsations	Abdomen #10, Figure 4.14. Palpitations or abdominal pulsations that occur in the upper abdomen just below the xiphoid process and are usually associated with patterns of *Ki Nobose*. Compare with *Do Ki* and *Ki*; here the term *Shin* does not refer to the area of the heart itself

Romaji	Kanji	Pinyin	English	Definition in this text
Shin Netsu	身熱	Shen Re	Body Fever	A fever that sweeps across the body, not accompanied by chill or sweating; usually designating the Bright Yang Stage (Yo Mei Byoh)
Shin No Hon So Kyo	神農本草経	Shen Nong Ben Cao Jing	The Divine Husbandman's Classic of Materia Medica	The oldest surviving Chinese Materia Medica, compiled in the Eastern Han Dynasty (25–220 CE); recording 365 medicinal substances classified into three categories: high, medium and low grade according to their medicinal effects and toxicity
Shin Pan	心煩	Xin Fan	Troublesome Heart	A restless feeling (han) in the area of the chest; also called Heart Vexation
Shin Shi Jikken	親試実験	Qin Shi Shi Yan	Personal Examination and Actual Experience	The pragmatic philosophy seen as the hallmark of the Koho-Ha school of Kampo. Yoshimasu Todo and Yamawaki Toyo in particular dismissed what they saw as the unreliability of speculative theories in medicine in favor of actual direct clinical experience. Hence the importance to them of accurate anatomy based on cadaver dissection, abdominal palpation and Formula Patterns based on concrete clinical signs and symptoms
Shin Sui On	振水音	Zhen Shui Yin	Splash Sound	The sound of fluids in the stomach and intestines upon palpation; see Shin Ka Bu Shin Sui On (above)
Shinto	神道	Shendao	The Way of the Gods	Indigenous polytheistic religion of Japan
Shisei	姿勢	Zishi	Posture	How one carries oneself, bearing. Comprising two characters, the first meaning "shape," the second "function." The correct physical posture appropriate to a particular discipline within the martial, fine and healing arts in East Asia

Shi Shin	四診	Si Zhen	The Four Diagnostic Exams	Sometimes referred to as the 4 Pillars of Diagnosis including Observation, Touch, Listening/Smelling and Questioning. They are considered objective measurements in *Kampo*, although they are not measurable in Western methodology
Shi Un Ko	紫雲膏	Zi Yun Gao	Purple Cloud Ointment	Modified by *Hanaoka Seichu* from *Wai Ke Zheng Zong* compiled by *Chen Shi-Gong*
Sho	小	Xiao	Small	Used to describe a pulse or sensation or also a size such as the lower (or "small") abdomen (*Sho Fuku*)
Sho	証	Zheng	Sho	A collection of (practitioner) signs and (patient) symptoms, including pulse, tongue and abdominal findings, that point to treatment by a specific herbal formula
Sho	正	Zheng	Upright	"Correct" or "Upright" as in the example of the correct healthy Vital energy (*Sho Ki*)
Sho Ben Fu Ri	小便不利	Xiao Bian Bu Li	Urine does not flow	Urinary impairment, oliguria/anuria ("urine flow is scanty/infrequent")
Sho Ben Ji Ri	小便自利	Xiao Bian Zi Li	Incontinence	Urine flow is uncontrolled; spontaneous or incontinent urination
Sho Ben Nan	小便難	Xiao Bian Nan	Difficult Urination	Dysuria, impediment to urinary flow, or painful flow
Sho En	消炎	Xiao Yan	To Clear Inflammation	To extinguish an inflammatory process. An anti-inflammatory action
Sho Fuku	小腹	Xiao Fu	Lower abdomen	*Sho Fuku* (lesser abdomen) refers to the "smaller" or lower abdomen

Romaji	Kanji	Pinyin	English	Definition in this text
Sho Fuku Cho Man	小腹脹満	*Xiao Fu Zhang Man*	Lower Abdominal Distention and Fullness	*Sho Fuku* refers to the lower abdomen, whereas *Cho Man* refers to a feeling of distension and fullness which may be either *Kyo* or *Jitsu*. This is a subjective patient experience as opposed to: *Sho Fuku (Ko) Man*—Abdomen #12, Figures 4.17 and 4.18, which is a practitioner finding in *Fukushin*
Sho Fuku Fu Jin	小腹不仁	*Xiao Fu Bu Ren*	Lower Abdomen Lacking Benevolence	Abdomen #11, Figure 4.15. A softness and numbness in the lower abdomen (*Sho Fuku*), which can progress to the lower body. The midline below the navel feels empty and hollow to the touch
Sho Fuku Ko Kyu	小腹拘急	*Xiao Fu Ju Ji*	Lower Abdominal Tight Spasm	Abdomen #9, Figure 4.13. A cramp or spasm which pulls along the inguinal region like a coil or cable and includes the lower portion of the rectus abdominis muscle and across the entire lower abdominal areas
Sho Fuku Ko Man	小腹硬満	*Xiao Fu Ying Man*	Lower Abdominal Resistance and Fullness	Abdomen #11, Figure 4.17. Distension in the lower abdomen, which is full, hard and resistant to the touch. Usually a sign of *Oketsu*
Sho Fuku Ko Ren	小腹拘攣	*Xiao Fu Ju Luan*	Pencil Line	Abdomen #11, Figure 4.16. A finding in the abdominal exam in which firm pressure reveals a depression in the midline below the navel and within that depression is felt a rigid line, thin like a pencil
Sho Fuku Kyu Ketsu	小腹急結	*Xiao Fu Ji Jie*	Lower Abdomen Spastic Knot	Abdomen #14, Figure 4.20. A spastic knot in the lower abdomen, which rebounds and is painful upon pressure. Always indicative of *Oketsu Sho*

Sho Fuku Man	小腹満	*Xiao Fu Man*	Lower Abdominal Fullness	Abdomen #11, Figure 4.18. There is a fullness in the lower abdomen found during the abdominal exam which is distended but not altogether hard and resistant. This usually points to Fluid Pathology of some kind (*Tan In*)
Sho In	少陰	*Shao Yin*	Lesser *Yin*	The second of the *Yin* (*In*) stage patterns in the *Sho Kan Ron*
Sho In Byo	少陰病	*Shao Yin Bing*	Lesser *Yin* Diseaser	The symptoms and treatment (formulas) associated with the *Sho In* Stage
Sho Kan	傷寒	*Shang Han*	Damaging Cold	This is the disease pattern chronicled in the *Sho Kan Ron*, which begins with chills and fever and ends with a prolonged coma; it serves as a model for assessing all illness. It is thought the illness described at that time in the *Han* dynasty may have been typhoid
Sho Kan Ron	傷寒論	*Shang Han Lun*	*On Cold Damage*	*A Treatise on the Shang Han* (an acute febrile disease, or a Damaging Cold) written by *Zhang Zhong Jing* 張仲景 (150–219 CE) sometime in the 2nd century
Sho Katsu	消渇	*Xiao Ke*	Wasting Thirst	Diabetes mellitus
Sho Ken	所見	*Suo Jian*	Findings	Clinical findings including signs and symptoms making up the Pattern (*Sho*)
Sho Ki	正気	*Zheng Qi*	Upright *Ki*	The natural, healthy *Ki* that in its "correct" and "upright" state stands in natural opposition to Pathogenic Ki (*Jya Ki*) in defending the body against disease
Shoku	触	*Chu*	Touch (light)	To contact or touch something/someone as in the initial manner of contact pressure used at the beginning of the *Fukushin* exam. Contrast with *Setsu*

Romaji	Kanji	Pinyin	English	Definition in this text
Shomu Tenno	聖武天皇	*Sheng Wu Tian Huang*	Emperor *Shomu*	724–749 CE. Husband of Empress *Komyo*
Sho So Ho I Kai	蕉窓方意解	*Jiao Chuang Fang Yi Jie*	*Inspired Lessons on Formula from a Window Facing a Japanese Banana Plant*	By *Wada Tokaku* (1743–1803), a physician of the Compromise School, a student of *Todo Yoshimasu*. The *Sho* is a reference to the poet Basho; this text is from the *Bunsei* period (1818–1830)
Sho So In	正倉院	*Zheng Cang Yuan*	The Treasure House	Located within Todaiji temple 東大寺 in *Nara*, it housed a collection of 900 treasures, amongst them many samples of medicinal substances which survive to this day as national treasures in Japan
Sho So Zatsu Wa	蕉窓雜話	*Jiao Chuang Za Hua*	*Small Talks from a Window Facing a Japanese Banana Plant*	A text written by *Wada Tokaku* (1821), also known as a *Manual of Medical Practices*; see the notes above on *Sho So Ho I Kai*. Most of *Wada's* textbooks were written by his students after he died
Sho Yo	少陽	*Shao Yang*	Lesser *Yang*	The Lesser *Yang* Stage in the *Sho Kan Ron*
Sho Yo Byo	少陽病	*Shao Yang Bing*	Lesser *Yang* Disease	The symptoms and treatment (formulas) associated with the *Sho Yo* Stage
Shudo Denmei	首藤傳明	*Shou Teng Chuan Ming*	*Denmei Shudo*	Contemporary Japanese Acupuncturist, teacher and author currently living and practicing in Tokyo. The longest surviving member of the Meridian Therapy style of Acupuncture (*Keiraku Chiryo*). Author of the text *Japanese Classical Acupuncture: Introduction to Meridian Therapy*, publ. Eastland Press, 2011

So Ho	創方	Chuang Fang	Original formula	An invented or original formula, in contrast to a Classical Formula (*Jing Fang*)
So Mon	素問	Su Wen	*Plain Questions*	First volume of the *Ko Tei Nai Kyo*
Sotai Ho	操体法	Cao Ti Fa	Sotai Therapy	A form of Japanese muscular/movement therapy developed by *Hashimoto Keizo* (1897–1993), a medical doctor, proposing a natural method to balance and restore harmony to the body without strain in much the same way as Acupuncture and other disciplines in East Asian Medicine. In fact the word itself is a reversal of the same characters used to mean "exercise" in Japanese: *Taiso* 体操, a deliberate reference to the fact that his system was a natural, effortless system of movement designed, through the breath, to move toward comfort and away from pain, unlike some of the contemporary exercise systems of his time
Sugita Genpaku	杉田玄白	Shan Tian Xuan Bai	Dr. *Genpaku Sugita*	1733–1817. Japanese scholar who wrote the seminal anatomy textbook along with *Maeno Ryotaku*, "New Text on Anatomy" (*Kaitai Shinsho*) published in 1774. It was based on a translation of the Dutch version (1734) of the original German anatomical text (1722) written by Johann Adam Kulmus (1689–1745)
Sugiyama Waichi	杉山和一	Shan Shan He Yi	Waichi Sugiyama	1614–1694. Sometimes regarded as the "Father" of Japanese Acupuncture. Blind practitioner in the early *Edo* period credited with the invention of the guide tube (*Shinkan* 針管) and the use of Silver and Gold needles as well as multiple publications

Romaji	Kanji	Pinyin	English	Definition in this text
Sui	水	Shui	Water	From the theory of three substances (Ki Ketsu Sui), a primary body fluid
Sui Bun	水分	Shui Fen	Acupoint CV9	Area above navel; an Acupuncture point on the Nin Myaku, Ren.9
Sui Byo	水病	Shui Bing	Water Illness	Disease induced by water/fluid imbalance or pathology
Sui Doku	水毒	Shui Du	Water Toxins	Accumulation of pathogenic fluid
Suiko Tenno	推古天皇	Tui Gu Tian Huang	Empress Suiko	Reign: 564–628
Sumo	相撲	Xiang Pu	Sumo Wrestling	The characters 相撲 literally mean "striking one another." Sumo wrestling involves a contest between two wrestlers, Rikishi 力士, literally "men of power" (referring to the fact that the original contests were between Samurai warriors), in which one loses by either being forced out of the ring or by touching any part of the body (other than the soles of the feet) on the ground
Suzuki Shunryu	鈴木俊隆	Ling Mu Jun Long	Shunryu Suzuki	1904–1971. Author of Zen Mind, Beginner's Mind (see "Selected Bibliography")
Suzuki Takeo	鈴木竹雄	Mu Mu Zhu Xiong	Takeo Suzuki	Successor to Masunaga Shizuto at the Iokai Center in Tokyo in 1981, then started teaching independently. Principal Sensei of the author
Taga Hoin	多賀法印	Duo He Fa Yin	Hoin Taga	Teacher of Misono Mubunsai
Tai In	太陰	Tai Yin	Greater Yin	The wide, vast, greater In, the first of the Yin Stages from the "Treatise on Cold Damage" (Sho Kan Ron)
Tai In Byo	太陰病	Tai Yin Bing	Greater Yin Stage	The symptoms and formulas associated with Greater Yin (Tai In) Stage

Tai Kyoku Ken	太極拳	Taijiquan	Tai Chi	Chinese internal martial art also practiced for health cultivation
Tai Ryoku	体力	Ti Fang	Body Strength	A measure of constitutional strength, e.g. Strong (*Jitsu Tai Ryoku*) or Weak (*Kyo Tai Ryoku*)
Tai Shitsu	体質	Ti Zhi	Body Type	Constitutional type. Can be *Yang* or *Yin* types (*Yo/In Tai Shitsu Sho*); *Qi* Blood or Fluid types (*Ki Ketsu Sui Tai Shitsu Sho*); Cold types (*Hie Sho*); nervous types (*Shin Keishitsu Sho*); weak digestive function types (*Icho Kyo Jyaku Sho*), and so on
Tai Yo	太陽	Tai Yang	Greater *Yang*	*Tai Yo*, great or wide *Yang*; Greater *Yang* is the first stage of the six divisions (*Roku Byo Sho*)
Tai Yo Byo	太陽病	Tai Yang Bing	Greater *Yang* Stage	The symptoms and formulas associated with Greater *Yang* (*Tai Yo*) Stage
Tamai Tempeki	玉井天碧	Yu Jing Tian Bi	Tempeki Tamai	*Shiatsu* practitioner known for his seminal text: "Finger Pressure Method" *Shiatsu Ho* 指圧法 (1939), likely the very first historical reference to the term *Shiatsu*
Tamba Masatada	丹波雅忠	Dan Bo Ya Zhong	Dr. *Masatada Tamba*	A famous *Kampo* physician who wrote the preface to the 1060 CE *Kang Ping* edition of the *Sho Kan Ron*; the *Otsuka* modern *Koho-Ha* tradition is based on this *Kang Ping* edition, rather than the *Song* edition commonly used in China. Author of the text "Selected Therapies" (*Iryakusho*)
Tan	痰	Tan	Body fluids	Classically, *Tan* referred to all body fluids, but in modern usage refers only to sputum or phlegm
Tanden	丹田	Dantian	Cinnabar or Elixir Field	The energetic center where the "movement of *Ki* between the Kidneys" occurs. See *Saika Tanden* (above)

Romaji	Kanji	Pinyin	English	Definition in this text
Tan In	痰飲	*Tan Yin*	Pathological fluids	*Tan* and *In* together indicate body fluids plus dietary fluids; or diseases characterized by retention of body fluids; or diseases due to accumulation of pathological fluids
Tashiro Sanki	田代三喜	*Tian Dai San Xi*	Dr. *Sanki Tashiro*	Japanese *Zen* Monk (1465–1537) who lived and studied medicine in China for 12 years (1487–1498). Returned with two important texts: *Zenku Shu* 全九集 (1452) and *Saiin Ho* 済陰方 (1455) introducing the work of the "four great physicians" of *Jin-Yuan* China, in particular that of *Li Dong Yuan* 李東垣 (1180–1251) and *Zhu Danxi* 朱丹渓 (1281–1358). This became known as *Li-Zhu* medicine (*Li Zhu Igaku*) in Japan and focused on tonifying therapies (*Ho Zai* 補剤). Considered the pioneer of the [**AQ**]"Later Generation School" (*Gosei-Ha* 後世派) of *Kampo*
Tei Sui	停水	*Ting Shui*	Water Accumulation	An abnormal accumulation of water (in the stomach); a sign of *Tan In*
Tonisho	頓医抄	*Dun Yi Chao*	*Classification of Disease*	Written in 50 volumes in Japanese between 1302 and 1304 by the monk physician *Kajiwara Shozen* based on various *Song* dynasty (960–1279) texts from China, in particular those printed in *Fujian* in Southern *Song* (1147) and then imported to Japan, such as the *Taihei Seikei Ho* 太平聖恵方

Toyo Hari	東洋針	*Dong Yang Zhen*	*Toyo Hari*	A style of Acupuncture developed in the 20th century, inspired by *Fukushima Kodo*, using very gentle stimulation at times with no puncturing at all, known as Contact Needling. Practiced widely by blind Acupuncturists in Japan
Ukketsu	鬱血	*Yu Xue*	Depressed Flow of Blood	Stagnated blood, due to depression of flow. Compare with *Oketsu*
Un Yo	温陽	*Wen Yang*	Warm *Yang*	Treatment method of warming the *Yang* functional activities of the body
Ura	裏	*Li*	Hidden	Meaning "bottom," "interior" or "rear," implying that which is hidden or nuanced. What cannot be immediately perceived from the outside. Something that is deeply hidden within or underneath the surface
Uttai	鬱滞	*Yu Zhi*	Depressed and Slumped	A flow disturbed by depression plus slumped (has become sluggish)
Wada Keijuro	和田啓十郎	*He Tian Qi Shi Lang*	Dr. *Keijuro Wada*	1872–1916. A Western-trained doctor, wrote a text called "The Iron Hammer of the Western World" (*Ikai No Tettsui* 医界之鉄椎) in which he compared the relative merits of *Kampo* and the new "Western" medicine. His summary was controversial at the time as he claimed traditional medicine to be far superior in most aspects to its modern rival

Romaji	Kanji	Pinyin	English	Definition in this text
Wada Tokaku	和田東郭	*He Tian Dong Guo*	Dr. *Tokaku Wada*	1743–1803. Well-known member of the Eclectic School (*Secchu-Ha*) along with *Asada Sohaku* and a student of *Yoshimasu Todo*. He is remembered in particular for his work on the theory and treatment of emotional disorders. He famously ascribed all such illnesses as due to *Qi* Stasis (*Ki Utsu*)—not unlike *Goto Konzan* before him—in his case ascribing the etiology uniquely to the Liver (not unlike in modern TCM)
Wa Ho	和方	*He Fang*	Japanese Folk Medicine	To be contrasted with Chinese Medicine (*Kampo*) and Western (or Dutch) Medicine (*Rampo*)
Wa Kan Yaku	和漢薬	*He Han Yao*	Sino–Japanese Herbal Medicine	Japanese interpretation of Classical Chinese Herbal Medicine
Watanabe Kenji	渡辺賢治	*Du Bian Xian Zhi*	Dr. *Kenji Watanabe*	*Kampo* Medicine Specialist with an M.D. and Ph.D. in internal medicine from Keio University School of Medicine. Director of the Center for Kampo Medicine at *Keio* and director of the *Otsuka* Clinic in Tokyo
Yakazu Domei	矢数道明	*Shi Shu Dao Ming*	Dr. *Domei Yakazu*	1905–2002. Close friend and colleague of Dr. *Ostuka Keisetsu's* from the *Gosei-Ha* School (see Chapter 2, "Renaissance of *Kampo* in modern Japan" section)
Yaku Butsu	薬物	*Yao Wu*	Crude Drugs	Ingredients of *Kampo*; unprocessed pharmaceutically active natural ingredients. In modern Japan the term for *Yaku Butsu* in extract form is Ethical Drugs and they are licensed as such

Yakucho	藥徵	Yao Zheng	*Pharmacological Demonstrations*	Written in 1771 by *Yoshimasu Todo* based on prescriptions from the *Sho Kan Ron* and from his own experience. In particular he suggested his own interpretations of the functions of individual drugs used in the classical formulas mentioned from the *Sho Kan Ron* and *Kin Ki Yo Ryaku*
Yakusho	藥証	Yao Zheng	Formula Pattern	The clinical evidence in the form of signs and symptoms, including the pulse, tongue and abdomen, that characterize any given formula
Yamato Jidai	大和時代	Da He Shi Dai	*Yamato* period	250–710 CE
Yamawaki Toyo	山脇東洋	Shan Xie Dong Yang	Dr. *Toyo Yamawaki*	1705–1762. Well-known student of *Goto Konzan* in the *Koho-Ha* tradition. Famous for having witnessed a cadaver dissection in 1754 upon which his book *On the Viscera* (*Zoshi* 蔵志, 1759) was based. This book essentially helped change the course of basic medical thinking of the time
Yanagiya Sorei	柳谷素霊	Liu Gu Su Ling	Sorei Yanagiya	Founder of the Meridian Therapy style of Acupuncture; started the Society for the Study of Practical Acupuncture and established the school of Meridian Therapy (*Keiraku Chiryo*) along with cohorts such as *Okabe Sodo, Inoue Keiri, Honma Akimi* now all deceased, and by later disciples, still living, such as *Okada Akizo, Shudo Denmai, Kuwahara Kuei* and *Ikeda Masakazu*

Romaji	Kanji	Pinyin	English	Definition in this text
Yo	陽	*Yang*	*Yang*	*Yo*, the first three stages of the six divisions; the bright, hot, active primal energy, symbolized by the sunny side of the mountain (image contained in the ideogram) in contrast to *Yin* (*In*)
Yo Chu No In	陽中の陰	*Yang Zhong Zhi Yin*	*Yin* within *Yang*	The *Yin* aspect of a phenomenon that is classified as *Yang*, e.g. abdomen #2b *Yin* Full Abdomen in Figure 4.4
Yo Chu No Yo	陽中の陽	*Yang Zhong Zhi Yang*	*Yin* within *Yang*	The *Yang* aspect of a *Yang* phenomenon, e.g. abdomen #2a *Yang* Full Abdomen in Figure 4.3
Yo Fuku Man	陽腹満	*Yang Fu Man*	*Yang* Full Abdomen	This is abdomen #2a described in Figure 4.3. It is the *Yo Chu No Yo* abdomen above
Yokozuna	横綱	*Heng Gang*	*Yokozuna*	The highest rank in *Sumo* wrestling
Yo Mei	陽明	*Yang Ming*	Sunlight *Yang*	The Bright *Yang* or *Yang* Brightness Stage, from the six divisions (*Roku Byo Sho*)
Yo Mei Byo	陽明病	*Yang Ming Bing*	Sunlight *Yang* Stage	The symptoms and formulas associated with the Sunlight *Yang* (*Yo Mei*) Stage
Yoshimasu Todo	吉益東洞	*Ji Yi Dong Dong*	Dr. *Todo Yoshimasu*	This *Edo* period (*Edo Jidai*) *Kampo* physician lived from 1702 to 1773 and was a major force in the Classical School (*Koho-Ha*), of which Dr. *Otsuka* later became an eminent modern advocate. He wrote extensively on the use of the abdomen in practice and his insistence on "Matching Pattern and Formula" (*Ho Sho I Chi*) is still the mainstay of *Kampo* practice to this day. Best known for his texts: [AQ] *Ruijuho* (類聚方) and *Yakucho* (藥徵). Probably the most influential of all the *Edo* period *Kampo* doctors from the *Koho-Ha*, especially in regard to his work on the abdomen

Yo Sho	陽証	Yang zheng	Yang Pattern	A pattern of any one of the three Yang Stages; Yang pattern of disharmony
Yumoto Kyushin	湯本求真	Tang Ben Qiu Zhen	Dr. Kyushin Yumoto	Otsuka Keisetsu's Kampo teacher; a physician (1876–1941) of the Taisho (大正1912–1926) and Showa (昭和 1926–1989) periods noted for his role in the Kampo restoration movement. His text "Traditional Japanese and Chinese Medicine" (Kokan Igaku 皇漢醫學, 1927) contributed greatly to the 20th century Kampo revival in Japan
Zazen	座禅	Zuo Chan	Seated Meditation	The practice of "sitting" in Zen
Zen	禅	Chan	Zen Buddhism	Japanese form of Mahayana Buddhist practice transmitted originally from India, through China in the Tang dynasty and then to Japan in the 5th century CE. Two main currents emerged over time: Rinzai and Soto with distinct traditions and focus, though in modern times aspects of each school are often combined
Zen Shiatsu	禅指圧	Chan Zhi Ya	Zen Shiatsu	A style of Shiatsu developed by the late Masunaga Shizuto (1925–1991) focusing on natural bodyweight pressure applied without effort using the principles of perpendicular, continuous and equal pressure (see Chapter 3, "Pressure" section)
Zesshin	舌診	She Zhen	Tongue exam	One part of visual diagnosis in the Four Diagnostic Methods of Kampo

Romaji	Kanji	Pinyin	English	Definition in this text
Zo Fu Setsu	臓腑説	*Zang Fu Shuo*	*Zang Fu* Organ Theory	The theory of the solid (*Zo*) and the hollow (*Fu*) organs which constitutes the main physiological basis of Chinese Medicine
Zui Sho Chi Ryo	随証治療	*Sui Zheng Zhi Liao*	Treatment According to the Proof	Therapy based on Japanese *Kampo* diagnosis of the *Sho* or traditional diagnostic pattern
Zu Tsu	頭痛	*Tou Tong*	Headache	Pain in any part of the head

Subject Index

Author Index